D0927919

DATE DUE

Health Care Errors and Patient Safety

Dedication

For Ruth and Sangeeta, with love

Epigraph

But there exists a black kingdom which the eyes of man avoid because its landscape fails signally to flatter them. This darkness, which he imagines he can dispense with in describing the light, is error with its unknown characteristics, error which demands that a person contemplate it for its own sake before rewarding him with the evidence about fugitive reality that it alone could give. ... Error is certainty's constant companion. Error is the corollary of evidence. And anything said about truth may equally well be said about error: the delusion will be no greater. ... Light is meaningful only in relation to darkness, and truth presupposes error. It is these mingled opposites which people our life, which make it pungent, intoxicating. [Louis Aragon, Préface à une mythologie moderne. In: Louis Aragon. *Le Paysan de Paris*. Paris: Gallimard, 1926, 11–15. Transaltion by Simon Watson in *Paris Peasant*. London: Jonathan Cape, 1971, 20–24.]

Health Care Errors and Patient Safety

EDITED BY

Brian Hurwitz
Department of English Language and Literature
Schools of Humanities and Medicine
King's College
London, UK

and

Aziz Sheikh
Centre of Population Health Sciences
University of Edinburgh
Edinburgh, UK

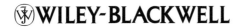

Library of Congress Cataloging-in-Publication Data

Health care errors and patient safety / edited by Brian Hurwitz and Aziz Sheikh.
 p. ; cm.
 Includes bibliographical references.
 ISBN 978-1-4051-4643-2
 1. Medical errors. 2. Hospital care—Safety measures. I. Hurwitz, Brian. II. Sheikh, Aziz.
 [DNLM: 1. Medical Errors. 2. Safety Management. WB 100 H434 2009]
 R729.8.H43 2009
 610—dc22

                          2008045731

A catalogue record for this book is available from the British Library.

Set in 9.5/12pt Palatino by Charon Tec (A Macmillan Company), Chennai, India (www.charontec.com)

Printed and bound in Singapore by Fabulous Printers Pte Ltd

1 2009

Contents

List of contributors

Anthony J. Avery
Professor
Division of Primary Care
Medical School
Queens Medical Centre
Nottingham NG7 2UH, UK

Richard Baker
Professor
Department of Health Sciences
University of Leicester
Leicester LE1 6TP, UK

Paul Barach
Associate Professor
Department of Anesthesiology
University of Miami Medical School
Miami, FL 33136, USA

Ruth Boaden
Professor of Service Operations
Management
Manchester Business School
University of Manchester
Manchester M15 6PB, UK

Stephen Buetow
Associate Professor and Director of Research
Department of General Practice and Primary
School of Population Health
University of Auckland
Auckland, New Zealand

Bernard Burnes
Professor of Organisational Change
Manchester Business School
University of Manchester
Manchester M15 6PB, UK

Tanya Claridge
Heaton Norris Health Centre
Heaton Norris
Stockport SK4 JXE, UK

Adrian Cook
National Patient Safety Agency
London W1T 5HD, UK

Angela Coulter
Chief Executive
Picker Institute Europe
King's Mead House
Oxford OX1 1RX, UK

Jo Ellins
Research Fellow
Health Services Management Centre
University of Birmingham
Birmingham B15 2RT, UK

Glyn Elwyn
Professor of Primary Care Medicine
Department of General Practice
Centre for Health Sciences Research
Cardiff University
Cardiff CF14 4YS, UK

Alan Forster
The Ottawa Hospital
Civic Campus
Ottawa
Ontario K1Y 4E9, Canada

Marshall F. Gilula
Director
Life Energies Research Institute
2510 Inagua Avenue
Miami, FL 33136, USA

Rachel L. Howard
Lecturer in Pharmacy Practice
Department of Pharmacy Practice
School of Pharmacy
University of Reading
Reading RG6 6AP, UK

Brian Hurwitz
Professor of Medicine and the Arts
Department of English Language and
Literature
Schools of Humanities and Medicine
King's College
London WC2R 2LS, UK

Olga Kostopoulou
National Primary Care Postdoctural Fellow
Department of Primary Care and General Practice
Primary Care Clinical Sciences Building
University of Birmingham
Birmingham B15 2TT, UK

Matthew Lawrie
School of Psychological Sciences
Coupland One
University of Manchester
Manchester M13 9PL, UK

Mavis Maclean
Joint Director
Oxford Centre for Family Law and Policy
Oxford OX1 2ER, UK

Alan F. Merry
Professor and Head of Department
Department of Anaesthesiology
University of Auckland
Auckland, New Zealand

Lesley Page
Visiting Professor in Midwifery
Nightingale School of Nursing and Midwifery
King's College London
London, UK

Dianne Parker
Head of Division of Psychology
School of Psychological Sciences
Coupland One
University of Manchester
Manchester M13 9PL, UK

Mike Pringle
Head of School of Community Health Sciences
Division of Primary Care
University of Nottingham
Nottingham NG7 2RD, UK

Alison Pryce
Senior Statistician
National Patient Safety Agency
London W1T 5HD, UK

Celia Roberts
Department of Education and Professional
Studies
Professor of Applied Linguistics
King's College London
Franklin Wilkins Building
Waterloo Bridge Annexe
London SE1 9NN, UK

John Sandars
Senior Lecturer in Community Based
Education
Medical Education Unit
University of Leeds
Leeds LS2 9JT, UK

Sarah Scobie
Head of Observatory
The National Patient Safety Agency
London W1T 5HD, UK

Aziz Sheikh
Professor of Primary Care
Research and Development
Centre of Population Health Sciences
University of Edinburgh
Edinburgh EH8 9DX, UK

Richard Thomson
Professor of Epidemiology and Public Health
Institute of Health and Society
Medical School
Newcastle upon Tyne NE2 4HH

Charles Vincent
Professor of Clinical Safety Research
Department of Biosurgery and Technology
10th Floor QEQM Building
St Mary's Hospital
London W2 1NY, UK

Geoff Watts
Science and medicine writer and broadcaster
London NW3 1LS, UK

Foreword

Healthcare professionals dedicate their working lives to improving the lives of others. It is a privilege to be in a position to cure, treat and support patients and their families, whether living or dying with disease. It is also a noble endeavour, driven by compassion and humanity. Yet the phrase 'only human' expresses a truth long understood in general but only relatively recently taken seriously within medicine: all human undertakings involve error. Despite the good intentions of motivated and caring healthcare professionals, one in three hundred hospital visits result in a death due to medical error. Patient safety has been most extensively studied in the secondary care setting, but is not limited to this field: it is universal.

This is by no means cause for despair. Although some error is inevitable, the rate can be reduced, and measures can be taken to prevent errors from being translated into harm to patients. If we learn effectively, the same errors need never recur. Opportunities to learn exist not only for individuals, but also for organisations.

Patient safety is rapidly evolving. Modern research provides new insights and solutions to increasingly recognised issues. Transmitting this information to all those who can benefit is now a major challenge. Gilula and Barach raise the important issue of patient safety education and curriculum design, and this is echoed by the work of the World Health Organization's World Alliance for Patient Safety to develop a curricular guide for medical students.

This book provides a theoretical groundwork on patient safety, but also practical advice for all those involved in healthcare: patients and their families, healthcare workers and institutions. I have long championed the involvement of patients and their families, and am delighted that their participation in patient safety is promoted here.

Avedis Donabedian famously said: 'Ultimately, the secret of quality is love… If you have love, you can then work backward to monitor and improve the system'. It is time that we channelled the real care and compassion of healthcare workers into frameworks which allow them to monitor, analyse, improve and re-evaluate systems to make care safer for patients.

To all those looking for an insight into recent developments in patient safety, thought-provoking discussions and advice on making care safer for patients: read on.

Sir Liam Donaldson
Chief Medical Officer
Department of Health

CHAPTER 1

Health care mistakes, violations and patient safety

Brian Hurwitz, Aziz Sheikh

Error is not something that is fallen into momentarily; it is omnipresent.

David Bates, 1996 [1]

Safety of health care today is at the nexus of empirical, ethical, legal and policy considerations worldwide. Concerns about safety originate in growing realisations which this volume charts, that health care provision is an industry that frequently, and, avoidably, harms vulnerable people. *Health Care Errors and Patient Safety* focuses on medical mistakes and violations, and what can be learnt from their intensive scrutiny in order to enhance patient safety [2,3].

Over the past two decades, aberrantly provided health care has become a major area of scientific investigation, public discussion and health policy formation. Enquiries into medical mistakes – their contexts, causes, consequences and costs – have widened in scope and deepened in conceptual grasp of error and violation [4–8]. Agencies and reporting mechanisms have been established to collect data on medical mishaps and safety incidents, to extract and promulgate lessons that can be learnt from them [9–11]. As a consequence, many more health care events and processes than in the past are today classified as mistakes. But as this book makes clear, many of these data suffer from biased numerators (from under-reporting of errors overall and a tendency to report the most dangerous or injurious incidents) and absent denominators (from lack of

---

Box 1.1: The underside of progress

To invent the sailing ship or steamer is to *invent the shipwreck*. To invent the train is to *invent the rail accident* of derailment. To invent the family automobile is to produce the *pile-up* on the highway.

Paul Virilio, 2007 [100]

Health Care Errors and Patient Safety. Edited by Brian Hurwitz and Aziz Sheikh.
© 2009 Blackwell Publishing, ISBN: 978-1-4051-4643-2.

> **Box 1.2: The relevance of Murphy's law according to Reason**
>
> 'Murphy's law says that if it's possible to do something wrong, people will.' That's why at least 50 patients worldwide have died such a horrible death from intrathecal vincristine. These deaths were certainly preventable, and design safeguards such as the new spinal-only connector will help. But safeguards do have a way of biting back, partly because new equipment tends to add to the complexity, opacity, and unfamiliarity of a situation. [101]

reliable information on how frequently relevant health care procedures are undertaken), which limits knowledge of error rates and curtails development of policies to improve health care safety [12,13].

The volume addresses the sparsely charted field of medical fallibility. In their planning and execution all human activities can inadvertently be misconstrued and mal-performed. The possibility of technological accidents, unintentional and unforeseeable occurrences that often (but not always) involve undesirable consequences, is woven into the design, operation and social relations of technology (Box 1.1). This represents the underside of progress: in parallel with exercising skill and know-how the possibility of error and violation is always present and nowhere more so than in provision of health care [14] (Box 1.2). In this chapter we sketch the origins and development of interest in medical error, violation and patient safety, and trace growing multidisciplinary recognition of fallibility in health care services.

Errors and mistakes

There is something bittersweet about human errors. Inadvertent and harmful they may be, but once recognised and understood utility can be rescued from them [15,16]. Much human learning is still undertaken by 'trial and error', through seeing and reviewing – kinaesthetically sensing – mismatches between intended and accomplished actions, processes captured in part by the saying *practice makes perfect*. But learning from health care errors is a far less individually centred activity than such an adage might imply.* In health care, learning from mistakes involves sharing and discussing them with patients and colleagues; it requires their accurate reconstruction and description, a taxonomy that can usefully categorise errors, a disciplined vocabulary and analytical framework that helps health care errors to be understood and communicated, and a medical culture capable of facing its own fallibility

---

*'Watch one, do one, teach one' might be considered a transformed version of this adage, which refers to how medical novices gain expertise 'on the job' – predominantly under pressure and by experiential learning and teaching with minimal guidance.

(see Chapter 14). Subjecting erroneous thought processes, procedures and techniques to review of this sort takes mental effort and moral bravery; it also demands health services structures that foster and support these processes [12] (see also Chapters 6 and 7).

At a time when the possibility of error pervades the health care enterprise, it has become apparent that the vast majority of errors, whether errors of health care planning or of execution [17], do not cause any harm directly. What is the significance of 'silent' errors, or 'near misses' as they are more commonly referred to, which in the past went frequently undocumented if not entirely unnoticed? Since errors appear to be a universal feature of health care processes, should they be viewed as (undesirable) norms? Should culpability be attached to harmless medical mistakes and, where errors are not injurious, can liability still be imposed [18,19]? If errors are forms of unintentional deviation from collectively agreed standards, should health care violations – *intentional* divergences from agreed procedures – fall within investigative frameworks designed to understand health care errors? These are just some of the questions which are explored in later chapters.

Violations

Deliberate deviations from rules or codes are known as violations and their variety and causes are considered from different perspectives in Chapters 2, 3 and 7. These health care actions are not described in manuals or rules of best practice but generally represent attempts to compensate for overcomplex, undependable systems – 'workarounds' that aim to achieve improvements [20]. Like errors, violations do not necessarily portend harm or a disregard of safety. The psychologist and student of error, James Reason, defines violations as 'deliberate – but not necessarily reprehensible – deviations from practices deemed necessary (by designers, managers and regulatory agencies) to maintain the safe operation of a potentially hazardous system' [21] – 'deviations from safe operating practices, procedures, standards, or rules' [17]. (Key terms in the study of health care safety are defined in Appendix 1.1, p.17.)

Violations are engendered in specific circumstances, for example, as a result of erroneous regulations or needlessly difficult operating procedures that lead operatives to take short cuts, ignore or deliberately bypass explicit rules and procedures, perhaps because of tiredness, which often lurks behind short cuts, perhaps because of time pressures, or as a result of rules and procedures that (appear to) lack rationale [22]. Violations differ from errors in stemming from deliberated choices, conscious decisions that seem to offer the transgressor some sort of benefit. However, the choices involved in health violations are not usually made entirely freely; they are often engendered by significant operating constraints and care system faults. For example, a doctor may decide to allow a relative to translate and interpret for an adult patient, a common violation of guidelines for employing interpreters [23], but because, at the time of a proposed consultation, no other alternative is really available, this should be attributed, at least in part, to an organisational failing or system error – the lack of accessible interpreters when needed in the health care system. In relation to the clinician, the decision can be seen as a violation of good practice guidelines, exercised with the aim of enabling the patient to consult there and then. But, in fact, such a decision may directly jeopardise clinical outcome and predispose to subsequent error because the patient may fail to disclose important information precisely because they are embarrassed to discuss health matters in front of a relative. This in turn may lead to delayed or faulty diagnosis; and the fact that the doctor has sanctioned a relative to interpret may mean the health service authorities to underestimate the need for more professional interpreters to be recruited by the service, thereby perpetuating the very system fault that engendered the violation in the first place.

As this example indicates, violations usually feature a rationale, the belief – sometimes mistaken – that transgression of a rule or regulation offers economy of effort without significantly threatening worse health outcomes. Because they involve conscious deliberated decisions, violations are generally believed to be avoidable by acts of will. However, we have seen that some violations may arise as compromises between best practice and what seems practicable in the circumstances. Custom and culturally reinforced mindsets influence decisions about whether or not to breach a regulation ('this is how I was taught to undertake this task, which was not according to a new rule set'). On the other hand, violations can stem from an attitude of recklessness on the part of a health carer who understands but chooses to ignore substantial risks that may be involved in transgressing a regulation.

Reason notes that industrial violations are more likely to be made by men than by women, and that their frequency declines with age [21]. Based on the type of transgression involved, violations are classified as routine, exceptional or criminal acts. Routine violations involve everyday breaches of rules, which typically consist of cutting corners, such as not always washing hands between examining patients. The consequences of this vary depending on the health care setting – in intensive care or infectious diseases units it may threaten life, whereas in general practice it may be relatively less dangerous. As Merry and McCall Smith point out [22, pp. 108–9], routine health care violations are legion, both in number and variety and include, for example:

providing patients with less information than certain regulatory bodies have prescribed for the purpose of obtaining informed consent; failing to check the results of clinical investigations (such as blood tests) in a timely manner; taking medical histories from patients in open ward situations which fail to provide adequate privacy; filling in labels incompletely; completing case notes inadequately …

Although violations are generally held to be avoidable, if they become a matter of habit or 'second nature' on the part of a health care grouping, such transgressions can become embedded in stereotypic actions undertaken without much conscious thought which then require special effort and training to prevent.

Exceptional violations occur in exceptional or extreme situations; for example, a sudden, unheralded clinical emergency that appears to necessitate breach of usual procedures. However, 'benevolent transgressions' are often subject to post hoc review and require explicit justification.

Criminal violations involve transgressions undertaken for deliberately harmful purposes, such as to defraud a patient or the health care system or, more rarely and bizarrely, to sabotage care and to injure patients [22] (see Chapter 3).

Others classifications of health care violations are possible. Reason, for example, divides them into 'routine', 'optimising' (those undertaken to further personal rather than task-related goals) and 'necessary or situational' violations (that appear to offer the only course available by which to get a job done in the circumstances, see also Chapter 2) [17].

Learning from errors and violations

Errors understood as unintentional divergences from desirable goals or standards have long been viewed as sentinel phenomena. 'Errors show us the way to truth' wrote the 16th century German astronomer, Johannes Kepler, when discussing observational errors and defects in instrumentation [24]. 'By far the most instructive part of a [military] campaign is to know why we fail' wrote George Scovell, a 19th century code-breaker in the Duke of Wellington's army during the Peninsular War [25, p. 47]. Mistakes, when recognised, require not only to be corrected but *corrected for*. Errors in thought or investigational procedure may lead to the construction of erroneous mental maps or models that embody faulty conclusions [26] that once identified, estimated, measured and taken into account, may lead to improved understandings [27]. Although generally identified retrospectively, the investigation of health care errors and violations can bring to light important misunderstandings about a situation and shortcomings of procedure which in turn, and when adjusted for, may lead to enhancements in patient safety [28].

Erring and moral judgment

In most walks of life error remains bound up with errancy, diverging from prescribed or recognised pathways – wandering fallibly off track. Where health care errors are in the frame, moral judgments keep close company [29] (Box 1.3). Those who err are generally characterised negatively, whether in psychological, attitudinal, character, knowledge-based or skills terms, because in this thought schema it is believed they should (and could) have done otherwise. Within such a schema, negative human traits operate not

---

Box 1.3: *The Mistake* by James Fenton

With the mistake your life goes in reverse.
Now you can see exactly what you did
Wrong yesterday and wrong the day before
And each mistake leads back to something worse

And every nuance of your hypocrisy
Towards yourself, and every excuse
Stands solidly on the perspective lines
And there is perfect visibility.

What an enlightenment. The colonnade
Rolls past on either side. You needn't move.
The statues of your errors brush your sleeve.
You watch the tale turn back – and you're dismayed.

And this dismay at this, this big mistake
Is made worse by the sight of all those who
Knew all along where these mistakes would lead –
Those frozen friends who watched the crisis break.

Why didn't they *say*? Oh, but they did indeed –
Said with a murmur when the time was wrong
Or by a mild refusal to assent
Or told you plainly but you would not heed.

Yes, you can hear them now. It hurts. It's worse
Than any sneer from any enemy.
Take this dismay. Lay claim to this mistake.
Look straight along the lines of this reverse.

The Mistake by James Fenton from *Out of Danger* (©James Fenton 1993) is reproduced by permission of PFD (www.pfd.co.uk) on behalf of James Fenton.

only to diminish the moral worthiness of the erring person, but also to help explain, at least in part, how a mistake may have come about: for example, by flawed reasoning, inattentiveness, absent mindedness, poor planning, poor memory, ignorance, arrogance, lack of insight, impatience, overambitiousness, hurriedness, lack of perspective, overconfidence, inability to listen, tiredness, laziness or clumsiness.

However, the modern perspective on errors conceptualises them as essentially, not merely definitionally, unintentional and therefore unavoidable by an act of will (and by use of foresight) on the part of the person who errs (see Chapter 6). On this account, judgmentalism towards someone who errs is an inappropriate and primitive attitude and response to a genuine error. Yet

---

Box 1.4: James Reason's parapraxia

One day in the late 1970s, James Reason was making tea, and the cat was clamouring to be fed. He efficiently opened the tin of cat food – and put it in his teapot. The two components got mixed up. Both the teapot and the cat's feeding dish afforded the same opportunity – putting stuff in. As a cognitive psychologist, Reason suddenly realised a new research topic was literally under his nose. In tracing the causes of absent-minded incidents, Reason began an exploration of human error. Three decades later, he has become a leading expert on error and one of the recognised architects of the tools used to improve patient safety.

R. Lertzman [103]

---

there remains a tension, as Judith André has noted, between lack of intention and avoidability: 'Mistakes are inevitable. On the other hand they are to be avoided; nothing counts as a mistake unless in some sense we could have done otherwise' [30]. It is 'avoidability in some sense' that grounds the moral disapprobation which modern students of error believe most usefully directs attention away from those who err towards identifying and improving poor design and 'latent errors' in health care systems and operations.

It is over a century since investigators began formally enquiring into human error non-moralistically. Sigmund Freud's *Psychopathology of Everyday Life* discussed everyday slips of the tongue and pen, misreadings, aberrant actions, forgetting names and muddling up of memories, which together he called 'parapraxes'. Freud believed their cognitive basis lay in intra-psychic conflicts with the unconscious; once repression fails, otherwise secret desires, ambitions, fantasies and fears erupt into waking life as perturbations of thought and action – slips, transpositions, substitutions and muddlements. This work was published in 1901 in the journal, *Monatsschrift für Psychiatrie und Neurologie*, appeared in book form in 1904 (in English in 1914) and was enormously influential in its naturalistic framing of the study of mistakes in showing that everyday errors might carry meanings that could be investigated empirically [31,32] (Box 1.4).

At the time that Freud's work was appearing in translation, a Hungarian psychiatrist, Jenö Kollarits, began observing his own and a smaller number of his wife and colleague's dyspraxias of speech, reading and writing ($n = 1100$). From these he constructed a fourfold phenomenological classification which comprised substitution (66% of the series), omission (21%), insertion (12%) and repetition (1%). Less concerned with psychological mechanisms than Freud [33], Kollarits recognised that in the commonest types of errors 'action is split away from intention by insufficient attention' [34] – a phenomenon recognised today in lapses ('glitches in cognition' such as failing to recall a drug name or not attending carefully to dosage) and slips (unintended acts arising from failures of selection or recognition such as writing the incorrect name or dosage of medications on prescriptions) [35–37].

Multidisciplinary perspectives

The multidisciplinary perspective on safety that this volume develops is rooted in a number of other 20th century health care developments which we consider briefly below. Firstly, there was a growing recognition throughout the century that iatrogenesis could be an important cause of serious patient harm: 'physicians, by ill-considered statements, are responsible for many a wrecked life, and … it is much easier to make a diagnosis than to unmake it', Francis Peabody wrote in a famous paper published in *JAMA* in 1927, clearly implicating misdiagnoses and poor communication in the genesis of patient harms [38,39]. In 1936, after the deaths of four patients who received mercuric oxicyanide instead of local anaesthetic injections in the Maria Hospital in Stockholm, medication-related harm was officially recognised in Sweden, which enacted legislation setting up a system of reporting of serious injuries related to medical treatment [40]. A clutch of post-War studies that sought to estimate the extent and variety of patient harms caused by hospital care [41–49] prompted Lucian Leape to encapsulate the magnitude of their significance visually, by comparing mortality from hospital-related harms to the death toll from three jumbo jets crashing every 2 days in the USA throughout the year. This startling image not only drew attention to the scale of the loss of life in hospitals from health related injuries, but to differences in the intensity and purpose of investigations that generally followed potentially avoidable deaths in the two sectors. Investigation into aeroplane crashes was rigorous and aimed at learning lessons wherever possible, whereas at the time of his comment, investigation into health care harms was generally less visible, less rigorous and relatively unsystematic. The Institute of Medicine's (IOM) report, *To Err Is Human*, extrapolated the findings of the same studies that Leape had referred to:

… at least 44,000 Americans die each year as a result of medical errors. The results of the New York Study suggest the number may be as high as 98,000. Even when using the lower estimate, deaths due to medical errors exceed the number attributable to the 8th-leading cause of death. More people die in a given year as a result of medical errors than from motor vehicle accidents (43,458), breast cancer (42,297), or AIDS (16,516). [50]

The title of the report, *To Err Is Human: Building a Safer Health System*, was plucked in part from Alexander Pope's 1711 poem, *An Essay on Criticism*. In penning 'To err is Human; to forgive, divine', Pope acknowledged that humans not only make mistakes but also crave forgiveness. But the highly influential systems approach which the IOM advocated did not engage

with forgiveness from patients harmed by health care [51] (see Chapter 13).[†]
Nevertheless, the IOM's synthesis of materials and concepts led to accelerated policy development in the field of patient safety worldwide.

Secondly, in the last quarter of the 20th century, psychologists interested in the cognitive origins of human error were joined by human factor engineers interested in the design of complex technologies and human–machine interfaces [21,52,53]. Meetings of psychologists, mathematicians, philosophers and engineers were sponsored by a variety of organisations (including the Science Committee of the North Atlantic Treaty Organization and the Rockefeller Foundation) to discuss human–machine interfaces, the concept of error in complex industrial settings, error recognition and taxonomies. These meetings marked the beginning of new cross-disciplinary interests in human errors [33,54]. Stimulated in part by industrial catastrophes that occurred in the 1970s and 1980s – the meltdown at Three Mile Island nuclear power plant near Harrisburg, USA, uncontrolled release of massive amounts of radiation from the Chernobyl nuclear power station in the Soviet Union, release of poisoned gas at Bhopal, India, extensive electrical power cuts in New York City, and uncontrollable conflagrations in the North Sea Piper Alpha oil rig and King's Cross underground station in London – engineers sought to discover what sorts of failures accounted for breakdowns on such a scale. Operator errors, small tolerance of error margins, too close coupling (i.e. direct transmission) of undesirable effects with insufficient buffering, and undetected failures in the organisation of plants meant that, in effect, accidents were waiting to happen: 'If interactive complexity and tight coupling – system characteristics – inevitably will produce an accident, I believe we are justified in calling it a *normal accident* or *system accident*. This is an expression of an integral part of the system, not a statement of frequency' wrote one influential errors analyst [52, p. 5]. Complex interacting defects – poor design embedded in layout or equipment, dysfunctional maintenance arrangements

---

[†]Alexander Pope penned this *Essay* in 1709 when he was only 21. It was published 2 years later and concerns the art of writing and criticism. In it, Pope identifies wit, a facility for subtlety in conceiving things – 'a perfect conception with an easy delivery' – as especially praiseworthy in a writer and pride the chief cause of judging ill of written works:

'Tis hard to say if greater want of skill
Appear in writing or in judging ill,
But of the two less dangerous is the offence
To tire our patience than mislead our sense:
Some few in that but numbers err in this,
Ten censure wrong for one who writes amiss,
A fool might once himself alone expose,
Now one in verse makes many more in prose.

The capacity to err that Pope had in mind is etched into our being. Humans are flawed, 'Born but to die, and reasoning but to err' he wrote in his later poem *Essay on Man* [1733].

and staff relations, pressure on profit to cost ratios and combinations of such 'sociotechnical factors' – in varying degrees were found to have predisposed to uncorrected (uncorrectable at the time) failings that caused colossal breakdown. Interest in defect latency in systems design arises from these meetings [33,55].

Thirdly, in the second half of the 20th century, sociological and ethnographic studies started to characterise how different subcultures within medicine handled medical mistakes, and which features of error the profession considered excusable and which blameworthy [56–59]. Medical etiquette generally forbade criticism of colleagues which meant that many health care errors (even when recognised) were handled by informal, ad hoc collegial processes dominated by the values and procedures of patronage common to clans rather than by the standards of civil scrutiny. Their findings uncannily reinforced concerns George Bernard Shaw had expressed more than half a century earlier in his preface to the play *Doctors' Dilemma* (1906):

Anyone who has ever known doctors well enough to hear medical shop talk, without reserve, knows that they are full of stories about each other's blunders and errors, and that the theory of their omniscience and omnipotence no more holds good among themselves than it did with Molière and Napoleon. But for this very reason no doctor dare accuse another of malpractice … the effect of this state of things is to make the medical profession a conspiracy to hide its own shortcomings. [60, p. 17]

Literary representations of medical mistakes and violations

Novelists and poets had depicted health care blunders and violations a good deal earlier. In *Madame Bovary* (1857), for example, Gustave Flaubert created a story that hinged on the character, education and practice of Charles Bovary, a French officier de santé (health officer), working in rural Normandy. A well meaning if not a particularly bright personal medical attendant, Charles Bovary clearly understands the boundaries of his knowledge and of his role, and initially has little interest in going beyond the level of his training and experience. In treating patients he successfully applies many of standard nostrums, external treatments, bleedings and ingeniously constructed splints; he engages with his patients' concerns and, in consequence, his reputation and practice grow. But Bovary lets himself be persuaded by Emma, his wife, and by the town's pharmacist, Homais, into operating on a patient's congenital clubfoot even though Bovary himself has had no formal surgical training in the procedure. Neither of his persuaders is motivated by concern for the patient's well being; Emma is bored with the domesticity of life with a provincial country doctor and longs for excitement, and the advancement that will ensue from her husband's surgical success which will propel her into the circle of the local aristocracy and point her towards Paris; Homais, on the other hand, believes himself to be an enlightened man of science. Inspired by reports of surgical progress he has read about only in newspapers and intoxicated by his own rhetoric, Homais spurs Charles on to perform surgery. Initially, at least, the procedure seems to take place uneventfully. But after 5 days of unremitting pain it is clear that the contraption used by Bovary to set the patient Hippolyte's foot postoperatively has caused severe pain and bruising. Gangrene sets in necessitating calling for a fully trained practitioner to amputate the leg. Charles recognises the damage he has caused Hippolyte and tries to make amends by buying him a wooden leg; and the resulting is that the clippity-clop of his patient's step forever reminds him of his professional blunder. The novel is an acute observation of provincial country doctoring in 19th century France, and a psychological study of a marriage between a naïve and gullible doctor which leads – in modern lingo – to a serious but unintended health care violation [61].

In the period after Shaw's *Doctors' Dilemma* many writers explored abuses and violations of medical practice. In A. J. Cronin's novel, *The Citadel* (1937), one surgical violation stands out; during an abdominal operation, Dr Charles Ivory incises rather than ligates a vascular lesion and as a result the patient bleeds to death on the operating table. There is no question of informing anyone, not least the patient's distraught widow – Ivory tells her that 'no power on earth could have saved him' – and in the novel no opportunity arises for anyone to learn from the mistake [62].

Years before sociologists began formally to study medical errors and violations, novelists and playwrights explored these phenomena – usually in terms of character and the closed culture of medicine and much earlier than clinicians themselves were able to acknowledge their own fallibility publicly. With only very occasional and sporadic exceptions, it was not until the 1980s that case histories written by clinicians disturbed by their own medical errors and unsure how best to advise patients of their occurrence, began to appear in print [63]. It is from this period that confessional, first-person accounts claim a place in medical journals and errors started to be discussed in professional (and increasingly public) fora [64]. These reports address questions such as: Can a doctor apologise without increasing medicolegal liability? Does apology vitiate medical indemnity insurance [65]? What effects do errors have on a clinician's self-esteem and practice [66,67]? What are the personal and institutional barriers to apologising [68]? Extended semi-fictionalised accounts of clinical cases allow in-depth exploration and discussion of the complexity of clinical errors [69], and book-length expositions by distinguished physicians and surgeons begin to be published featuring health care errors. These works explore the uncertain nature of clinical knowledge, the cognitive, emotional and interpersonal origins of diagnostic bias, the narrow scope and stereotypical nature of much clinical thinking, the relatively closed cultures of medical practice and the omnipresent need for 'common sense' and 'human touch' abilities in dealing with errors: capacities to listen attentively and to empathise with patients, which in the pages of some of these works, can only be achieved by heroic doctors [70,71].

Medical heroism triumphs in *Bodies* (2003), a disturbing novel by a former junior hospital doctor, Jed Mercurio, featuring a doctor who for a while is also a heroin user who gets caught up in a dizzying array of medical errors and violations that are dealt with by colleagues and the hospital authorities by denial, rationalisation, confabulation and cover-up. Towards the end of the book its unnamed doctor soliloquises:

I'm ashamed of medicine, the profession I once held above all others. But more I'm ashamed of myself. I'm ashamed of having approved of this secret society because it granted me a second chance after I killed the Breathless Lady. Now I see it acts without discrimination between error and negligence, between inexperience and incompetence, between remorse and arrogance. The code of silence is absolute. It shields us all alike. [72, p. 170]

The narrator of *Bodies* manages to redeem himself only when he summons up the courage to blow the whistle on colleagues and to apologise to the relatives of a patient who had died as a result of a medical mistake that had taken place months previously and about which the dead patient's relatives knew nothing. The dramatised version of the novel brought medical errors and violations into the homes of a large television audience. According to the network that screened the TV series, such dramas concerned not just 'heroic, handsome doctors and pretty nurses', but 'the truth about a group of stressed-out professionals doing a sometimes impossible job while confronting all-too-real dilemmas' [73].

Today, the public image of medicine conspicuously encompasses fallibility: late 20th century Hollywood films which feature medical roles no longer only depict stereotypes of the dedicated, compassionate doctor. A new zone of medical work is becoming visible, which reveals the lives and experience of doctors who feel conflicted about careers that are at odds with their personal lives, who make errors, commit violations and face litigation [74].

Patient safety

The moral imperative that generations of students and doctors have taken to be an ethical foundation to their practice – 'first do no harm' – is one that is flouted inadvertently or deliberately on a daily basis. Whether or not this motto should be taken to be ethically aspirational rather than a principle of practice [75], the need is pressing to develop insights from the study of errors and violations which can help us to lower the hazards of health care and enhance patient safety [76]. Until recently, a significant impediment has been lack of an agreed definition of patient safety, and how to recognize the myriad threats to it. The National Patient Safety Agency's current definition,

'A patient safety incident is any unintended or unexpected incident which could have harmed or did lead to harm for one or more patients being cared for by the NHS' is becoming widely used in the UK and elsewhere [9]. It offers an inclusive starting point matched by the World Health Organization's World Alliance for Patient Safety map and classification scheme, which provides five complementary root nodes, or primary classifications, for use in analysis of safety incidents:

1 Impact: the outcome or effects of medical error and systems failure, commonly referred to as harm to the patient.

2 Type: the implied or visible processes that were faulty or failed.

3 Domain: the characteristics of the setting in which an incident occurred and the type of individuals involved.

4 Cause: the factors and agents that led to an incident.

5 Prevention and mitigation: the measures taken or proposed to reduce incidence and effects of adverse occurrences [77–79].

Agreement on conceptual and organisational factors is a prerequisite for making sense of international incident data on patient safety, which reporting systems now collect [9]; it also aids understanding of how to translate the descriptive insights these systems offer into tangible improvements in patient care.

An area of patient safety that is attracting scrutiny in the UK relates to the effectiveness of medicines regulation at a national level. Failure of the Medicines and Healthcare products Regulatory Agency (MHRA) to recognise and warn in a timely manner of an increased likelihood of suicidal and violent behaviour, and of the existence of a dependence syndrome, associated with prescribing some selective serotonin reuptake inhibitor drugs, reflects potentially serious system defects in the post-licensing surveillance of drugs [80–83]. There appears to have been insufficient awareness within the MHRA of the severe limitations of relying on clinical trials when assessing benefits and harms of medicines in routine medical practice (most trials are underpowered to detect important, unwanted, rare medication effects), and failure to appreciate the extent of the bias in favour of benefit that stems from non-publication of negative trial results [84]. Feedback from the users of these drugs, supporting concerns about the existence of these negative effects, was not incorporated into the MHRA assessment of medication, which skewed perceived benefit versus risk for these drugs [85].

The other area in health care safety that is gathering importance is the role that patients can play in helping to avoid errors and minimise hazard [86] (see Chapter 12). The US Agency for Healthcare Research and Quality (AHRQ) now posts a patient fact sheet on its website entitled *20 Tips to Help Prevent Medical Errors* prefaced by reference to the IOM's estimates of yearly mortality from current health care provision (its tips are summarised in Box 1.5) [87,88]. Jerome Groopman, a Harvard oncologist, exhorts patients to help doctors to avoid errors. In his view, patients themselves offer the final defence against misdiagnosis and medical mismanagement:

Box 1.5: AHRQ patient fact sheet *20 Tips to Help Prevent Medical Errors* [87]

1 The single most important way you can help to prevent errors is to be an active member of your health care team.

2 Make sure that all of your doctors know about everything you are taking. This includes prescription and over-the-counter medicines, and dietary supplements such as vitamins and herbs.

3 Make sure your doctor knows about any allergies and adverse reactions you have had to medicines.

4 When your doctor writes you a prescription, make sure you can read it.

5 Ask for information about your medicines in terms you can understand – both when your medicines are prescribed and when you receive them:
- What is the medicine for?
- How am I supposed to take it, and for how long?
- What side effects are likely? What do I do if they occur?
- Is this medicine safe to take with other medicines or dietary supplements I am taking?
- What food, drink or activities should I avoid while taking this medicine?

6 When you pick up your medicine from the pharmacy, ask 'Is this the medicine that my doctor prescribed?'

7 If you have any questions about the directions on your medicine labels, ask.

8 Ask your pharmacist for the best device to measure your liquid medicine. Also, ask questions if you are not sure how to use it.

9 Ask for written information about the side effects your medicine could cause.

10 If you have a choice, choose a hospital at which many patients have the procedure or surgery you need.

11 If you are in a hospital, consider asking all health care workers who have direct contact with you whether they have washed their hands.

12 When you are being discharged from the hospital, ask your doctor to explain the treatment plan you will use at home.

13 If you are having surgery, make sure that you, your doctor and your surgeon all agree and are clear on exactly what will be done.

14 Speak up if you have questions or concerns.

15 Make sure that someone, such as your personal doctor, is in charge of your care.

16 Make sure that all health professionals involved in your care have important health information about you.

17 Ask a family member or friend to be there with you and to be your advocate (someone who can help get things done and speak up for you if you cannot).

18 Know that 'more' is not always better.

19 If you have a test, do not assume that no news is good news.

20 Learn about your condition and treatments by asking your doctor and nurse and by using other reliable sources.

For three decades practicing as a physician, I looked to traditional sources to assist me in my thinking about my patients: textbooks and medical journals; mentors and colleagues with deeper or more varied clinical experience; students and residents who posed challenging questions. But after writing this book, I realized that I can have another vital partner who helps improve my thinking, a partner who may, with a few pertinent and focused questions, protect me from the cascade of cognitive pitfalls that cause misguided care. That partner is my patient or her family member or friend who seeks to know what is in my mind, how I am thinking. [89, p. 268]

Groopman wants people worried about being misunderstood or incorrectly diagnosed in future to be helped to prompt doctors to rethink the nature of their possible problems, by posing questions, such as: What else could it be? Is there anything that doesn't fit? Is it possible I have more than one problem?

How active a role patients can be expected to take in ensuring the safety of health care at times of physical and psychological impairment, or moments of particular vulnerability, is considered in detail in Chapter 12. Other high-risk industries ask (or demand that) their users play a role in ensuring better safety, such as by using seat belts in cars, helmets on motor cycles and pedal cycles, and by not using mobile phones in aeroplanes. But the knowledge and interpersonal confidence required to optimise the safety of health care far exceeds use of relatively simple, reliable, fail-safe gadgets such as seat belts and cycle helmets which help protect from harm [90,91], through actions which are generally backed by legislation, surveillance and some form of enforcement. Nevertheless, such measures posit a degree of partnership between high-risk industries and their users that health care is beginning to emulate [92,93].

When accounting for patients harmed by health care, doctors tend to rationalise what has happened. This displaces moral responsibility away from those who may have caused harm and provides those confronted with consequent injury with some degree of psychological defence against their own emotions. John Banja notes that narcissistic needs on the part of many health carers, who are often motivated by unconscious desires to gain the praise and love of their patients, can easily be transformed when mistakes become apparent, into controlling behaviour, emotional distance and lack of empathy. Rationalisation not only carries a risk of distorting what may have happened (see Chapter 14), but also serves the emotional function of relieving anxiety and helping to maintain moral self-worth [94].

However, it is not only clinicians who feel guilty about medical mistakes (see Chapter 13):

family members frequently experience similar or even stronger feelings of guilt. Patients and their families may fear further harm, including retribution from health care workers, if they express their feelings or even ask about the mistakes which they perceive. And clinicians may turn away from patients who have been harmed, isolating them at moments when they are most in need [95].

There is no 'master method' for comprehending the array of possible health care mistakes and violations that can lead to improved safety in health care [96]. Some approaches to health care hazards stress flawed human agency, culpability and the potential for human perfectibility through training, life-long education and technology; other approaches give primacy to understanding natural science and complex systems in health care whilst stressing room for continuous improvement.

Health Care Errors and Patient Safety offers a multilayered contribution to understanding aberrantly provided health care arranged in three sections. **Part 1, Understanding patient safety**, contains six chapters that explore theories, concepts and cultures central to a better understanding of health care safety. Chapter 2 outlines the cognitive basis of different sorts of clinical errors and violations. Chapter 3 argues the case for treating the worst sort of violation, unlawful healthcare killing, as a safety incident as well as a serious crime. Chapter 4 delineates the rationale for including errors by patients within overall concerns of safety in health care, whilst Chapter 5 focuses on the role of organisations and organisational culture when making changes to health care systems that are designed to benefit safety. How the law recognises and deals with medical errors is examined in Chapter 6, which argues that it generally makes moral culpability too closely dependent on a harmful health outcome and is inefficient in compensating patients. The final chapter in this section echoes Chapter 6 in considering the many advantages (and some disadvantages) of instituting a no-blame culture in health care.

Part 2, Threats to patient safety, focuses on areas of health care that are especially hazardous to patients. The cognitive components of diagnostic errors, one of the most frequent and potentially serious types of clinical errors, are carefully dissected in Chapter 8, and miscommunications in the context of a linguistically diverse society are set out and analysed in Chapter 9. Chapter 10 highlights points of transition in health care between different health jurisdictions such as hospital wards, primary and secondary care, night and day shifts and across staff handovers – that are especially hazardous to patients, and Chapter 11 documents effective programmes of medicine management which improve patient safety. Chapter 12 reviews and reinforces the huge role that patients have to play in prevention of health care errors at policy, information and individual levels.

Part 3, Responses to health care errors and violations, examines approaches to handling errors and violations at individual, data collection and educational health care levels. Chapter 13 outlines the suffering that is compounded by inadequate explanation and apology after safety incidents, which good practice can alleviate. The benefits of disciplined team reflection offered by root cause analysis are set out in Chapter 14. Chapter 15 reviews sources and methods to estimate the frequency of health care safety events and Chapter 16 sets out the challenges posed by collecting and analysing reports of health care errors on a national scale. How to design and teach patient safety curricula in medical schools in North America and the UK are the subjects of Chapters 17 and 18, and the final chapter zooms in on media representations of health care safety, and the drives and constraints on how journalists frame reports on medical errors.

Contributions to this volume range widely across health care and policy terrains and collectively reveal the extent to which safety issues ramify throughout health service provision. 'Narratives rather than numbers are the primary data of the safety sciences' writes James Reason, and this volume contains many vignettes that encapsulate errors, violations and safety incidents. But, in the safety sciences, Reason cannily adds 'numbers have their place' [97] too, and the volume embraces a strong focus on incident analysis of conventional and new safety data (Chapters 15 and 16).

Towards the close of the 19th century an anonymous reviewer in *The Lancet* noted that 'knowledge grows but mistakes recur' [98]. In seeking to build greater awareness and insight into medical fallibility, health care mistakes and violations, we hope that *Health Care Errors and Patient Safety* will help to interrupt this sad succession.

Appendix 1.1: Glossary of key terms in health care safety

Adapted from appendix 1 of Runciman et al. [99].

Adverse event: an incident in which a person receiving health care is harmed.

Adverse reaction: an adverse event where the correct process is followed for the context in which the event occurs but unexpected harm results.

Error: a mistake – an unintentionally wrong conduct or judgment that usually manifests as doing the wrong thing (commission) or not doing the right thing (omission), may or may not result in harm, and is not the result of the operation of chance.[‡]

Event: something that happens to or with a person.

Health care incident: an event or circumstance, which could have or did have or resulted in unintended or unnecessary harm to a person and/or complaint, loss or damage.

Health care outcome: the health status of an individual, a group or population, which is wholly or partially attributable to a health care action, event or circumstance.

Health care safety: hazards from health care processes.

[‡] Reason defines error as a generic notion that 'encompasses all those occasions in which a planned sequence of mental or physical activities fails to achieve its intended outcome, when these failures cannot be attributed to the intervention of some chance agency' [21, p. 9].

Health care system: the structures, procedures, policies, culture and organisation of a health care facility.

Health care violation: a deliberate deviation from accepted rules, procedures or standards that may be intended to benefit (rarely to harm) patient care, but which may be culpable and reprehensible.

Iatrogenic: arising from or associated with health care rather than an underlying disease or injury.

Liability: responsibility for an action according to law or in a legal sense.

Mistake: an error – an unintentionally wrong conduct or judgment that usually manifests as doing the wrong thing (commission) or not doing the right thing (omission).

Near-miss: an incident that did not cause harm.

Negligence: an incident causing harm, damage or loss to an individual as a result of substandard care where a duty exists to provide care of a reasonable standard (as decided by due legal process).

Quality of health care: the extent to which a health care process or product produces a desired specifiable outcome.

Risk (of an intervention): generally the chance of harm, whether by commission or omission.

Risk management: (i) design and implementation of a programme to identify and avoid or minimise risks to patients, staff or visitors of health care facilities; (ii) design and implementation of a programme to identify and avoid or minimise risks of financial losses including legal liability of health care staff or institutions; and (iii) design and implementation of a programme to identify and transfer risks to others by payment of insurance premiums.

Root cause analysis: a systematic investigative process that identifies factors contributing to a health care incident.

Side-effect: an effect, other than that intended, produced by an agent; in pharmacology this term refers to an undesirable effect that generally has dose–response characteristics (although this seems not to be the case in anaphylaxis).

References

1 Bates D. The epistemology of error in late Enlightenment France. *Eighteenth-Century Studies* 1996; **29**: 307–27.

2 Tonks A. Patient safety. Safer by design. *British Medical Journal* 2008; **336**: 186–8. Available at http://www.bmj.com

3 National Patient Safety Association, Saferhealthcare: http://www.saferhealthcare.org.uk/ihi.

4 Institute of Medicine. To err is human: building a safer health system. *In*: Kohn LT, Corrigan JM, Donaldson MS, eds. *Errors in Health Care: A Leading Cause of Death and Injury.* National Academy Press, Washington, 1999: 160–84.

5 Department of Health. *An Organisation with a Memory: Report of an Expert Group on Learning from Adverse Events in the NHS.* HMSO, London, 2000.

6 Department of Health. *Building a Safer NHS for Patients – Implementing an Organisation with a Memory*. HMSO, London, 2001.

7 Donaldson L. *Building a Safer NHS for Patients: Improving Medication Safety. A Report by the Chief Pharmaceutical Officer*. Department of Health, London, 2004. Available at http://www.dh.gov.uk/en/Publicationsandstatistics/Publications/PublicationsPolicy AndGuidance/DH_4071443.

8 Agency for Healthcare Research and Quality. *Medical Errors and Patient Safety*. AHRQ, London, 2003. Available at http://www.ahrq.gov/qual/errorsix.htm.

9 National Patient Safety Agency, NHS Safety Division, UK: http://www.npsa.nhs. uk/patientsafety/.

10 Institute for Safe Medication Practices, USA: http://www.ismp.org/.

11 National Coordinating Council for Medication Error Prevention and Reporting, USA: www.nccmerp.org.

12 Leape LL. Error in medicine. *Journal of the American Medical Association* 1994; **272**: 1851–7.

13 Royal S, Smeaton L, Avery AJ, Hurwitz B, Sheikh A. Interventions in primary care to reduce medication related adverse events and hospital admissions: systematic review and meta-analysis *Quality and Safety in Health Care* 2006; **15**: 23–31.

14 Berger J. *Signatures of the Invisible*. A conference convened by the European Organisation for Nuclear Research, the London Institute and the Gulbenkian Foundation, Lisbon, 2002. (Quoted in Virilio P. *The Original Accident*. Polity Press, London, 2007: 12.)

15 Hurwitz B. Erring and learning in clinical practice. *British Journal of General Practice* 2002; **52**: S26–S30.

16 Horton R. The uses of errors. *Lancet* 1999; **353**: 422–3.

17 Reason J. Understanding adverse events: the human factor. *In*: Vincent C, ed. *Clinical Risk Management*, 2nd edn. BMJ Books, London, 2001: 9–30.

18 Gorovitz S, MacIntyre A. *Toward a Theory of Medical Fallibility*. Hastings Center Report Vol. 5, No. 6. 1975: 13–23.

19 Quick O. Outing medical errors: questions of trust and responsibility. *Medical Law Review* 2006; 14 (1): 22–43.

20 Besnard D, Baxter G. *Human Compensations for Undependable Systems*. Technical Reports Series No. CS TR 819. University of Newcastle upon Tyne, Newcastle, 2003. Available at http://rogue.ncl.ac.uk/file_store/trs/819.pdf.

21 Reason J. *Human Error*. Cambridge University Press, Cambridge, MA, 1992.

22 Merry A, McCall-Smith A. *Errors, Medicine and the Law*. Cambridge University Press, Cambridge, 2001.

23 Irshad T, Worth A, Sheikh A. Are translation and interpretation services a necessity or a luxury? *Diversity in Health and Social Care* 2007; **4**: 87–9.

24 Hon G. On Kepler's awareness of the problem of experimental error. *Annals of Science* 1987; **44**; 545–91.

25 Urban M. *The Man who Broke Napoleon's Codes*. Faber and Faber, London, 2001.

26 Hacking I. *Representing and Intervening*. Cambridge University Press, Cambridge, 1984.

27 Hon G 'If this be error': probing experiment with error. *In*: Heidelberger M, Steinle F, eds. *Experimental Essays – Versuche zum Experiment*. Nomos, Baden Baden, 1998: 227–48. (Cited in Schickore J. (Ab)using the past for present purposes: exposing contextual and trans-contextual features of error. *Perspectives on Science* 2002; **10**: 433–56.)

28 Allchin D. Error types. *Perspectives on Science* 2001; **9**: 3858.

29 Frader JE. Mistakes in medicine: personal and moral responses. *In*: Rubin SB, Zoloth L, eds. *Margin of Error*. University Publishing Group, Hagerstown, MD: 2000: 113–29.

30 André J. Humility reconsidered. *In*: Rubin SB, Zoloth L, eds. *Margin of Error*. University Publishing Group, Hagerstown, MD, 2000: 59–72.
31 Freud S. *The Psychopathology of Everyday Life*. Penguin Freud Library (Richards A, ed.). Penguin Books, Hamondsworth, 1976.
32 Strachey J. Introduction. *In*: Freud S. *The Psychopathology of Everyday Life*. Penguin Freud Library (Richards A, ed.). Penguin Books, Hamondsworth, 1976: 31–6.
33 Senders JW, Moray NP, eds. *Human Error*. Lawrence Erlbaum Associates, Inc., NJ, 1991.
34 Kollarits J. *Observations on dyspraxias (errors of action). Comparing errors in speaking, reading and writing*. Manuscript, 1937 (Personal communication from John Senders 2006.)
35 Anonymous. *Unit 5: Medication Errors*. Available at http://www.mindspring.com/~mgilula/Unit5.pdf (accessed January 2008).
36 Dean B, Schacter M, Vincent C, Barber N. Causes of prescribing errors in hospital inpatients: a prospective study. *Lancet* 2002; **359**: 1373–8.
37 Cresswell KM, Fernando B, McKinstry B, Sheikh A. Adverse drug events in the elderly. *British Medical Bulletin* 2007; 1–16.
38 Peabody F. The care of the patient. *Journal of the American Medical Association* 1927; **88**: 877–82.
39 Sharpe VA, Faden AI. *Medical Harm*. Cambridge University Press, Cambridge, 1998.
40 Ödergård S. From punishment to prevention? *Safety Science Monitor* 1999; **3**: 1–10.
41 Schimmel EM. The hazards of hospitalization. *Annals of Internal Medicine* 1964; **60**: 100–10.
42 Mills DH, ed. *Report on the Medical Insurance Feasibility Study*. Sutter Publications, San Francisco, 1977.
43 Steel K, Gertman PM, Crescenzi C et al. Iatrogenic illness on a general medical service at a university hospital. *New England Journal of Medicine* 1981; **304**: 638–42.
44 Lesar TS, Briceland LL, Delcoure K et al. Medication prescribing errors in a teaching hospital *Journal of the American Medical Association* 1990; **263**: 2329–34.
45 Clasen DC, Pstonik SL, Evans RS, Burke JP. Computerised surveillance of adverse drug events in hospital patients. *Journal of the American Medical Association* 1991; **266**: 2847–51.
46 Brennan TA, Leape LL, Laird N et al. Incidence of adverse events and negligence of hospitalized patients: report of the Harvard medical practice study I. *New England Journal of Medicine* 1991; **324**: 370–6.
47 Leape LL, Brennan TA, Laird N et al. The nature of adverse events in hospitalized patients: report of the Harvard medical practice study II. *New England Journal of Medicine* 1991; **324**: 377–84.
48 Baker GR, Norton PG, Flintoft V et al. The Canadian Adverse Events Study: the incidence of adverse events among hospital patients in Canada. *Canadian Medical Journal* 2004; **17** (11): 1678–86.
49 Vincent C, Neal G, Woloshynowych M. Adverse events in British hospitals: preliminary retrospective record review. *British Medical Journal* 2001; **322**: 517–19.
50 Kohn LT, Corrigan JM, Donaldson MS, eds. *To Err Is Human: Building a Safer Health System*. Committee on Quality of Health Care in America, Institute of Medicine, 1999. Available at http://www.nap.edu/catalog/9728.html.
51 Berlinger N. *After Harm*. Johns Hopkins University Press, Baltimore, 2005.
52 Perrow C. *Normal Accidents – Living with High Risk Technologies*. Basic Books, New York, 1984.

53 Rasmussen J. *Information Processing and Human–Machine Interaction: An Approach to Cognitive Engineering*. New Holland, New York, 1986.
54 Bento JP. *Man Technique Organization. Course for MTO analysis for National Board of Health and Welfare. Kurs I MTO-analys for Socialstyelesen* (in Swedish). Kärnkraftsäkerhet och Utbildnings AB, Studsvik, Nyköping. (Cited in Ödergård S. From punishment to prevention? *Safety Science Monitor* 1999; **3**: 1–10.)
55 Runciman B, Merry A, Walton A. Health care: a dysfunctional system. *In*: Runciman B, Merry A, Walton M. *Safety and Ethics in Health Care*. Ashgate, Aldershot, 2007: 59–82.
56 Light D. Psychiatry and suicide: the management of a mistake. *American Sociological Review* 1972; **77**: 821–38.
57 Friedson E. *The Profession of Medicine*. Harper and Row, New York, 1970.
58 Bosk CL. *Forgive and Remember: Managing Medical Failure*. University of Chicago Press, Chicago, 1979.
59 Rosenthal M. *The Incompetent Doctor*. Open University Press, Buckingham, 1995.
60 Shaw GB. *The Doctor's Dilemma*. Penguin Books, London, 1946.
61 Flaubert G. *Madame Bovary*. Translated by Geoffrey Wall. Penguin Books, London, 1991.
62 Cronin AJ. *The Citadel*. Gollancz, London, 1937.
63 Hilficker D. Facing our mistakes. *New England Journal of Medicine* 1984; **310**: 118–22,
64 Horton R. We all make mistakes: tell us yours. *Lancet* 2001; **357**: 88.
65 Cuzner E. Safety in health care. Saying sorry is not admission of liability. *British Medical Journal* 2008; **336**: 291. Available at http://www.bmj.com/cgi/content/full/336/7639/291-b?hits=10&FIRSTINDEX=0&HITS=10&searchid=1&resourcetype=HWCIT.
66 Hobbs R. Checks and balances. *Lancet* 2002; **360**: 254.
67 Poulter NR. Suppositions and surprises. *Lancet* 2001: **358**: 1448.
68 Flyn G. Oh no, not again? *BMJ Careers*. 21 January 2006: gp27.
69 Rothman MD. The error. *Yale Journal of Medical Humanities* May 2003. Available at http://yjhm.yale.edu/essays/mrothman1.htm.
70 Gawande A. *Complications*. Picador, New York, 2002.
71 Groopman J. *How Doctors Think*. Houghton Mifflin Company, Boston, 2007.
72 Mercurio J. *Bodies*. Vintage, London, 2003.
73 *Bodies*. http://www.bbc.co.uk/bbcthree/programmes/bodies/.
74 Welsh JM. Strong medicine and the movies: a review. *Literature and Medicine* 1993; **12**: 111–20.
75 Smith CM. Origin and uses of *Primum non Nocere* – above all, do no harm! *Journal of Clinical Pharmacology* 2005; **45**: 371–7.
76 Provonost P. *The Science of Patient Safety: From Rhetoric to Reality.* Video available at http://distance.jhsph.edu/trams/index.cfm?event=training.playSection&sectionID=69.
77 World Health Organisation. *International Classification for Patient Safety*. Version 1.0 for use in field testing, 2007–2008.
78 Chang A, Schyve PM, Croteau RJ, O'Leary DS, Loeb JM. The JCAHO patient safety event taxonomy: a standardized terminology and classification schema for near misses and adverse events. *International Journal for Quality in Health Care* 2005; **17**: 95–105.
79 World Health Organisation. *Towards a Common International Understanding of Patient Safety Concepts and Terms: Taxonomy and Terminology Related to Medical Errors and System Failures*. Department of Health Service Provision, World Health Organisation, Geneva, 2003.
80 Herxheimer A. Turbulence in UK medicines regulation: a stink about SSRI antidepressants that isn't going away. *In*: Glavanis K, O'Donovan O, eds. *Power, Politics and Pharmaceuticals*. Cork University Press, Cork, 2008: 171–82.

81 Medawar C, Hardon A. *Medicines out of Control? Antidepressants and the Conspiracy of Goodwill*. Aksant, Amsterdam, 2004.

82 Herxheimer A. Pharmacovigilance needs a complete rethink (abstract). Available at http://www.socialaudit.org.uk/6080327.htm#winners (posted 28 March 2008).

83 Lumley CE, Walker SR, Hall C, Staunton N, Grob PR. The under-reporting of adverse drug reactions seen in general practice. *Pharmaceutical Medicine* 1986; **1**: 205–12.

84 Chalmers I. The lethal consequences of failing to make full use of all relevant evidence about the effects of medical treatments: the importance of systematic reviews. *In*: P. Rothwell (ed). Treating individuals: From Randomised Trials to Personalised Medicine. London: Elsevier, 2007: 37–58.

85 Medawar C, Herxheimer A. A comparison of adverse drug reaction reports from professionals and users, relating to risk of dependence and suicidal behaviour with paroxetine. *International Journal of Risk and Safety in Medicine* 2003/4; **16**: 3–17.

86 Senders JW. My adventures as a hospital patient. *Quality and Safety in Health Care* 2002; **11**: 365–8.

87 Agency for Healthcare Research and Quality. *20 Tips to Help Prevent Medical Errors Patient Fact Sheet*. AHRQ, London, 2000. Available at http://www.ahrq.gov/consumer/20tips.htm.

88 Berntsen KJ. *Fatal Care and the Patient's Guide to Preventing Medical Errors*. Praeger, New York, 2004.

89 Groopman J. *How Doctors Think*. Houghton Mifflin Company, Boston, 2007.

90 Lyons M. Should patients have a role in patient safety? A safety engineering view. *Quality and Safety in Health Care* 2007; **16**: 140–2.

91 Entwistle VA. Differing perspectives on patient involvement in patient safety. *Quality and Safety in Health Care* 2007; **16**: 82–3.

92 Patients for Patient Safety, London: http://www.nc-hi.com/pdf%20files/London_Declaration_EN.pdf.

93 World Health Organisation, Patients for Patient Safety: http://www.who.int/patientsafety/patients_for_patient/en/.

94 Banja J. *Medical Errors and Medical Narcissism*. Jones and Bartlett Publishers, Sudbury, MA, 2005.

95 Delbanco T, Bell SK. Guilty, afraid, and alone – struggling with medical error. *New England Journal of Medicine* 2007; **357**: 1682–3.

96 Chambers T. Framing our mistakes. *In*: Rubin SB, Zoloth L, eds. *Margin of Error*. University Publishing Group, Hagerstown, MD, 2000: 13–24.

97 Reason J. Foreword. *In*: Runciman W, Merry A, Walton M. *Safety and Ethics in Health Care*. Ashgate, Aldershot, 2007: xiv.

98 Anonymous. Scientific error. *Lancet* 29 January 1898: 320–2.

99 Runciman W, Merry A, Walton M. *Safety and Ethics in Health Care*. Ashgate, Aldershot, 2007.

100 Virilio P. *The Original Accident*. Polity Press, London, 2007.

101 Quoted in Tonks A. Patient safety. Safer by design. *British Medical Journal* 2008; **336**: 186–8. Available at http://www.bmj.com/cgi/content/full/336/7637/186.

102 Lertzman R. From absent minded to error wise: a conversation with James Reason. Saferhealthcare. Available at http://www.saferhealthcare.org.uk/IHI/Topics/AnalysisandTheory/Features/AbsentMinded.htm.

PART 1

Understanding patient safety

CHAPTER 2

When is an 'error' not an error?

Dianne Parker, Tanya Claridge, Matthew Lawrie

Background

Over the last decade, health care professionals, politicians and the public have begun to appreciate the scale and the human and fiscal impact of medical error. Findings from epidemiological studies around the world are consistent [1–8]; an assimilation of the results of all these studies led the World Health Organization (WHO) to conclude that one in 10 people receiving health care worldwide will suffer preventable harm from it [9]. The minimisation of error, and the promotion of patient safety is, therefore, of great human, academic and commercial interest, as well as a prime focus for health care delivery organisations, the media, patient groups and the public.

In the United Kingdom (UK) consideration of patient safety in the National Health Service (NHS) has been embedded in all government reports related to quality of care since 1998 [7,10,11]. Indeed patient safety was the first of the core developmental health care standards developed and published by the Healthcare Commission in 2004. Moreover, in 2001, the UK Department of Health created a new national body, the National Patient Safety Agency (NPSA), in an attempt to consolidate the previous fragmented and unsystematic approach to the consideration of patient safety (see Chapter 16 for a consideration of how to analyse NPSA data).

Academic interest in patient safety has also grown exponentially across a range of medical and academic disciplines. One research approach to the issue has been to carry out epidemiological studies investigating the frequency and nature of patient safety incidents, an effort in which the NPSA's National Reporting and Learning System has played a key role. Many researchers have attempted to apply lessons to health care organisations related to risk management derived from experience and research in other high-risk industries [12–15].

Use of rules

Many high-risk industries tackle safety issues systematically, developing a safety management system (SMS) that integrates the organisation's efforts in

---

Health Care Errors and Patient Safety. Edited by Brian Hurwitz and Aziz Sheikh.
© 2009 Blackwell Publishing, ISBN: 978-1-4051-4643-2.

Box 2.1: Rules to control behaviour – on the road

All learner drivers in the UK are trained to drive on the left hand side of the road. This rule is enforced both formally (the police would stop a car driving on the wrong side of a road) and informally (other road users would let their disquiet be known!). There is nothing intrinsically safer about driving on one side of the road compared to the other. The safety benefits are achieved through standardisation of individuals' behaviour, which increases predictability within the system.

Box 2.2: Rules to control behaviour – in the military

Safety is of utmost importance on the deck of an aircraft carrier. While jets are taking off and landing all personnel are required to stand on a painted line on the deck. This ensures that everyone is in a safe place on the deck during the operations where risk is highest. It also ensures that all personnel can see any potential hazards that may arise and can alert the crew quickly.

Box 2.3: Rules to control behaviour – in health care

The consistent implementation of a protocol covering patient identification processes would prevent all instances of wrong site, wrong procedure, wrong person surgery. Preoperative verification processes, standard operation site marking and final verification processes should be specified and standardised across health care organisations.

---

the identification and management of hazards [16]. One crucial aspect of an SMS is the use of rules to control behaviour. The underpinning assumption is that rules, in the form of protocols or guidelines, can be developed that document best practice, compliance with which will increase standardisation of activities in complex and dynamic systems. Examples of rules from driving, the military and healthcare can be found in Boxes 2.1, 2.2 and 2.3.

Safety procedures in most organisations are designed in broadly the same way. They set out best practice – the safest way to carry out a task. Procedures can be used as training/educational tools and/or for competency assessment, and are designed with intelligent compliance in mind.

Compliance with rules: error or violation?

In health care contexts the use of procedures to manage behaviour is made more complex by the nature of the work and the demands of the working environment. Health care professionals frequently have to deal with non-standard, novel situations. This means that developing procedures and guidelines to standardise their behaviour is challenging. Moreover, the principles of health care practice are regulated both distally by professional bodies (e.g. General Medical Council, Nursing and Midwifery Council) and proximally, as day-to-day health care practice is managed by the employing organisation. The monitoring typically used to ensure compliance with procedures in other industries is simply not feasible in most health care environments given the fase pace, variety and complexity of day-to-day healthcare delivery. It is not surprising, therefore, that the research evidence suggests that compliance with clinical guidelines is inconsistent [17–19].

In attempting to understand the reasons for non-compliance with rules designed to ensure safe practice it is useful to consider a different strand of research. In recent years, a great deal of interest has been shown in the broad concept of human error by both academics and health care practitioners [20–22]. However, until now, scant attention has been paid to the distinction between error and violation, which has been shown to be axiomatic in other areas of human factors safety research (with some notable exceptions [23,24]). James Reason has offered formal definitions of error and violation that highlight the conceptual distinctions between them. Errors occur when 'a planned sequence of physical or mental activities fails to achieve its intended outcome' [25]. They arise from individual information-processing problems, in terms of attention, memory or performance or some combination of all three. Violations, on the other hand, can be defined as 'deliberate – but not necessarily reprehensible – deviations from those practices deemed necessary (by designers, managers and regulatory agencies) to maintain the safe operations of a potentially hazardous system' [25]. Violations are not mistakes, and are best understood as intentional failures to comply with a rule. In a situation where two conflicting rules exist, a violation may be unavoidable. Where no rules exist, a violation is not possible. To understand non-compliant behaviour with rules the social context within which violations occur also has to be considered. For instance, in a situation where rules are routinely broken by a work group, managers may turn a blind eye, so that violations become acceptable behaviour.

In health care those charged with the development and implementation of protocol-based care (standards, guidelines, protocols, integrated care pathways) expect that the rules they have developed will be followed. Additionally, they assume those using the rules to have both the competence to avoid making an error and the motivation not to commit a violation. There is also some research evidence to suggest that resistance to standardisation is an issue. Some health care professionals, especially doctors, seem prepared to accept the evidence base for some guidelines but resent the restriction imposed by protocols on their clinical freedom [26]. Clearly, no system of rules in health care should preclude the exercise of professional judgment. It should be acknowledged from the outset that questioning rules that are inappropriate, unworkable or conflicting can lead to improvement in rule development and, ultimately, the safety of patients.

It might be argued that the error–violation distinction is not important in health care. This is partly because the culture of clinical practice traditionally focuses on patient outcomes rather than clinician behaviour [27,28]. While this patient-focused approach is commendable in many ways, it can disadvantage the clinician. To illustrate this, consider the following. One doctor has acted contrary to protocol and saves a seriously ill patient, while another has followed all the best practice guidelines but nevertheless the result is an adverse outcome for the patient. The non-compliance of the first doctor is unlikely to be sanctioned, whereas the second doctor may be held to account for his/her actions due to the outcome for the patient. A shift in focus from patient outcomes to clinician behaviour would be useful both in avoiding unfair scrutiny of clinicians doing their best for sick patients, and in demonstrating the importance of the error–violation distinction.

Error types

Two basic error types have been distinguished:
1 *Skill-based errors* (*slips and lapses*) occur when planning is adequate but the planned actions do not go as intended. They are skill-based failures of execution, such as misconnecting oxygen tubing to intravenous (IV) tubing or forgetting to pass on essential details of a patient's treatment plan at shift handover. (See Chapter 10 on transitions in health care.)
2 *Mistakes*, or rule- or knowledge-based errors, are failures of intention which occur when actions may go entirely as planned but the plan is inadequate to achieve its intended outcome, a rule is applied incorrectly or the actions do not achieve the intended outcome due to knowledge deficits.
• *Rule-based mistakes* occur in relation to pre-learned solutions, for instance in terms of training or protocols. They can involve the misapplication of a good rule (in the wrong circumstance), the application of a bad rule or the non-application of a good rule.
• *Knowledge-based mistakes* occur in novel situations where a solution has to be developed on the spot. This involves the use of slow, resource-limited but computationally powerful conscious reasoning using an often inaccurate and incomplete 'mental model' of the problem.

Violation types

Four types of violation have been described (Box 2.4) [29]:
1 *Routine violations* are those that are widespread and frequent. If perpetrators are not 'punished' by the system (perhaps by an adverse event or peer disapproval) these violations become part of the normal way of working. As an example from health care, it is accepted practice in some departments that part of the required documentation is not completed.
2 *Optimising violations* alleviate boredom on the job, or work round a rule to give the perpetrator a sense of achievement. The perpetrator cuts a corner, or completes the task in a non-standard way, in order to achieve a better outcome

---

Box 2.4: Types of violation and suggested solutions

1 *Routine violation*: a doctor doing ward rounds does not clean his/her hands between touching patients.
Solution: the NPSA's 2004 'Cleanyourhands' campaign has achieved good results via a combination of providing alcohol-based rubs to facilitate hand cleaning, using posters in situ as reminders, and empowerment of patients to question hospital staff.
2 *Optimising violation*: the reconnection by an anaesthetist of a partially-used bag of fluid.
Solution: education to raise awareness about the risk of air entrainment (this violation is usually committed to avoid wasting a partially used bag of fluid) and the development of single-use connectors to prevent re-use.
3 *Situational violation*: a nurse on night shift lifts an elderly patient who has fallen back into bed, without using a hoist.
Solution: provision of hoists on every ward would prevent the need for violations based on lack of equipment.
4 *Exceptional violation*: five minutes before the hospital pharmacy is due to close, a pharmacist is required to dispense a new drug which is not yet on the computer system. The case is urgent and the patient's notes are unavailable. The pharmacist goes ahead and dispenses the drug without checking for potential interactions.
Solution: make sure that information about new drugs is available to pharmacists in written form for use until it is entered in the pharmacy computer system. Reinforce the protocol of checking for interactions.

---

for him/herself, for the organisation or, in a health care setting, for the patient. Staff who move from one organisation to another in the same sector may commit this type of violation, by bringing 'better' ways of working from their previous experience.

3 *Situational violations* are provoked by the system. They occur when a rule cannot be followed, given the local circumstances. For instance, the equipment required to follow a rule is not available.

4 *Exceptional violations* occur in exceptional circumstances, where extreme time pressure or stress may prevent people from following even the most basic rules. Although the precise conditions that provoke exceptional violations are not well understood they are generally associated with resistance to change and motivational problems (low morale, the failure to reward compliance or to sanction non-compliance) occurring in a regulated social context.

Managing error and violation

A further crucial aspect of the distinction between error and violation is the fact that the strategies required to reduce these two types of aberrant behaviour differ considerably. In general terms, error minimisation requires the provision of adequate information, credentialing and monitoring of skills. On the other hand, the reduction of violations can only be achieved by changing the attitudes of violators and/or the culture in which they work. In order to reduce either, the situation in which they occur must be taken into account. High workload, time pressure and poor design make both error and violation more likely. Helpful interventions are likely to include an assessment and, if necessary, adjustment of staffing level and workload, and ergonomic analysis and improvement of the working environment.

However, some interventions target errors alone. These include assuring individuals' competency for their posts, and ensuring they have up-to-date training and development in core skills.

Those dealing with routine violations should consider the removal of rules that are routinely ignored, and involve staff in the development, monitoring and evaluation of new rules. If that is not feasible, then improved supervision, incorporating clear consequences for the individuals and their managers is a possibility. It is important to investigate the reasons for routine violations, including a consideration of staff attitudes and possible underlying organisational factors.

To minimise optimising violations, management should set clear expectations and be seen themselves to comply with rules they have set. The provision of a robust, transparent evidence base for each rule implemented, together with high level endorsement of the rules (e.g. by Royal Colleges and the trust's executive team) are also helpful. An alternative would be to incentivise compliance with rewards or public recognition – to some extent this already happens in the NHS, e.g. with the Quality and Outcomes Framework of standards and targets on which a significant proportion of UK general practitioners' (GPs') income is now based.

To reduce the occurrence of situational violations it is vital to undertake a needs assessment, to identify the resources required to follow the rule. It must be acknowledged from the outset that the rule may be changed following the risk assessment. This process involves ensuring that the patient safety measures in place are adequate and that all involved are aware of any variance made to the procedure. The staff expected to follow the rule should be involved in developing a process map to support its use. Once the rule has been revised, teams should be encouraged to ensure compliance with their own rules.

Exceptional violations cannot readily be planned for. Helpful approaches include training for unexpected situations, using role play and emergency/crisis planning, developing situation awareness skills and team skills for those who regularly have to confront novel situations.

Conclusion

The development of rules is not sufficient to ensure the quality and safety of health care. In order to have an effect such rules have to be followed. There is currently a tendency in health care to assume that non-compliance with rules is the result of human error. In this chapter, the differences between error and violation, and their subtypes, have been explored. It has been suggested that since error and violation have different psychological origins, they require different remediation strategies, making a deeper exploration of non-compliant behaviour essential.

For rules to be followed they must be appropriate and as simple and easy to apply as possible. Given the complexities of modern health care, it must be accepted that it will not always be feasible to develop a rule to prescribe the correct course of action ahead of time. It is also important to acknowledge that conditions at the patient interface may make it difficult or impossible to access and apply the relevant protocol appropriately.

The implementation of a safety management system that incorporates the use of rules to manage behaviour requires careful management if compliance levels are to be improved. Factors for consideration include local ownership, resources, evaluation, feedback, education and training. The implementation of rules without educating and resourcing the health care professionals expected to follow them is unlikely to lead to success. In real terms, adoption of the approach suggested here for assessing and improving patient safety could represent the low hanging fruit in the orchard of patient safety initiatives.

References

1 Thomas EJ, Studdert DM, Burstin HR et al. Incidence and types of adverse events and negligent care in Utah and Colorado (abstract). *Medical Care* 2000; **280**: 261–71.
2 Brennan TA, Leape LL, Laird NM et al. Incidence of adverse events and negligence in hospitalized patients. Results of the Harvard Medical Practice Study. *New England Journal of Medicine* 1991; **324**: 370–6.
3 Institute of Medicine (1999) *To Err Is Human: Building a Safer Health System*. National Academies Press, Washington.
4 Sox H Jr, Woloshin S. How many deaths are due to medical error? Getting the number right. *Effective Clinical Practice* 2000. (Accessed 22 June 2006 at www.acponline.org/clionical-information/journals-publications/ecp/novdec00/sox.htm)
5 *HealthGrades Quality Study: Patient Safety in American Hospitals*. 2004 accessed at http://66.102.9.104/search?q=cache:PvBu2IpQNoUJ:www.healthgrades.com/media/english/pdf/hg_patient_safety_study_final.pdf+healthgrades,com&hl=en&ct=clnk&cd=2&gl=uk.
6 Wilson RMcL, Runciman WB, Gibberd RW et al. The quality in Australian Health Care study. *Medical Journal of Australia* 1995; **163**: 458–71.
7 Department of Health Expert Group. *An Organisation with a Memory*. Department of Health, London, 2000.
8 Baker R, Norton P, Flintoff V et al. The Canadian Adverse Events Study: the incidence of adverse events among hospital patients in Canada. *Canadian Medical Association Journal* 2004; **170**: 1678–85.
9 World Alliance for Patient Safety (2004) Patient safety. A global priority (editorial).
10 Donaldon L and Philip P. *National Standards, Local Action*. Bulletin of World Health Organisation, 2004; **82**: 891–970.

11 Smith J. *Building a Safer NHS for Patients: Improving Medication Safety.* Department of Health, London, 2004.

12 Helmreich R. On error management: lessons from aviation. *British Medical Journal* 2000; **320**: 781–5.

13 Kirk S, Parker D, Claridge T, Esmail A, Marshall M. *Patient Safety Culture in Primary Care: Developing a Theoretical Framework for Practical Use. Quality and Safety in Healthcare,* 2007; **16**: 313–320.

14 Patterson ES, Roth EM, Woods DD, Chow R, Orlando J. Handoff strategies in settings with high consequences for failure: lessons for health care operations. *International Journal for Quality in Health Care* 2004; **16**: 1–8.

15 Gaba DM, Singer SJ, Sinaiko AD, Bowen G, Ciaveralli AP. Differences in safety climate between hospital personnel and naval aviators. *Human Factors* 2003; **45**: 173–85.

16 Health and Safety Executive (1997) *Successful Health and Safety Management.* HSG No. 65. HSE Books, London.

17 Grilli R, Lomas J. Evaluating the message: the relationship between compliance rate and the subject of a best practice guideline. *Medical Care* 1994; **32**: 202–13.

18 Pathman DE, Konrad TE, Freed GL et al. The awareness-to-adherence model of the steps to clinical guideline compliance: the case of paediatric vaccine recommendations. *Medical Care* 1996; **34**: 873–89.

19 Grol R, Grimshaw J. From best evidence to best practice: effective implementation of change in patients' care. *Lancet* 2003; **362**: II46–II54.

20 Vincent C, ed. *Clinical Risk Management.* BMJ Publishing Group, London. 1995.

21 Weingart SN, Wilson RM, Gibberd RW, Harrison B. Epidemiology of medical error. *British Medical Journal* 2000; **320**: 774–7.

22 Walton M. Creating a no-blame culture: have we got the balance right? *Quality and Safety in Healthcare* 2004; **13**: 163–4.

23 Neale G. Reducing risks in medical practice. *In:* Vincent C, ed. *Clinical Risk Management.* BMJ Publishing Group, London, 1995; 253–76.

24 Alamberti R, Vincent C, Auroy Y, de Saint Maurice G. Violations and migrations in healthcare: a framework for understanding and management. *Quality and Safety in Health Care* 2006; **15**: 66–71.

25 Reason JT. *Human Error.* Cambridge University Press, Cambridge, 1990.

26 Claridge T, Parker D, Cook G. Pathways to patient safety: the use of rules in healthcare. *In:* Walshe K, Boaden R, eds. *Patient Safety: Research into Practice.* Open University Press, Milton Keynes, 2006; 198–208.

27 Ashcroft D, Morecroft C, Parker D, Noyce P. Likelihood of reporting adverse events in community pharmacy: an experimental study. *Quality and Safety in Health Care* 2006; **15**: 48–52.

28 Lawton RL, Parker D. Judgements of rule-related behaviour in health care professionals: an experimental study. *British Journal of Health Psychology* 2002; **7**: 253–65.

29 Lawton R. Not working to rule: understanding procedural violations at work. *Safety Science* 1998; **28**: 75–95.

CHAPTER 3

Intentionally harmful violations and patient safety: the example of Harold Shipman

Richard Baker, Brian Hurwitz

Harold Shipman was an English doctor who killed around 250 of his patients during a career that began in 1970 and ended in 1998 [1]. Whilst working as a junior hospital doctor he killed approximately 15 patients and another 235 or so when working as a general practitioner. More dreadful behaviour by a doctor is difficult to imagine. Serial murder on this scale by anyone is exceptionally rare and it is reasonable to ask whether it is possible to learn anything from such events that can help to improve patient safety.

In this chapter we put the case for viewing Shipman's professional 'life course' as a series of inter-related patient safety events. We argue that it is not possible fully to understand how Shipman came to be such a successful and prolific serial killer nor learn how the safety of health care systems can be improved unless his appalling activities are studied using approaches developed to investigate patient safety. And if the case can be made successfully for identifying lessons for patient safety from such heinous events, it follows that health professionals should also seek lessons from more common and less extreme events.

The World Health Organisation (WHO) defines a patient safety occurrence as 'an event which resulted in, or could have resulted in, unintended harm to a patient by an act of commission or omission, not due to the underlying medical condition of the patient' [2]. Whatever the complexity of his actual motives – and they will almost certainly never be known [3] – when Shipman administered massive doses of diamorphine he clearly intended harm, as he was fully aware of the lethal consequences of such actions. He aimed (and was almost 100% successful) at terminating the life of his victims and he knew that in doing so he transgressed ethical, professional and legal prohibitions (this is evidenced by his attempts to conceal these activities). But on the WHO's definition Shipman's practice falls outside questions about patient safety. We argue that the WHO definition stands in need of revision precisely because it excludes Shipman's case (and others like his), which we argue require

Health Care Errors and Patient Safety. Edited by Brian Hurwitz and Aziz Sheikh.
© 2009 Blackwell Publishing, ISBN: 978-1-4051-4643-2.

pre-eminently to be understood within a patient safety framework (in addition to relevant legal and criminal frameworks).

The Shipman story: a brief outline

A detailed investigation of the deaths of Shipman's patients has been undertaken by a public inquiry. After meticulous review of all the surviving material, it was possible to piece together with reasonable confidence the key events in Shipman's career, to identify most of the murders, and estimate the total number of patients who were killed. It is clear that he began to kill patients from very early in his career, and continued to do so until he was arrested. After graduating from Leeds University Medical School in 1970, Shipman began a variety of posts as a junior doctor at a nearby hospital, Pontefract General Infirmary. The first certain killing occurred in 1972 (paragraph 7.47 of the Inquiry's sixth and final report) [1]. On leaving the Infirmary in 1974, he became a GP at a practice in Todmorden in Yorkshire. The Inquiry concluded that he had unlawfully killed one patient and it suspected him of the unlawful killing of six others in 1976 (appendix F of the first report) [4], but by September of that year he had been discovered by his GP colleagues in the practice to have been abusing pethidine, an opiate analgesic drug. He was ejected from the partnership and practice, and following a police investigation was convicted of dishonestly obtaining drugs, forgery of NHS prescriptions and unlawful possession of pethidine, and was fined £600. After spending a short period in a private hospital where Shipman was treated for his addiction, the General Medical Council (GMC) accepted the advice of a medical report about his recovery from addiction and allowed Shipman to resume practice with a warning – that these offences would be taken into account by the GMC if he were to offend again.

After undergoing assessment and withdrawal from pethidine at The Retreat in York, Shipman took up a post as a clinical medical officer; then, in 1977, he was appointed as a partner in a group practice in Hyde, Greater Manchester. During 1978, he killed at least four patients and is suspected of killing five others [4], and he continued to kill patients throughout his time as a partner in the practice, reaching a total of at least 71 deaths before he left that practice. In 1992, he moved to a single-handed practice where he was able to accelerate the rate of killing, so that by 1997 he was killing at a rate of one patient every 10 days. No one raised questions about what he had been doing until March 1998, by which time Shipman had murdered more than 240 people. In that month, on the basis of her own concerns about the number of cremation certificates she had been asked to sign, reinforced by the concerns of a local funeral director (the Inquiry's second report, paragraphs 1.20–1.36) [5], a general practitioner in a neighbouring practice raised the issue with the coroner, who asked the police to investigate. After a cursory investigation, the police concluded there were no grounds for concern. The last murder took place in July 1998, and Shipman was arrested in September of that year, after suspicions that he had forged the will of a patient were reported to the police by a relative.

Shipman killed patients with intravenous injections of diamorphine. Typically, the patient was alone at home in the afternoon, and Shipman made a home visit on some pretext and whilst there he administered a lethal injection. Shipman would either report the death as occurring in his presence, for example from a heart attack or stroke, or would leave the body to be found by a relative or friend later in the day. He would complete the death certificate and cremation form, giving a plausible but often fabricated story of pre-existing disease. The patient group in which most of the deaths occurred was women aged 75 years or over, although Shipman also killed men and people aged under 65 (and there is significant suspicion that he killed a 10-year-old child when working on a paediatric hospital ward [1]).

Errors and violations

Violations are deliberate deviations from proper procedures or rules, whereas errors are unintentional deviations [6] (see Chapter 1). The violation of rules or procedures can sometimes lead to major accidents, as in the case of the sinking of the boat, *The Herald of Free Enterprise*, when to save time, the bow doors of the cross-channel ferry were not fully closed before leaving harbour, as a result of which 187 people died [7]. Patient safety processes rightly focus more commonly on errors and the creation of a culture in which errors are reported, but if health care is to be safe we also need to appreciate that violations occur, why they occur and how to prevent them. Whilst most violations are used as short cuts and do not arise from harmful intentions, Shipman's actions were intentionally lethal, and errors by others sometimes assisted his purposes, as did defective systems and procedures for monitoring the activities of GPs.

The distinction between errors and violations is not always clear-cut. In some bureaucratised but low-risk situations, low-risk violations may be tolerated as the only way to get a job done on time. At the time of the sinking of *The Herald of Free Enterprise*, it was believed that allowing the doors of car ferries to remain open when the ship was within the port's outer seawalls was safe, this being near universal practice at the time, and this formed part of the defence mounted by the captain who survived the ship's capsize. The captain claimed that no violation (deviation from a professional standard) had taken place, a prerequisite for a legal finding of negligence, but the judge condemned the usual standard that was in place at the time as being high risk and an 'obvious folly' [7,8]. In effect, the judge declared the prevailing professional standard of the time to be defective, which can be understood to be a latent systems failure in maritime procedures and practices.

The origins of violations that are not intended to be harmful may be understood in different ways. They may arise from the motivation of individuals and their beliefs of the likely risks and benefits of committing a violation. Alternatively, organisational and cultural factors may operate as, for example, in the vulnerable system syndrome in which blame of front-line workers, denial of system weaknesses and single-minded adoption of financial targets make health care violations more likely. In a third model, external pressure on the organisation promotes gradual migration from safe practices to minor violations that become more extreme as tolerance of violations develops, and as violations cease to be recognised [9].

Patient safety also distinguishes between active and latent failures. Active failures are the immediate causes of the safety incident, which in this case were Shipman's unlawful violations. The latent failures rest in the systems, procedures and culture of the organisation or organisations in which Shipman worked. James Reason expressed this as follows [6]:

Latent failures are created as the result of decisions taken at the higher echelons of the organisation. Their damaging consequences may lie dormant for a long time, only becoming evident when they combine with active failures and local triggering factors to breach the system's many defences.

Interactions between active and latent failures and errors or violations are well illustrated by the classic Swiss cheese diagram. However, in this case the hazard was not a chance occurrence depicted by an arrow passing through holes that just happen, on rare occasions, to be aligned throughout all the layers of cheese (Figure 3.1). Shipman, snake-like, was able to slip through non-aligned holes. Following Figure 3.1, the hazard – Shipman – might have been prevented from killing patients by a variety of systems (e.g. different death certification procedures, better systems for monitoring controlled drug prescribing and other aspects of GPs' clinical practice, and postmortems that include routine toxicology for common poisons) and by individuals working alongside Shipman and responsible for cooperating with him in such systems. If the systems are poorly designed ('full of holes'), latent failures are likely to occur when the coincidence of several independent factors takes place (or is engineered by a violator). Individuals will make errors, but the errors will be more common and more difficult to identify and remedy if the systems themselves are poor. The interaction between latent and active failures leads to breakdown in the defences or layers of the cheese.

As with errors, in preventing violations we need to appreciate how the underlying systems failed to prevent or expose the violation, and learn how to minimise these latent failures. In the case of violations, blame and punishment may be necessary, but either way, to develop safer systems, the latent failures should be identified and dealt with. The experience of the airline, railway and oil industries shows how the investigation of violations to discover the latent failures can improve safety [9–12].

The Shipman Inquiry was instructed by Parliament to conduct an investigation that recognised the principles underlying the safe management of high-risk industries. It was established under the Tribunals of Inquiry (Evidence) Act 1921, and the terms of reference are shown in Box 3.1.

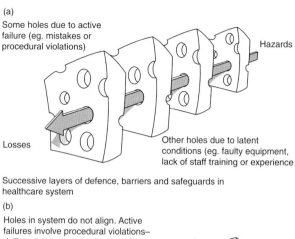

(a)

Some holes due to active failure (eg. mistakes or procedural violations)

Hazards

Losses

Other holes due to latent conditions (eg. faulty equipment, lack of staff training or experience

Successive layers of defence, barriers and safeguards in healthcare system

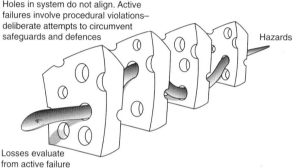

(b)

Holes in system do not align. Active failures involve procedural violations– deliberate attempts to circumvent safeguards and defences

Hazards

Losses evaluate from active failure

Successive layers of defence, barriers and safeguards in (better designed) healthcare system

Figure 3.1 (a) The defences, barriers and safeguards against errors and violations. (b) Replacement of arrow with a snake that finds a tortuous route though a series of non-aligned holes. (Reproduced with permission). Reason J, Managing the Risks of Organizational Accidents. Ashgate, 1997.

Box 3.1: Terms of reference of the Shipman Inquiry [4]

- after receiving the existing evidence and hearing such further evidence as necessary,
- to consider the extent of Harold Shipman's unlawful activities;
- to enquire into the actions of the statutory bodies, authorities, other organisations and responsible individuals concerned in the procedures and investigations which followed the deaths of those of Harold Shipman's patients who died in unlawful or suspicious circumstances;
- by reference to the case of Harold Shipman to enquire into the performance of the functions of those statutory bodies, authorities, other organisations and individuals with responsibility for monitoring primary care provision and the use of controlled drugs.

Following those enquiries, to recommend what steps, if any, should be taken to protect patients in the future, and to report its findings to the Secretary of State for the Home Department and to the Secretary of State for Health.

The Inquiry therefore had authority to investigate the layers of defences, barriers and safeguards designed to protect patients, in addition to merely investigating the actions of Shipman himself. The outcome has been the most searching public investigation into the regulation and monitoring of doctors that has been undertaken in the last 100 years.

Inevitably some doctors have felt uncomfortable about the intensity of the Inquiry's scrutiny and the recommendations it has put forward. It may have seemed that the investigation of aspects of clinical practice and of the workings of the GMC was based on an assumption that doctors were collectively partly responsible for what had happened, and that the introduction of new intrusive and demanding procedures to eliminate risk would be the result. Shipman's actions were as abhorrent to doctors as to everyone else, indeed probably more so since they constituted a breach of the principles of care that the medical profession collectively holds dear. How could such deviant and unusual behaviour have broad lessons for all doctors? The reactions of many doctors to Shipman and the Inquiry and its recommendations reflect this understandable point of view. Yet, although killing by doctors is very rare, it is not unknown. In a recent review of doctors charged with manslaughter in medical practice in Britain between 1795 and 2005, 85 cases were identified [13]. Sixty were acquitted, 22 convicted and three pleaded guilty. Of the 25 found guilty, 10 were classified as mistakes, four as slips or lapses, one as unknown and 10 were violations. There has been an increase in such charges, with 44 of the 85 taking place in the years 1975–2005, of which 14 (32%) resulted in convictions. The nurses Beverley Allitt [14] and Benjamin Green [15] are additional examples of murder of defenceless patients by health professionals in Britain. (At the time of writing, a Glasgow nurse, Collin Norris, is standing trial accused of murdering four elderly hospital patients with insulin [16].)

An element of fatalism can be detected in some of the reactions to Shipman. Editorials in both the *British Medical Journal* (*BMJ*) and *The Lancet* shortly after Shipman's conviction accepted that the detection of a doctor determined on criminal action is difficult [17,18]. 'It is difficult to envisage any set of laws or regulations that will guarantee that the acts of a criminal as experienced, knowledgeable, cool, and determined as Shipman can be prevented in the future' said Bill O'Neill in the *BMJ* [17]. It has also been argued that lessons from Shipman have little to do with medicine and its practice because he was a killer who just happened to be a doctor [19]. Consequently – it is argued – an inquiry may tell us something about such a killer but will tell us little about UK medicine or health care generally. Doctors are certainly not collectively responsible for Shipman and his crimes; they could not have foreseen the possibility that one of their number could be such a determined serial killer. But doctors, along with others, are responsible for investigating the latent failures that enabled Shipman to operate so lethally for so long. They are also responsible for acting on the findings of the Inquiry.

The latent failures

There were failures in several fields [20,21], but here we concentrate on four: the handling of complaints, monitoring of general practitioners, controlled drug procedures and cremation certification.

Complaints

The system for dealing with complaints failed to trigger an investigation of Shipman's clinical performance even though several complaints were made. These included formal complaints by patients to the local health authority in 1985, 1990 and 1992 (he was also reported to the GMC about the third complaint). The complaint in 1985 that reached the health authority concerned alleged inadequate care of a patient who died from a rare respiratory illness. After investigation, the complaint was dismissed by the health authority (the Inquiry's fifth report, paragraph 6.30 [22]). The complaint to the health authority in 1990 related to the prescription of the wrong dose of medication for epilepsy. Shipman admitted the error and was found in breach of his terms of service (he was also found negligent in an associated civil action [23]). The complaint in 1992 related to failure to attend a patient who had requested a visit, and again Shipman was found in breach of his terms of service and a fine of £800 was imposed. The GMC was informed of the outcome of this case and of the case from 1990, but no disciplinary action was taken by it. Whilst individually none of these complaints were sufficient to suggest the true nature of Shipman's activities, none involved careful review of Shipman's performance, and collectively they failed to trigger such a review. Further, the system failed to ensure that the additional past drug abuse was in fact taken into account in deciding whether additional checks were needed.

The weaknesses of the system for handling complaints extended further than the failure to document them in a single record. There were also inhibitions to the reporting of concerns. The manager of a sheltered housing development noticed that the deaths of Shipman's patients were different to the patients of other doctors (the Inquiry's fifth report, paragraphs 8.17–67 [22]). With other doctors, patients gradually increased in frailty and dependence, needing greater support up to the time of death. With Shipman's patients, death was sudden and Shipman was either present or had been present shortly before death. By 1995–1996, the manager had become convinced that Shipman was responsible for the deaths and on one occasion called the police after a patient had been found dead. However, Shipman reassured the police that the death was natural. One of the deceased patient's relatives discussed the possibility of murder by Shipman with the manager. The manager attempted to bring her concerns to the attention of the housing officer but was not taken seriously. In talking with the housing officer, it appears that the manager referred to Shipman as 'Dr Death' (a term also used about Shipman by some of his practice staff (the Inquiry's fifth report, paragraph 9.76) [22]).

Similar suspicions about Shipman's activities occurred to John Shaw, a taxi driver in Hyde (the Inquiry's fifth report, paragraphs 8.68–76 [22]). His customers included many elderly people who were patients of Shipman, and he observed that several apparently well women had died suddenly. He had a card index of his customers and began to note down details of suspicious deaths. However, he did not know to whom he should report his concerns and did not expect to be believed even if he did report them. Two home helps also developed concerns following the sudden deaths of patients of Shipman, but they also felt that their concerns about a doctor would not be believed (the Inquiry's fifth report, paragraphs 8.77–2 [22]). In 1996–1997, two funeral directors working in their family business noticed that Shipman's patients often died alone, sitting up, dressed in their day clothes and showing no signs of having been ill (the Inquiry's fifth report, paragraphs 8.93–97 [22]). Shipman was often present when the patient died. The funeral directors felt that no one would believe them if they raised their concerns, and that they might be regarded as 'mad'. Eventually, however, in early 1998 they did report their concerns to a local GP and this helped to trigger the initial police investigation that concluded there was no problem.

The health professionals working with Shipman in general practice did not have information available to them to generate concerns, and the practice nurse who worked with him in the single-handed practice was dominated by Shipman and reliant on him for explanations about patients' deaths (the Inquiry's fifth report, paragraph 9.100 [22]). There was, however, an opportunity for some hospital doctors to raise the alarm (the Inquiry's third report, paragraphs 13.1–246 [24]). In 1994, Shipman was called to a patient who had asthma. He administered diamorphine, allegedly for chest pain caused by a heart attack, but the patient's daughter was in the house and an ambulance was called and resuscitation was commenced. The patient was transferred to hospital. Diamorphine should not be given to someone with acute asthma because it depresses respiration, which could lead to death. The administration of diamorphine in this case was dangerously bad clinical practice at best and the patient suffered brain damage and lingered in a persistent vegetative-like state as a result. Although the hospital doctors were aware that the patient had suffered a respiratory arrest caused by diamorphine, this knowledge did not lead them to make contact with Shipman, or to refer the issue to an authority such as the GMC with powers of investigation. When the patient eventually died some 15 months later, the information conveyed to the coroner did not adequately make clear that Shipman's actions were at fault.

Monitoring of general practitioners

Shipman was known to be an expensive prescriber but was resistant to encouragement to prescribing more economically [23]. At the time, information would have been available about achievement of a limited number of targets – immunisation and cervical cytology screening rates for example. Profiles of numbers of patients referred to specialists would have been available towards the end of Shipman's career. Shipman's practice premises were subject to inspection to ensure the facilities were adequate. During the 1990s, Shipman undertook a number of clinical audits, reporting the findings to the local medical audit advisory group (one of the audits undertaken in 1997 studied the reasons for patients leaving the practice; deaths accounted for 27.9% of patients leaving the practice [23]). There was little other information available to the health authority or his colleagues about his performance. For example, the group practice in which he worked from 1977 to 1992 did not have information about the numbers of deaths and was therefore unable to discover that death rates were relatively high. Shipman's medical records were of poor quality; they were often illegible and were usually brief and incomplete. They were never inspected and neither his GP partners nor locums covering for his absences or holidays seem to have raised concerns about the quality of his records. There was also no broad, objective assessment of Shipman's clinical performance. Since he had qualified as a doctor in 1970, no individual or agency had conducted a formal assessment to determine whether he remained fit to practise. The assumption in those days appears to have been that a doctor was fit to practise unless something serious was discovered to have gone wrong.

Controlled drug procedures

Diamorphine and pethidine are controlled drugs, and therefore subject to specific regulations. The regulations in force in Shipman's working lifetime required that doctors in possession of controlled drugs should maintain a register recording the day on which the drugs were obtained and supplied. The registers should be available for inspection by authorised inspectors. In addition, the regulations specified the arrangements for safe storage of controlled drugs and disposal of any unused drugs.

In view of the fact that Shipman had been convicted of drug offences involving pethidine – in 1976 he had pleaded guilty to three charges of obtaining ten ampoules of 100 mg pethidine by deception, three charges of unlawful possession of pethidine, and two charges of forgery of NHS prescriptions [20,25] – it might be expected that particular attention would be paid to his subsequent prescribing of controlled drugs. In fact, this was not the case. Shipman did not maintain a controlled drugs register, claiming that he did not carry controlled drugs because of his past addiction. If he needed to administer diamorphine to a patient, he would write a prescription and collect the drug from a pharmacist. He did indeed collect diamorphine prescriptions, as inspection of the pharmacy registers would have revealed. However, the frequency with which he did this was not identified as a matter of concern, neither by an inspector nor by the pharmacist herself. Shipman obtained most of his supplies of diamorphine by over-prescribing the drug to patients with terminal illnesses, and collecting the unused drug after the patient had died. On one occasion, a district nurse noticed that Shipman had purloined several ampoules of morphine prescribed for the care of a terminally ill patient, but she accepted the explanation he offered at the time, that he owed the ampoules to another doctor, and the matter was not taken any further (the Inquiry's fourth report, paragraph 12.30 [25]).

Furthermore, the system of inspection of GPs' controlled drug registers, and discussion with them of their use of these drugs, fell into a state of suspension or confusion following the disbanding of the regional medical officer service that had responsibility for this task up until 1990. Weaknesses in the systems for monitoring controlled drug use by GPs were not limited to Shipman's locality. A survey of GPs in Leicestershire showed that their registers were infrequently or never inspected, and many GPs were unclear about the rules governing registers and the disposal of drugs. Their confusion was evident in the mix of different types and quality of registers being maintained [26]. General practitioners' variable use of controlled drugs registers at this period is an example of how errors can become endemic in a poorly maintained system.

Cremation certification

In England, before a body can be cremated, approval must be obtained from a doctor (the medical referee) authorised by the Home Office to grant this approval. The process centres on the completion of a set of forms. Form A is completed by the deceased's relative who is requesting cremation, Form B by the doctor who attended the deceased during the final illness, Form C by a second doctor who confirms he or she is satisfied with the statement provided by the doctor completing Form B, and Form F which is completed by the medical referee and which supplies the legal authorisation for cremation. The process dates from the cremation regulations of 1903, although there have been a number of modifications in the intervening years. Nevertheless, the system is broadly the same as when it was introduced at the beginning of the 20th century.

The Shipman Inquiry found that cremation forms were often poorly completed by doctors and, in particular, the intention that the doctor completing Form C should independently take steps to verify the circumstances of death reported by the doctor completing Form B was not being fulfilled. Many doctors, the Inquiry concluded, regarded the completion of Form C as a technical requirement only, and did not see themselves as conducting an independent investigation into the cause and circumstance of death. The Inquiry decided that, as presently carried out, the cremation certification procedures were of very little value [24]. Reform of the system was recommended, above all making it mandatory for the Form C doctor to question at least one person who is independent of the Form B doctor and who has some knowledge of the circumstances of death.

Discussion

The pain and suffering caused to patients and families by the activities of Harold Shipman, initially as a hospital doctor and later as a GP, are incalculable. These people put their trust in an apparently bona fide member of the medical profession who was in fact an intentional serial violator of absolute professional and legal prohibitions—a health care saboteur (see Chapter 6). His violations involved serial murder and disposal of victims' bodies under the aegis of publicly funded systems of professional registration and regulation, health care provision, deaths registration and mortality monitoring, all of which failed to bring his activities to light over a period of more than two decades. Morally, the very least his victims and their families deserve is that the full exposure of Shipman's activities should lead to detailed, no-stones-unturned scrutiny of how he operated within these everyday structures unhindered for so long.

In outlining the context in which Shipman was able to murder 250 people before detection, we have drawn on the reports of the Inquiry, to which witnesses gave evidence under oath, and which involved study of contemporaneous documentary evidence when available. Much of the evidence, including transcripts of the hearings, can be found on the Inquiry's website (http://www.the-shipman-inquiry.org.uk/). Other evidence is taken from a review conducted by one of us of Shipman's clinical practice based on direct inspection of his clinical records, cremation certificates and other material [23]. The Inquiry's reports and the associated transcripts and documentary evidence are voluminous, and many commentators are unlikely to have studied them in depth; we have not, therefore, drawn on other, often poorly informed secondary sources. The basis for our case is therefore founded on reliable sources.

As a hospital doctor, Harold Shipman appears initially to have killed people occasionally and opportunistically, but as a GP he subsequently found he could murder relatively freely and effortlessly. He could obtain supplies of diamorphine easily and as a doctor with domiciliary care responsibilities, he could gain access to the privacy of peoples' own homes by self-invitation. In these comfortable, private and domestic circumstances patients held out their arms to be 'given' an injection which, unbeknownst to them, would kill them, after which Shipman lied plausibly to their families, saying he had called for an ambulance but had cancelled it when it became clear the death of their relative was irreversible. As the official custodian of their loved one's medical history, Shipman could persuade shocked relatives that the victim had died both expectedly and understandably of natural causes, which he would certify.

A marginally higher proportion of deaths certified by Shipman was followed by cremation in comparison with patients of local practitioners (75.2% vs 70.6%), and it is possible that he sometimes encouraged relatives to choose cremation for the deceased [23]. He was certainly successful in gaining the necessary cremation authorisation from other local doctors. He also knew that he could rely on a lack of any routine toxicology, not to bring to light the true cause of death – diamorphine poisoning – in the case of the few victims whose sudden deaths resulted in postmortems.

The point that needs to be emphasized is that for Shipman, serial murder was not actually difficult. He sometimes killed two people on the same day and on several occasions he was able to follow the murder of one member of a longstanding couple with subsequent killing of their surviving spouse – again undetected. The chilling truth is, that over the years, murder for Shipman had become a routine. Yet serial killing can only ever become routine where obstacles to its accomplishment have been fully and comprehensively overcome and where all, or almost all, health service and civil systems for monitoring a doctor's activities – especially around the time of a patient's death – are so inadequate (in systems terms, so full of latent defects) as to allow murder in the same way, by the same means, by the same man, to become repeated and established over decades.

The Inquiry revealed the ways Shipman operated and brought to light a series of latent safety failures in several UK systems of regulation, some of which have been the subject of further investigation and inquiry. For example, new procedures for handling controlled drugs are being introduced [27], proposals to reform medical regulation are under debate and are likely to be included in early legislation [28] and there are plans (albeit rather modest and currently postponed [29]) for reform of the coroner service system and death certification system [30]. It is our contention that the techniques developed to ensure patient safety should be deployed in response to egregious violations as well as in response to much commoner medical errors. Much in patient safety, however, rests on encouragement for reporting errors, with mistakes regarded as opportunities for learning rather than transgressions that demand punishment. Would inclusion of malicious violations as a category of patient safety event deter reporting? We think not, for the following reasons.

First, the overwhelming majority of health professionals do not commit malicious violations. Reporting offers a way of helping professionals, concerned about the care of their patients, to identify such events. Had a functioning reporting scheme been in operation during Shipman's career, the GPs, nurses, pharmacists and hospital doctors who noticed peculiarities in his clinical behaviour would have had a means of reporting them. Methods for involving patients in reporting safety incidents are in their infancy, and we do not yet know how this can be implemented as a routine. For example, the completeness and accuracy of patient reporting remains to be established. Nevertheless, a patient safety system that allowed reports from patients and the public might have enabled the home helps, taxi driver and housing officer to draw attention to their concerns, a possibility that should encourage investigation of practical ways of involving patients in safety systems.

Second, doctors can take important lessons from such events, and in response to Shipman, some have done so. For example, doctors in Hyde have introduced for themselves tighter systems for cremation certification, taking a lead in a field where policy makers have yet to act [31]. Doctors in local practices – including those caring for Shipman's patients – have taken a lead in developing and testing systems for patients to gain electronic access to their own clinical records, a scheme that is now being extended to a large sample of practices in the UK. The system allows patients to scrutinise their own medical record, and to question and request corrections where they believe there to be errors in their records. It is not intended as a method for 'preventing a Shipman', but it has potential to foster greater openness and improved communication between patients and their general practitioners, something that is desirable in itself and which also should deter the occasional untruthful doctor from fabricating record entries. It is a development that is attracting intense interest among policy makers and health service leaders, and the doctors involved find themselves at the forefront of an international movement to improve doctor–patient relationships and the quality of care through patient access to their own records. If you talk to patients at these practices, some of whom were patients of Shipman, you will encounter a vision of what partnership between doctor and patient in the future could be like.

Third, doctors and other health professionals are already participants in systems to minimise the dangers of malicious staff. They are governed by, and report individuals to, their respective regulatory bodies (in the case of medicine in the UK, the GMC). The improvements to these regulatory bodies in recent years and better systems at local level to ensure identification, investigation and reporting, have led to more consistent approaches. Consequently, the risk of a poor or malicious performer remaining undetected is, arguably, smaller today than it was 5 years ago. In practice, therefore, we argue that no practical distinction should be drawn between the obligation to report an error committed and the obligation to report a violation observed. Patient safety demands a just rather than a blame-free culture; if after proper investigation blame is appropriate, blame is required (see Chapters 6 and 7). The medical associations, colleges and academies have a responsibility for fostering a just culture through leadership that emphasises doctors' responsibilities rather than concentrating on defence of doctors' interests.

The WHO definition of a patient safety event discussed above should be broadened to include health care violations. Although little is known about the extent and frequency with which health care violations are committed on a daily basis, they should be classed as safety events. By definition, violations are intentional transgressions of rules, regulations, policies or agreed procedures undertaken, for the most part, to achieve beneficial and positive ends as seen from the perspective of the violator. Although deliberately performed, violations are usually not intended to have a harmful outcome. Yet there is a category of violations that is clearly intentionally harmful and which carries lessons for patient safety in the same way that errors and other violations do. It is not sufficient to rely on criminal or regulatory investigation procedures to identify and respond to these lessons. Health professionals and organisations share responsibility for learning from intentionally harmful violations, and the involvement of patient safety systems by the relevant health care organisations' provides the right mechanism.

References

1 The Shipman Inquiry. *Sixth Report: Shipman, the Final Report.* The Shipman Inquiry, Manchester, 2005. Available at http://www.the-shipman-inquiry.org.uk/case_decision. asp?idx=pc&id=DG&fn=26&from=r.

2 World Health Organisation World Alliance for Patient Safety Project to Develop an International Patient Safety Event Classification. *The Conceptual Framework of an International Patient Safety Event Classification.* WHO, Geneva, 2006.

3 Soothill K, Wilson D. Theorising the puzzle that is Harold Shipman. *Journal of Forensic Psychology and Psychiatry* 2005; **16**: 285–98.

4 The Shipman Inquiry. *First Report. Death Disguised.* The Shipman Inquiry, Manchester, 2002.

5 The Shipman Inquiry. *Second Report.* The Shipman Inquiry, Manchester, 2003.

6 Reason J. Safety in the operating theatre. Part 2: Human error and organisational failure. *Quality and Safety in Health Care* 2005; **14**: 56–61.

7 Health and Safety Laboratory. *The Causes of Major Hazard Incidents and How to Improve Risk Control and Health and Safety Management: A Review of the Existing Literature.* HSL/2006/117. Buxton Health and Safety Executive, 2006 (www.hse.gov.uk/research/hsl_pdf/2006/hsl06117.pdf).

8 Holyoak J. Raising the standard of medical care. *Legal Studies* 1990; **10**: 201–11.

9 Amalberti R, Vincent C, Auroy Y, de Saint Maurice D. Violations and migrations in health care: a framework for understanding and management. *Quality and Safety in Health Care* 2006; **15** (Suppl I): i66–i71.

10 Helmreich RL. On error management: lessons from aviation. *British Medical Journal* 2000; **320**: 781–5.

11 Rt Honorable Lord Cullen PC. *The Ladbroke Grove Rail Inquiry Report*, Part 1. HSE Books, Norwich, 1999. Available at www.hse.gov.uk.

12 Step Change Group. *Step Change in Safety* Aberdeen 2007. Available at http://www.stepchangeinsafety.net/stepchange/AboutUs.aspx.

13 Ferner RE, McDowell SE. Doctors charged with manslaughter in medical practice 1795–2005: a literature review. *Journal of the Royal Society of Medicine* 2006; **99**: 309–14.

14 Allitt Inquiry. *Independent Inquiry Relating to Deaths and Injuries on the Children's Ward at Grantham and Kesteven General Hospital during the Period February to April 1991 (The Clothier Report).* HMSO, London, 1994.

15 Alexander Harris Solicitors. *Nurse convicted of murder of two patients by lethal injection.* Available at http://alexanderharris.co.uk/article/Nurse_convicted_of_murder_of_two_patients_by_lethal_injection_2588.asp (accessed 7 Nov. 2007).

16 Chamberlain G, McBeth J. Scots nurse charged with four murders. *The Scotsman* 7 Nov. 2007. Available at http://news.scotsman.com/index.cfm?id=1655132007 (accessed 7 Nov. 2007).

17 O'Neill B. Doctor as murderer. Death certification needs tightening up, but it still might not have stopped Shipman. *British Medical Journal* 2000; **320**: 329–30.

18 Anonymous. Effect of Shipman case on family practice. *Lancet* 2000; **355**: 421 Editorial.

19 Wyndham BMA Second Opinion. *News Review* March 2000; page 35.

20 Hurwitz B. *Many of Shipman's bizarre and divergent practices were detected but were neither properly registered nor investigated.* Available at http://bmj.bmjjournals.com/cgi/eletters/331/7513/411#114726 (accessed 6 Nov. 2007). Electronic publication only…

21 Hurwitz B. Murder most medical, disposal most discreet. *Lancet* 2004; **364**: Suppl 1: s38–9. Available at http://image.thelancet.com/extras/04sup_18_webversion.pdf 5 (accessed 7 Nov. 2007).

22 The Shipman Inquiry. *Fifth Report – Safeguarding Patients: Lessons from the Past, Proposals for the Future*. The Shipman Inquiry, Manchester, 2004. Available at http://www.the-shipman-inquiry.org.uk/reports.asp.

23 Baker R. *Harold Shipman's Clinical Practice 1974–1998*. Department of Health, London, 2001.

24 The Shipman Inquiry. *Third Report. Death Certification and the Investigation of Death by Coroners*. The Shipman Inquiry, Manchester, 2003. Available at http://www.the-shipman-inquiry.org.uk/reports.asp.

25 The Shipman Inquiry. *Fourth Report. The Regulation of Controlled Drugs in the Community*. The Shipman Inquiry, Manchester, 2004. Available at http://www.the-shipman-inquiry.org.uk/reports.asp.

26 Baker R, Moss P, Upton D, Pankhania J. Investigation of systems to prevent diversion of opiate drugs in general practice in the UK. *Quality and Safety in Health Care* 2004; **13**: 21–5.

27 Department of Health. *Safer Management of Controlled Drugs: Changes to Requirements for Requisitions for the Supply of Schedule 1, 2 and 3 Controlled Drugs (interim guidance, England)*. Department of Health, London, 2007. Available at http://www.dh.gov.uk/en/Publicationsandstatistics/Publications/PublicationsPolicyAndGuidance/DH_079571.

28 Chief Medical Officer. *Good Doctors, Safer Patients. Proposals to Strengthen the System to Assure and Improve the Performance of Doctors and Protect the Safety of Patients*. Department of Health, London, 2006.

29 Baker R, Cordner S. Reform of investigations of deaths. *British Medical Journal* 2006; **333**: 107–8.

30 Department for Constitutional Affairs. *Coroner Service Reform*. Department for Constitutional Affairs, London, 2006.

31 Tanna V. Moving on from Shipman. *British Medical Journal* 2005; **331**: 411.

CHAPTER 4

Patient safety and patient error

Stephen Buetow, Glyn Elwyn

This chapter was previously published in *The Lancet* (2007) vol. 369; January 13th and is reproduced with permission.

Do patients make errors? Of course they do, according to the Institute of Medicine [1], which reports that 'patients make errors too'. Indeed, at first glance it seems nonsensical to suggest otherwise, not least since the same observation has been made several times over the past half century [2–4]. Yet the contribution of patients (and their care givers) to medical error has been discussed only rarely. This reluctance to consider patient fallibility and, as a result, to identify and manage the errors that patients make, could threaten patient safety.

Does this silence indicate an unwillingness to analyse such a sensitive issue? Or, despite claims to the contrary, is patient error merely a false construction: can patients, by definition, not make mistakes? In this chapter, we discuss, and draw attention to, the concept and context of patient errors. We also consider how analysis of the errors to which patients contribute could aid in the development of strategies to avoid such mistakes, and consider whether such processes could benefit from active participation by patients. We focus on concerns raised by consumer groups about the quality and safety of health care [5], and on the action areas targeted by the World Alliance for Patient Safety [6] such as clinical risk management and patient involvement in improving patient safety.

Patient errors

What does it mean to say that patients make errors, and why does this concept matter? We used the framework developed by James Reason, who defined errors as actions not completed as intended (errors of execution) or as actions proceeding as intended but failing to achieve the outcome intended because the plan was wrong (errors of planning, also called mistakes). Errors can be attributable to systems, people or settings. Systems theory suggests that most errors result from the convergence of many factors, which interact

Health Care Errors and Patient Safety. Edited by Brian Hurwitz and Aziz Sheikh.
© 2009 Blackwell Publishing, ISBN: 978-1-4051-4643-2.

to produce an error-prone environment [7]. These so-called latent errors occur upstream, where they are out of the direct control of the people making the errors. Latent errors are thought to pose the main threat to patient safety [1]. Systems theory states that people can also contribute directly or via systems deficiencies, indirectly contributing to making or avoiding errors. Individuals tend to make these so-called active errors at their point of contact with the health system. The concept of medical error emphasises the medical settings, such as hospitals [8,9] and primary care clinics [10,11], where both latent and active errors take place. Patient error more often consists of active errors than of systems error. From the premise that direct errors by people are less important than errors caused by deficiencies in the system, the idea of patient error might not be useful. However, this premise has not been proven for patient error. The prevalence of active errors by patients is unknown.

The concept of medical error fails to acknowledge that patients can contribute to, or avoid, errors both in and out of these settings. Whereas the accepted view of medical error depersonalises error by attributing it to groups of professionals or health care organisations, a new focus on patient error would ascribe active errors to the actions of patients. Such a concept would need to distinguish between people and their settings, not only because the current concept of medical error is clinician centric, but because it does not clearly acknowledge that people, as autonomous entities, produce active errors wherever they come in contact with the health system. Specific attributions of error – for example to patients acting outside a medical setting – would help to clarify the question of who contributes to such errors, whether directly or via systems deficiencies. And, despite debate about how to identify a patient, it might be more feasible to identify the errors made by patients than those made by the many types of interacting clinical providers. The different types of error are not mutually exclusive: an error such as refusal of clinical investigations, which originates in the process of patient–clinician interaction, could be attributed to both a patient and a clinician.

Reason [7] emphasises that error is not useful without a clear understanding of intention. Patient error should be predicated on the intention of the patient rather than that of the clinician. On this basis, we can avoid questions about who determines the right outcome for a patient, and acknowledge that a patient should be entitled to err. The application of Reason's [7] concept of error to patient error would exclude patient actions that almost produce unwanted consequences (near-misses), and would distinguish patient error from a patient's choice or decision to behave in a certain way (e.g. non-adherence to treatment, medical advice or medical appointments) [12]. Intentional non-adherence by a patient, even if seen as errant by health providers, could be a reasoned choice [13] rather than an error – unless it fails to achieve the patient's intended health outcome. For example, a patient might decide not to take a non-steroidal anti-inflammatory drug, which has been prescribed with her agreement to treat her back strain, after learning about the drug's possible side effects. Even if the patient's back problem persisted, her non-adherence would not be classified as an error, since she achieved the health outcome she intended – of avoiding side effects. However, if she also expected to recover quickly despite not taking treatment, her non-adherence would be classified as a knowledge-based error, since her intended health outcome was not achieved.

The context of patient errors

Patient error should be understood with respect to the personhood and social roles of patients. As people, patients should be free to make decisions, consciously or otherwise, and to retain the moral agency to err. Another important context is the variety of roles of patients, which help to define their capacity and opportunity to make or avoid errors. As consumers and co-producers of care [14], competent patients have their own experiential and embodied knowledge. Indeed, modern consumerism, improvements in public access to education and advances in information technology have progressively narrowed the gap between professional and patient knowledge [15]. Since patients' knowledge enables them to understand, reason and share decision making, they are also at increased risk of fallibility. Another context for error is that because patients adopt the so-called sick role – the expected behavioural norms and values that are appropriate to individuals who become temporarily sick – their propensity to make errors could increase [16]. Hibbard [14] has identified two further roles for patients – in informed choice and evaluation of health care – in which patients are able to avoid or reduce error.

Patient error can have important, and potentially avoidable, consequences. Patients' errors could harm their own health care (e.g. by damaging patient–clinician relationships) or compromise their health (e.g. by delaying clinic attendance, or not providing pertinent information to clinicians). Patient errors can also affect other people in their social network or impose economic costs on families, colleagues and employers. Since patient errors will probably increase in frequency in the context of 'greater emphasis on community-based long-term care, increased ambulatory surgery, shorter hospital lengths of stay, and greater reliance on complex drug therapy' [1], the challenge will be to reduce these negative consequences of patient error.

Patients' errors also occur in the context of factors that limit their capacity and opportunity to avoid contributing to error. For example, patients might agree to actions that they prove unable to achieve because of constraints such as access to money, health, knowledge and physical resources (including transportation). An agreed action might represent an unreasonable burden for a particular patient. Other constraints include power differences between patients and providers, which often, if not usually, favour medical professionals. A power difference could trigger patient error by limiting a patient's opportunity to act in an autonomous capacity (e.g. a patient might choose to ignore a plan if they felt powerless to challenge or modify it during their clinical visit).

Some of the constraints that predispose patients to making errors could be altered. But many active errors by patients result from unavoidable human fallibility, and would be impossible to eliminate without trespassing on personal autonomy. Yet errors have consequences for everyone involved in the delivery of care. The respect due to a competent patient requires that they be granted the capacity to help shape the conditions that predispose to errors and make informed choices that could contribute to avoiding errors. As Kennedy [17] states, to suggest that the principle of autonomy imposes a burden of participation that disadvantaged patients cannot bear 'is as offensive as it is untenable'.

Mechanisms and types of error

Most patient errors result from their own behaviour [18]. Table 4.1 shows examples of errors attributable to patients in the planning or execution of actions necessary for their own health care. Patients often consciously neglect their needs and responsibilities in their own health care – whether through choice, or because of competing priorities and constraints [19]. Patients can also forget to take treatment, or may not have appropriate resources to access it [20]. Although some errors might originate in patients' interactions with others, such errors could be correctly attributed to both patient error and medical error (as noted, these are not mutually exclusive). Table 4.1 shows that patients can make or avoid errors as producers of health care before visits to medical settings and as consumers and co-producers during and after such visits. The errors of planning are especially diverse, but common themes are decisions not to access care that is needed to improve health, decisions to access the wrong care or the wrong level of care, and agreement with plans that patients cannot deliver.

Patients can also contribute to errors through their role in underlying failures within health care systems. Patients can influence organisational cultures and system characteristics that might indirectly trigger errors. For example, if a patient has an unrealistic expectation that clinical performance will be error-free, they might reduce their own personal vigilance. The desirability of patient vigilance (when feasible) has been illustrated by a malpractice case [21] in which a patient discovered cancer during breast self-examination, and successfully sued her radiologist for not detecting the cancer in her mammograms. A patient's level of vigilance is part of the context for potential error, and relates to the social role of being a patient and the patients' own agency and initiative.

Promotion of patients' safety

In speculatively opening a debate on the issue of patient error, we have identified a need for empirical work on patients' contribution to error and for the development of a taxonomy of error, perhaps by using formal consensus-building methods (J. Reason, University of Manchester, personal communication). This theoretical foundation should facilitate the

Table 4.1 Examples of active errors by patients, by phase of illness trajectory.

	Domain	Error of planning (wrong plan to achieve aim)	Error of execution (action does not go as intended)
Pre-consultation	Attendance	Deliberately avoids or delays attendance for formal clinical care	Forgets to attend for planned consultation
		Makes inappropriate demands for care (e.g. home visit)	Does not notify clinical provider of expected late arrival for consultation
		Refuses to use booking system for non-urgent primary care	Does not use telephone services according to clinic protocol
		Chooses not to notify clinical provider about inability to attend or lateness	Forgets to cancel appointment if unable to attend
Consultation	Information giving and coordination	Chooses not to offer clinical provider certain information (e.g. symptoms, personal or family history, lifestyle behaviours or drug use)	Forgets to report certain information or ask prepared questions
		Distorts information given to clinical provider	Fails to state information clearly (e.g. preferences)
		Does not check understanding when uncertain	
	Manner and attitude		Adopts disrespectful manner and attitude
	Investigations	Refuses clinical investigations (e.g. laboratory tests or referrals)	Forgets to bring relevant items to consultation
		Does not attend for clinical investigations	Forgets to attend for investigations
		Does not follow instructions for clinical investigations (e.g. does not fast for a fasting blood sugar test)	Does not follow instructions for investigations (e.g. owing to misunderstanding)
	Diagnosis	Rejects diagnosis offered by clinical provider	
	Treatment	Refuses treatment offered by clinical provider	Forgets to take treatment
		Overestimates ability to do agreed clinical tasks	
		Pushes clinical provider for inappropriate treatment	
Post-consultation		Chooses not to adhere to treatment plan	Fails to read medication labels and instructions carefully

construction of priorities for action to support patient safety. For health care providers, continuing actions to promote patient safety might be extended to include working cooperatively with patients and the public to recognise, understand and manage the various types of patient error. For example, providers could engage with the public through childhood education programmes, and try to gather the insights of several different groups into how patients can contribute to error. Action to manage these sources of error would need to target both patients' participation in the systems that make them susceptible to error and their contributions to the cause of active errors at their point of contact with the health system. Providers might need to develop programmes to teach patients to be more effective participants in their own health care and to ensure their own safety by prioritising their needs and responsibilities as consumers and co-producers of health care.

Patients could certainly have a role as a resource in systems-wide approaches to promote patient safety. Such approaches have focused on reporting, analysing and managing risks, but could also include policies to synchronise patients' expectations of organisational safety with what is achievable. Assessments of the so-called safety culture of health care organisations have tended to ignore the perspectives of laypeople such as patients [22], and will be compromised in their aims unless they involve patients and other stakeholders in developing an understanding of how patients and providers interact with their health systems. With patient participation, health care systems could be better designed to avoid and manage errors from all sources, including patients. In turn, we need to enable patients to keep their active errors controlled to a minimum, which will need recognition, support and education of patients for their active participation in, and control over, their own health care. Patients have a role, for example, in monitoring adverse health events [23], reporting errors [24] and meeting the responsibilities they agree with their health care provider.

What is the appropriate response when patients' responsibilities are persistently unmet, or their attitudes and behaviours are consistently poor? Attribution of blame has been reported to shackle patient safety initiatives [25], for example, if it discourages people with good intentions from open discussion of errors. However, such blame might be deserved (merit-based view) or might lead to the desired change in patient safety (consequentialist view) [26]. We suggest that patients are morally responsible for avoidable errors that they make, contribute to or can influence [27]. However, errors should be viewed as shared opportunities to learn from experience and to prevent recurrence. (Chapter 12 explores the many ways in which patients can help to prevent health care errors.)

Conclusion

Patient error can be overlooked by a narrow focus on the complex conditions under which health care professionals contribute to system errors and medical errors. Patient errors are an important part of the patient safety puzzle, and will probably increase in frequency [1]. Patients' errors not only endanger their own health but also adversely affect family, friends and communities. It would be impossible to avert all these consequences, or to forestall all of the antecedents of patient errors, because they are part of the conditions of care. However, we have suggested how safety plans could include patients' participation to keep patient error to a minimum. We have also discussed the concept of how patients contribute to error and the context in which they do so. The scarcity of published scientific work on this subject can probably be explained by the tendency to confuse the recognition of patient error with attribution of blame. But the danger of unfair accusation of patients should not prevent analysis of the issue or attention being given to the risks identified. Clinicians need to think about patients' contribution to error because patients should be acknowledged in theoretical thinking.

Acknowledgments

We thank James Reason, who provided helpful feedback on this chapter.

References

1 Kohn L, Corrigan J, Donaldson M. *To Err is Human: Building a Safer Health System.* National Academy Press, Washington, 2000.
2 Osserman K. Common errors by patients in the management of diabetes. *New York State Journal of Medicine* 1953; **53**: 1637–9.
3 D'Arcy PF. Iatrogenic disease: a hazard of multiple drug therapy. *Royal Society Health Journal* 1976; **96**: 277–83.
4 Lundeen J, Souba W, Hollenbeak C. Sources of error in delayed payment of physician claims. *Family Medicine* 2003; **35**: 355–9.
5 Kinney E. Tapping and resolving consumer concerns about health care. *American Journal of Law and Medicine* 2000; **26**: 335–400.
6 World Health Organisation. *World Alliance for Patient Safety: Forward Programme 2005.* WHO, Geneva, 2004.
7 Reason J. *Human Error.* Cambridge University Press, Cambridge, 2002.
8 Brennan T. The Institute of Medicine report on medical errors – could it do harm? *New England Journal of Medicine* 2000; **342**: 1123–5.
9 Thomas E, Petersen L. Measuring errors and adverse events in health care. *Journal of General Internal Medicine* 2003; **18**: 61–7.
10 Ely J, Levinson W, Elder N, Mainous AI, Vinson D. Perceived causes of family physician errors. *Journal of Family Practice* 1995; **40**: 337–44.
11 Rubin G, George A, Chinn DJ, Richardson C. Errors in general practice: development of an error classification and pilot study of a method for detecting errors. *Quality and Safety in Health Care* 2003; **12**: 443–7.
12 Barber N. Should we consider non-compliance a medical error? *Quality and Safety in Health Care* 2002; **11**: 81–4.
13 Donovan JL, Blake DR. Patient non-compliance: deviance or reasoned decision-making. *Social Science and Medicine* 1992; **34**: 507–13.

14   Hibbard J. Engaging health care consumers to improve the quality of care. *Medical Care* 2003; **41** (Suppl 1): 61–70.

15   Elwyn G, Edwards A. Evidence-based patient choice? *In*: Edwards A, Elwyn G, eds. *Evidence-based Patient Choice – Inevitable or Impossible?* Oxford University Press, Oxford, 2001.

16   Parsons T. *The Social System*. Free Press, Glencoe, IL, 1951.

17   Kennedy I. Patients are experts in their own field. *British Medical Journal* 2003; **326**: 1276–7.

18   Hardmeier B, Braunschweig S, Cavallaro M et al. Adverse drug events caused by medication errors in medical inpatients. *Swiss Medical Weekly* 2004; **134**: 664–70.

19   Zaghloul SS, Goodfield MJ. Objective assessment of compliance with psoriasis treatment. *Archives of Dermatology* 2004; **140**: 408–14.

20   Loh CY, Chao SS, Chan YH, Wang DY. A clinical survey on compliance in the treatment of rhinitis using nasal steroids. *Allergy* 2004; **59**: 1168–72.

21   Steinberg A. Carol Fubini, attorney, cancer patient advocate. *The Boston Globe* 30 May 2005.

22   Nieva V, Sorra J. Safety culture assessment: a tool for improving patient safety in healthcare organizations. *Quality and Safety in Health Care* 2003; **12** (Suppl 2): 17–23.

23   Vincent C, Coulter A. Patient safety: what about the patient? *Quality and Safety in Health Care* 2002; **11**: 76–80.

24   Meyer G, Battles J, Hart J, Tang N. The US Agency for Healthcare Research and Quality's activities in patient safety research. *International Journal for Quality in Health Care* 2003; **15**: 125–30.

25   Leape L, Berwick D. Safe health care: are we up to it? *British Medical Journal* 2000; **320**: 725–6.

26   Hussain-Gambles M, Neal R, Dempsey O, Lawlor D, Hodgson J. Missed appointments in primary care: questionnaire and focus group study of health professionals. *British Journal of General Practice* 2004; **54**: 108–13.

27   Buetow S, Elwyn G. Are patients morally responsible for their errors? *Journal of Medical Ethics* 2006; **32**: 260–2.

CHAPTER 5

Health care safety and organisational change

Ruth Boaden, Bernard Burnes

Any views on what needs to change within organisations in terms of patient safety, and the process by which such change will take place, are dependent how the organisation, and the individuals within it, are viewed. This chapter outlines a wide range of perspectives on both organisational change and on patient safety, and identifies their implications for the improvement and study of, patient safety.

'Change management' is not a distinct discipline but one that draws on a number of social science perspectives and traditions [1]; its definition is further complicated by the inter-relationships of many traditions within social science. 'Patient safety' by its nature is multidisciplinary, although much of the literature in this area does not explicitly acknowledge the perspective from which it has been written. A review of the key perspectives can be found in [2].

Schools of thought regarding organisational change

There are three main schools of thought within organisational change. The individual perspective school comprises two types: the behaviourists and the Gestalt-field psychologists. Behaviourists view behaviour as resulting from the interaction of the individual with the environment, whilst this is viewed as only a partial explanation by the Gestalt-field psychologists, who argue that behaviour is a result of both the environment and human reason. This leads to differing views about how organisational change can then be achieved: by modifying the external stimuli acting on the individual, or by helping individuals to change their understanding of themselves and their situation. This contrast is reflected in the difference between internal and external approaches to performance – and patient safety – improvement for organisations as a whole [3]. External approaches, such as regulation, primarily focus on external issues through,

Health Care Errors and Patient Safety. Edited by Brian Hurwitz and Aziz Sheikh.
© 2009 Blackwell Publishing, ISBN: 978-1-4051-4643-2.

for example, inspection. Internal approaches tend to focus on internal systems of operation through, for example, self-assessment.

The group dynamics school has a long history, originating with the work of Kurt Lewin, and it emphasises change through teams and work groups, rather than individuals – because individuals work in groups and therefore individual behaviour 'must be seen, modified or changed in the light of groups' prevailing practices and norms' [1, p. 263]. This view has been very influential, since most organisations would now view themselves not simply as comprising individuals but groups or teams. The focus of change is at the group level, and attempts to influence group norms, roles and values.

The open systems school considers the organisation as a whole, being comprised of a number of subsystems which are interconnected so that changes to one will have an impact on other parts of the overall system. Systems are 'open' in that they interact with their external environment and also with each other internally. The principal systems typologies [4] are often viewed as:
• The organisational goals and values subsystem.
• The technical subsystem (knowledge, techniques and technologies needed for the organisation to function).
• The psychosocial subsystem (climate and/or culture).
• The managerial subsystem.

The open systems school has been very influential, with support from a range of theorists [5,6], although its critics claim that it 'does not comprise a consistent, articulated, coherent theory. Much of it constitutes a high level of abstraction' [7, p. 138]. The systems view is very relevant to patient safety with some authors arguing that we need to 'make sure we see safety as a systems property, and build patient safety deeply into the designs of care' [8, p. 254]. The implication of this view of safety as a property of the system is that organisations should 'stop relying on exhorting the workforce to give safe care; we have a healthcare workforce already trying very hard not to harm anyone' [8, p. 254].

Elements of these schools of thought can be seen in the wide variety of approaches to organisational change, although there is general agreement that the two dominant approaches are the planned and emergent approaches [1,9–15].

Planned change

The planned approach dominated from the 1950s until the early 1980s, and comprised four complex elements [1]:
1 *Field theory*: an approach to understanding group behaviour by mapping out the totality and complexity of the field in which the behaviour takes place [16].
2 *Group dynamics*: Lewin's view was that it was not possible to change the behaviour of a group successfully unless one understood the interactions (dynamics) between its members [17,18].

3 *Action research*: a two-pronged process which would allow groups to identify and achieve change. It emphasises that change requires action, and is directed at achieving this, and also recognises that successful action is based on analysing the situation correctly, identifying all the possible alternative solutions and choosing the one most appropriate to the situation at hand.

4 *Three-step model*: Lewin [19] argued that a successful change project involved three steps:

- Step 1: *Unfreezing*. Lewin argued that equilibrium needs to be destabilised (unfrozen) before old behaviour can be discarded (unlearnt) and new behaviour successfully adopted.
- Step 2: *Moving*. Unfreezing is not an end in itself; it 'creates motivation to learn but does not necessarily control or predict the direction' [20, p. 62]. Instead, one should seek to take into account all the forces at work and identify and evaluate, on a trial and error basis, all the available options [19].
- Step 3: *Refreezing*. Seeking to stabilise the group at a new equilibrium in order to ensure that the new behaviours are relatively safe from regression.

Lewin saw these elements as being used and working together rather than being seen as separate theories. In order to achieve successful change, he believed it was necessary [1]:

- To analyse and understand how social groupings were formed, motivated and maintained. This requires the use of both field theory and group dynamics.
- To change the behaviour of social groups. This requires the use of both action research and the three-step model of change.

Planned change was viewed as primarily aimed at improving the operation and effectiveness of the human side of the organisation through participative, group- and team-based programmes of change [1,21]. Lewin died in 1947, but his approach to planned change was broadened out and updated by the organisation development movement and was applied to organisation-wide initiatives [9]. Nevertheless, by the early 1980s, it became clear that many organisations needed to transform themselves rapidly and often brutally if they were to survive [1,22–24], and given its group-based, consensual and relatively slow nature, planned change was not seen as appropriate to such situations [1].

Emergent change

The rationale for the emergent approach stems [25, p. 37] from the belief that:

… the key decisions about matching the organisation's resources with opportunities, constraints and demands in the environment evolve over time and are the outcome of cultural and political processes in organisations.

From the emergent perspective, change is seen as being continuous, dynamic and contested and emerges both unpredictably and in an unplanned way. Its supporters stress five features of organisations that promote or obstruct success:

- Organisational structure.
- Organisational learning.
- Managerial behaviour.
- Power and politics.
- Organisational culture.

Proponents of the emergent approach argue that, in particular, planned change has ignored or cannot deal with power and politics and organisational culture. In terms of the latter issue, there has been a growing understanding over the last two decades of the importance of organisational culture to organisational performance. This has been led by the culture-excellence school which argued that success stemmed from organisations adopting flexible cultures that promote innovation and entrepreneurship and that encourage bottom-up, continuous and cooperative change [24,26].

Organisational culture

This is seen as providing the context within which decisions are made about what and how to change. Interest in organisational culture has a long history in disciplines such as sociology and organisational studies [20,27] and there is now increasing interest in applying and extending their insights to the health care sector [28]. Most fundamentally, the concept of an organisation having a 'culture' is contested and there is an ongoing polarised debate between those who see culture as a variable that can be manipulated and measured ('what an organisation has') and those who see it as a descriptive metaphor ('what an organisation is') [28]. Despite this philosophical tension, there is agreement that culture can be conceptualised as the shared beliefs, norms and values of the people that work in an organisation and it is generally accepted that organisational culture has the potential to influence actions and patterns of communication [15,28–30].

A safety culture

We are now seeing an increasing emphasis being placed on organisational culture to explain how people perceive and act on safety issues within their organisations, and therefore how fundamental and sustained changes to patient safety can be made [29] – sometimes referred to as the 'safety culture' of an organisation [31]. There appears to be no one approach to creating a patient safety culture, as six case studies of organisational culture change related to patient safety show [32]. Some of the six organisations tried to change culture directly, others used more indirect approaches, 'by relying on particular reforms in the structure or process of care, such as promoting teamwork to improve safety vigilance or introducing methods to reduce variability in the processes of care, and hoping that attitudes would change as behavior changed' [32, p. 170], and some were using both. In all cases it was identified that leadership commitment was essential to success. As Box 5.1 shows, both top-down and bottom-up approaches can be successful.

Box 5.1: Top-down and bottom-up approaches to implementing a patient safety culture [32]

• *The top-down approach*: Sentara Norfolk General Hospital had a comprehensive change strategy that seemed to help accelerate the pace and scope of organisational change, although this approach required much more up-front investment of staff time and resources than other bottom-up approaches. The hospital also found that flexibility was needed – corporate principles had to be adapted and embedded in each unit's specific work.

• *The bottom-up approach*: Kaiser Permanente instituted a programme of organisational learning to promote teamwork and communication in high-risk areas such as surgery and labour and delivery, which included preoperative briefings that were shown to improve safety culture, teamwork and staff turnover rates. These briefings were described as 'a powerful way to change the way that people think about and practice teamwork' leading ultimately to organisational change. Kaiser Permanente believes that 'effective change requires a "bottom-up approach" supported by leadership and physician involvement, combined with ways of inculcating expected behaviours in everyday practice'. Comparison of those cases taking a unit-based approach to change showed that discrete achievements build interest and momentum for introducing change in other units, although it was recognised that change may be uneven across units and leaders may need to take specific action to ensure consistent change across the organisation.

There are a number of approaches that can be taken to assess safety culture: some take a typological approach assessing results in reference to one or more 'types' of cultures (e.g. the Manchester Patient Safety Assessment Framework). Other tools take a dimensional approach, with safety culture being described in terms of its position on a number of continuous variables. The majority of safety culture assessment tools are survey questionnaires that assess the opinions of individual members of staff on a series of predetermined statements about safety. The resultant 'scores' are said to indicate the strength of the safety culture present in the organisation. However, this approach only evaluates individual attitudes and opinions, rather than their shared beliefs, values and assumptions and fails to evaluate the 'deeper – and probably more important – manifestations of the culture of an organisation … the complexity of interactions between staff members within organisations, the differing influence of individuals and professional groups on culture and the emergent nature of safety culture' [33].

Power and politics

A consideration of culture may lead to the conclusion that organisations are 'essentially political entities whose decisions, actions and major developments are influenced and determined by shifting coalitions of individuals attempting to protect or enhance their own interests' [1, p. 168]. This is certainly the view of both post-modernists and processualists, who draw attention to the role of power and politics in decision making [15,34,35]. The post-modernists argue that:

In a socially-constructed world, responsibility for environmental conditions lies with those who do the constructing. … This suggests at least two competing scenarios for organizational change. First, organization change can be a vehicle of domination for those who conspire to enact the world for others … An alternative use of social constructionism is to create a democracy of enactment in which the process is made open and available to all … such that we create opportunities for freedom and innovation rather than simply for further domination. [34, pp. 367–8]

The processualists take a similar view, stating that:

The processual framework … adopts the view that change is a complex and dynamic process which should not be solidified or treated as a series of linear events … central to the development of a processual approach is the need to incorporate an analysis of the politics of managing change. [10, pp. 3–4]

The sociological writings on patient safety have also drawn attention to the importance of power and politics [36]. However, only in a few instances has much been written to date about the politics of managing change in the context of patient safety, and this work tends to focus on the power of the medical profession and the challenges which approaches to managing patient safety bring to this power: 'the "patient safety" agenda challenges the technical … domains of medical practice, which have typically remained outside the scope of political and managerial reform in healthcare' [37, p. 164]. The same author concludes that findings 'highlight the potential for doctors to resist, subvert and capture managerial prerogatives [i.e. patient safety policy] in order to maintain professional authority' [37, p. 164]. It is therefore possible that in attempting to improve patient safety, the power relationships between doctors and managers will be challenged.

A framework for change

Whilst the planned and emergent approaches to change have tended to vie with each other as to which is most appropriate, there are many other approaches as well. There is also a growing view that one approach to change cannot be applicable to all organisations and all change situations, and that a more contingency-based model is required [13]. This view is illustrated in the framework for change (Figure 5.1), which seeks to show the situations in which particular approaches to change are most appropriate.

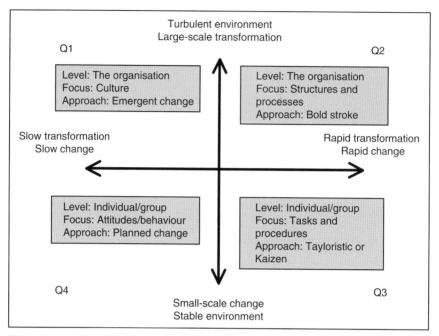

Figure 5.1 A framework for change [1].

Change and patient safety

Improving patient safety has often been seen as requiring changes to individuals' behaviour through the application of relatively small-scale and incremental change initiatives, rather than as requiring an organisation-wide transformation [38]. However, the distinction between the individual (what they do and how they do it – the bottom two quadrants of the framework in Figure 5.1) and the organisation (its culture and structure – the top two quadrants of the framework in Figure 5.1) are not always clear [39]. Nor is it clear, in seeking to improve patient safety, if those involved understand the range of approaches to change on offer and which would be most appropriate in their situation. To understand these issues further, it is necessary to identify the key perspectives on patient safety.

The individual perspective: the contribution of psychology

Psychology has produced many insights into the nature and causes of human error. Initially these insights were applicable to high-risk industries where up to 80% of accidents and incidents are caused by human error [40], but more recently they have also been applied in the medical field. Research has led [41] to several important distinctions in terms of error:

1 *Slips/lapses and mistakes.* Error can be defined as 'the failure of planned actions to achieve their desired ends – without the intervention of some

unforeseeable event' [42], with a 'slip' then being a problem with the execution of a good plan, whilst a mistake is an inappropriate or incorrect plan that is correctly executed.

2 *Error and violations.* Slips, lapses and mistakes are all unintentional and arise from information-processing problems. Their frequency can be reduced by skills training, improving knowledge, workplace information and redesign. However, violations often have to do with motivation, and can be described as deliberate deviations from normal or recommended practice that are, at least in part, intentional. Reducing violations is linked to aspects of the organisation such as morale, attitudes, beliefs, norms and organisational safety culture [43] rather than to competence assessment or training.

There is also a perspective on the understanding of accidents which focuses attention and blame on the individual involved, by considering 'accident proneness' (some individuals have personality characteristics that make them more prone to accidents [44]). This can lead, however, to individual blame, and perhaps dismissal or retraining, leading to the view that the risk of another accident has disappeared. However, this approach can sometimes be seen as somewhat simplistic, given that adverse incidents in most systems have multiple causes. Nevertheless, there are instances, as Box 5.2 shows, where the cause of errors can be attributed to the attitudes and actions of individuals. Though these are often seen as being difficult to change, there are occasions when they are the product of poor or inadequate communication. Once the relevant information is given and understood, individuals can quickly and permanently change their behaviour.

The group perspective: the contribution of sociology

A sociological perspective suggests that things that go wrong are due to failures of the system rather than individual failures. This view is justified by arguing that 'complex organisations have both the capacity to achieve goals that individuals cannot achieve and to introduce sources of error that are similarly not directly attributable to the behaviour of individuals' [45]. Organisational sociology has a long tradition of studying mistake, misconduct and disaster – 'the dark side of organisations' [46], because of its acceptance that mistakes of all kinds are a common, even normal, part of work. A review of the extensive but often unconnected literature in this area [46] showed causal relationships between:

• The *environment* in which organisations operate.
• Organisational *structures* (including complexity, centralisation and formalisation).
• *Processes* (informal organisation, power and learning).
• *Tasks* (level of skill, technology and the role of knowledge).

Following from this, West [45] describes four intrinsic characteristics of organisations that are relevant to the level of risk and danger in health care settings:

1 *The division of labour*, where it is argued that specialisation brings problems of coordination, communication and cooperation and therefore increases

---

Box 5.2: 'Don't distract me, I'm administering medicines': taking steps to tackle interruptions

At Bradford Teaching Hospitals they identified a risk in the administration of medicines in that nurses are interrupted and distracted when involved in giving medicines to patients. Two attempts were made to address this: introducing coloured aprons for nurses to wear when giving medicines and designating responsibility for medicines to an allocated nurse on each shift. However, in the long term, neither of these measures seemed to work. More investigation into the root cause of the problem revealed that:

One day while I was undertaking a medicines assessment for a qualified nurse on a busy care of the elderly ward, we were interrupted by a physiotherapist who wanted a list of patients she needed to see that day. When I asked the physio why she'd interrupted us, she was genuinely confused about why that could be a problem. Realising that what was obvious to me wasn't obvious to her, I asked other ward staff (porters, domestics and ward clerks) and – to my surprise – got the same reaction. They were all aware that they shouldn't interrupt other staff, but didn't really know why. Most suspected it was related to productivity and to make sure work got done quickly.

In Lewin's work on change management, part of the process of implementing change involves helping people to understand the need for change. This incident showed that many staff did not understand why nurses should not be interrupted when administering medicines. So the Trust then gathered data on the extent of the issue of interruption, and provided staff interrupting the nurses' administration of medicines with a short burst of information to help them understand the importance of allowing nurses to work uninterrupted. The effect of this is being reviewed at two time points, including at least 6 months after the intervention, in the hope of finding evidence for the effectiveness of intervention in encouraging staff to sustain changes in their behaviour. It is hoped that raising staff awareness about medication errors will help stop them distracting nurses while they are giving medicines to patients. The manager running this programme says that 'changing behaviour isn't easy but that doesn't mean it shouldn't be done'.

Developed from material available at http://www.saferhealthcare.org.uk/IHI/Topics/ManagingChange/SafetyStories/DontDistractMe.htm (accessed 18 June 2007).

---

the likelihood of adverse events. Whilst standardisation and formalisation of tasks may reduce the complexity of work, they can have negative effects. Rules, standard operating procedures, guidelines, protocols and role specifications may become out of date, unless regularly reviewed.

2 *Social structural barriers to communication.* The tendency to form relationships with other people who are like ourselves (the homophily principle) is one of the few ideas in sociology for which there is overwhelming empirical support. In health care it is argued that 'barriers to communication are erected by the hierarchical nature of hospital organisations, by the importance of professional allegiances, and by the gendered nature of work in healthcare settings' [45]. There is evidence to suggest that is particularly so with doctors [47], implying there is still a very strong professional boundary around medicine – 'adverse events can happen simply because individuals of lower status experience difficulties in challenging the decision of a person of higher status' [45].

3 *Diffusion of responsibility* means it is very hard to ascertain who is responsible for what in a large organisation [47]. Mistakes are often associated with a particular decision and it is often then assumed that the decision maker was 'at fault'. However those in the middle – 'sufficiently senior to make important and visible decisions but insufficiently senior to be cloaked by the diffusion of responsibility that lies over senior managers' [45] – are often blamed. The distinction between active and latent failures is relevant here: latent failures (also sometimes known as error-provoking conditions) are likely to be removed in time and space from the 'event', but act as contributory factors. West [47] argues that 'In health care we are acutely aware of the behaviour of individual decision makers but we often fail to follow the causal chain back to the managers, civil servants, or politicians who may have failed in repeated decisions over many years to provide an environment conducive to patient safety'.

4 *The environment of organisations* is shown by many examples in literature to be influential: for example, organisations set up for one purpose come to strive for other, very different, goals. Health care in particular is vulnerable to wider socioeconomic and political pressures that can divert attention to goals that are not directly related to patient care so that the sources of danger to patients are removed from the organisation itself.

As the above discussion indicates, improving the operation and safety awareness of groups is a difficult and complex process. However, there are a number of tried and tested approaches that have shown real benefits. Box 5.3 shows the benefits that can be gained by the use of one such approach, crew resource management (CRM), which has a long history as a valuable safety tool, with its study and practice being a mandatory requirement (by the Civil Aviation Authority in the UK) for all holders of professional flying licences. There are an increasing number of examples of this being used to break down barriers to communication between team members, with a resulting impact on patient safety.

The systems perspective: the contribution of quality improvement

The quality improvement perspective views organisations as systems, or series of processes. It does, however, by its nature, draw on a variety of academic perspectives including services marketing, organisation studies, human resource management and organisational behaviour, especially

---

Box 5.3: Crew resource management at University Hospitals Coventry and Warwickshire NHS Trust (UHCW)

A variant of CRM, developed by a training company, was an element of a package of measures to address a variety of direct issues and underlying causes at UHCW identified in an external review in 2002, which reported that the Trust did not learn from errors because staff felt they would be unfairly blamed for mistakes they reported. A group was established to review all serious incidents and ensure that they were systematically managed and acted on. Training for staff was developed to promote incident reporting as well as promoting personal responsibility and a team approach to safety.

The major outcome from the training was an increase in incident reports from 50 per month in June 2002 to an average of 700 per month (including slips, trips and falls) in 2005. This figure represents a rate of about 8.5% of inpatient admissions. There were also improvements in the Clinical Negligence Scheme for Trusts ratings and external performance review ratings – to a three star rating in 2005, to which this training was seen to contribute. The Trust recognised that without organisational systems and processes to extract, evaluate and implement the learning from incident reporting, sustainable change would not occur.

Developed from material available at http://www.saferhealthcare.org.uk/IHI/Topics/ManagingChange/SafetyStories/8268_humanfactorsapproachat UniversityHospitalsCoventry.htm (accessed 18 June 2007).

---

change management [48]. Whilst there has been considerable diversity in terminology about quality improvement, both in industry at large and in terms of its application within health care, many accept that it is based on the following change principles [49]:

- Focus on work processes.
- Analyse variability.
- Manage by 'fact', i.e. systematically collected data.
- Learning and continuous improvement.

Comparisons between a variety of quality improvement and safety perspectives [48] show that they all focus on the motivation and beliefs of individuals in the organisation, which define the culture as well as the behaviour that results from this. The requirement to obtain and analyse appropriate data is clear in all perspectives, although safety perspectives focus on reporting rather than 'measurement for improvement', which is key for quality. All perspectives do, however, emphasise the role of learning and sharing lessons. However, the role of leadership is not explicit in all cases of either quality or safety, and the assumption that the organisation consists of a series of interdependent processes is also not mentioned in all perspectives.

As with improving group performance, there are also a number of tried and tested approaches to improving the performance of systems within organisations. Box 5.4 shows the benefits that can be gained from adopting the six sigma approach which, though originally developed for use in manufacturing organisations, is now widely used in the service sector.

The clinician's perspective: an individual, part of a team and working within an organisational system

Whilst the clinical perspective may be one of the key ones in terms of change to improve safety it is also complex, since those describing it argue that both

---

Box 5.4: Using six sigma to measure, control and improve processes to manage hospital-acquired pressure ulcers

OFS St Francis Medical Center (OSF), Peoria, Illinois, aimed to decrease the number of hospital acquired pressure ulcers by 50% in 6 months primarily by using the six sigma methodology. The aims were to:
• Define the opportunity to decrease hospital-acquired pressure ulcers.
• Measure the process performance and rates of pressure ulcers using a prevalence and incidence study.
• Analyse the information obtained from data collection, benchmarking and from literature searches.
• Improve the processes by implementing changes.
• Control (sustain) the gain made over the course of the project and into the future.
A variety of changes were made to practice, with organisational changes including:
• Clear definition of the role and responsibility of the charge nurse, Registered Nurse (RN) team and patient care techniques.
• Weekly process performance data collection until levels of greater than 75% compliance were reached, when data collection could become monthly.
• A unit champion was created with the responsibilities of data collection, resources, encouraging unit compliance, making recommendations for improvement, and helping quarterly prevalence and incidence study.
• A process of accountability and responsibility was developed for the unit manger as the process owner.
• Quarterly prevalence and incidence study was conducted. Results were reported to the National Center for Nursing Quality, the process owner, nursing director and chief nursing officer.
The results of the initiative are shown in Figure 5.2.
   Developed from material available at http://www.ihi.org/IHI/Topics/PatientSafety/SafetyGeneral/ImprovementStories/MemberReportDecreasingHospitalAcquiredPressureUlcers.htm (accessed 18 June 2007).

(Continued p. 68)

Box 5.4: (Continued)

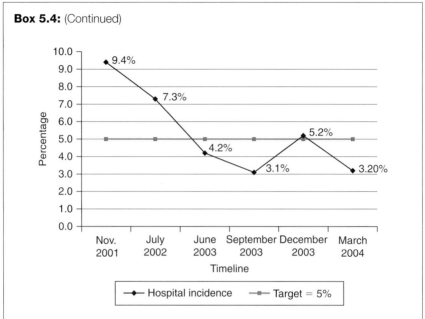

Figure 5.2 Incidence of hospital-acquired pressure ulcers in a programme using the six sigma methodology.

individual and group factors are influential. Here we consider the perspective of the doctor, whilst recognising that other clinical professions might have alternative perspectives.

Esmail [50] provides an account of the clinical perspective from a family physician, and argues that clinical practice is inherently unsafe – decisions are regularly made where the potential for something going wrong is significant. He describes the contrast between how such practice appears to outsiders and how it appears internally:

It might seem that I do this with an air of confidence brought about by the apparent knowledge and experience that I have as a member of the medical profession. But scratch below the surface of what I do and you will see the doubts and mistakes, failures as well as successes and how uncertain and messy it all is.

Medical uncertainty is one of the core characteristics of medical culture. Fox [51] describes and analyses how training for uncertainty takes place in medical practice by identifying three categories of uncertainty:
• The limitations and gaps in medical knowledge.
• The incomplete mastery of medical knowledge.
• The difficulty in differentiating between personal ignorance and limitations in medical knowledge.

The view that the practice of medicine is always going to be fallible [52] proposes that there is so much uncertainty in medicine because of the following:
• *Ignorance*: science can only ever give a limited understanding of how things happen.
• *Ineptitude*: the knowledge is available but doctors fail to apply it correctly (both of which can be overcome).
• *'Necessary fallibility'*: there are some kinds of knowledge that science will never deliver, often around predicting how an individual will behave – 'No patient is quite like any other patient' [50]. This limitation cannot be overcome. Box 5.5 shows that what one clinician defines as a medical error may not be seen as such by a clinician from a different medical discipline, complicating further the uncertainty around medical practice.

Esmail [50] argues that 'With everything we know about people and diseases and how to diagnose and treat them, it is difficult especially for non physicians to understand how deeply this uncertainty runs'. The consequence of this training for uncertainty is that when things go wrong there is a tendency to concentrate on process and for clinicians to blame themselves or patients. However, this is not to imply that there is a lack of concern for risk within medical practice or a lack of focus on ensuring that knowledge is up to date and that every possibility is considered.

Every time I see a patient I convince myself that I will offer the best treatment, drawing on my knowledge and my diagnostic skills. It is not vanity and I would argue that it is a necessary part of good medicine. It is true that things can go wrong quite easily sometimes but it is also true that effort does matter; diligence and attention to detail can make a difference. [50]

Many doctors do not appear to recognise approaches labelled 'continuous quality improvement' or 'process re-engineering' because it is 'the dry language of structures not people' [50]. However, by whatever systems measures are used, doctors will sometimes make mistakes and it does not seem

---

Box 5.5: Differing clinical perspectives on medical error

Different clinical professionals have been shown to identify activities as errors differently depending on their particular discipline [53]. A study of a range of examples included case analysis of 'near-miss' vignettes and showed that 'The identification of a physician error may become ambiguous because observers cannot readily determine whether the questionable event reflects an innovative attempt to expand patient treatment, a difference of professional opinion or a lack of professional judgment' [53]. A series of medication-error near-miss vignettes had the same patient outcome (no harm), but varied in whether the wrong medication was attributed to the actions of the nurse, pharmacist or physician, depending on who was classifying the error.

reasonable to ask that doctors achieve perfection, although 'they should never cease to aim for it and take personal responsibility for the errors that they make' [50]. One of the key issues with regard to patient safety is the need to have a commonly agreed set of definitions as to what constitutes medical error but, as Box 5.5 shows, clinical professionals can find it difficult to agree upon what is and what is not a medical error.

Is there evidence about what works?

There is currently very little empirical research investigating the efficacy of organisational level interventions in reducing error in health care. A review of 42 health care research studies [54] identified seven controlled experimental studies but 80% of them provided insufficient detail of the method or findings to allow the strength of the relationship between organisational factors and error to be determined, and only 38% of the studies reviewed were underpinned by a theoretical framework. The authors concluded that 'there is little evidence for asserting the importance of any individual, group or structural variable in error prevention or enhanced patient safety at the present time'. However, they attributed some of the deficiencies in the quality of research to the fact that the field is relatively new. They recommend that managers should:
• Prioritise the safety issues which the organisation needs to address.
• Specify what outcomes they would like to see for each issue and ensure that accurate data are collected.
• Implement different interventions and compare their costs and benefits.

So what can be done?

It should also be recognise that some 60–80% of all change initiatives, of whatever type, fail [1]. Though this may seem dispiriting, if we reverse these figures, we can see that 20–40% succeed. The question, therefore, is how can organisations put themselves into the 20–40% category when attempting to improve patient safety? The key is to choose an approach that is suitable for the type of change being undertaken [1]. If we take the five examples of change cited in this chapter (see Boxes 5.1–5.5) and link them to the framework for change shown in Figure 5.1, we can see that they can be placed in different quadrants:
• *Example 1* (Box 5.1): Culture change clearly falls into quadrant 1 and, whether approached from a top-down or bottom-up perspective, would tend to be most appropriately undertaken through an emergent approach.
• *Example 2* (Box 5.2): This involves changing attitudes at the individual/group level and, therefore, falls into quadrant 4 and is best achieved by planned change.
• *Example 3* (Box 5.3): This involves changing attitudes and behaviours at the individual/group level and falls into quadrant 4 and is best achieved by planned change.
• *Example 4* (Box 5.4): This concerns system-level change and tends to be more about collecting and analysing data than changing attitudes and

behaviour per se. Depending on the size and nature of the system involved, this could either fall into quadrant 2 or quadrant 3. Therefore, it could be achieved by a bold stroke or Tayloristic/Kaizen approach.
• *Example 5* (Box 5.5): This involves the attitudes and behaviour of individuals and groups. Consequently it falls into quadrant 4 and might best be undertaken using a planned approach to change.
It follows from the above that, if they wish to increase their chances of achieving successful change in relation to patient safety, organisations must identify the type of change which is required (individual, group, organisation-wide, etc.) and choose the most appropriate approach to achieving that type of change. Therefore the first step in tackling suboptimal performance is to understand the cause of the problem [1]. Does it lie with the individual, group or organisation as a whole? Is it primarily a behavioural/cultural issue or to do with the design of jobs/processes or the overall structure of the organisation? Only when these questions have been answered satisfactorily is it possible to choose an appropriate approach to change and to design an effective change.

Conclusion

Just as there exist a number of approaches to organisational change, so there is more than one approach to improving patient safety. Consequently, where concerns over patient safety arise, the key issue is to understand where the problem lies (whether it be at the individual, group or organisational levels) and to apply an appropriate approach to change. This is likely to require a multidisciplinary/multiprofessional group who possess the sufficient understanding and skill to conduct such an exercise. It will also need the involvement of those with experience in areas where patient safety concerns are most pronounced. As Shapiro [51, p. 3] notes, simplistic approaches to change management in the health care context are 'naïve and will fail' [55, p. 3].

Achieving successful change requires an understanding of the basic principles and approaches to change, rather than just attempting to apply a particular technique or approach: 'If you understand the theory behind the tools and realities of your own situation, you will then have a better chance of understanding the appropriate techniques and of knowing how to tailor them to the unique needs and opportunities facing your organisation' [56]. The dangers of a top-down rational approach to policy making and implementation with regard to patient safety are already documented [57].

Only when there is an understanding of and broad agreement on the factors that give rise to patient safety concerns can an organisation move forward to plan and implement changes which will resolve those issues. Crucial to this is the need to recognise that the approach to change which the organisation adopts must arise from an understanding of the changes it wishes to make rather than a preference for a particular approach to change. In order to achieve this, the dominance of the medical perspective with regard to patient safety needs to be recognised and resolved, which will almost certainly involve difficult challenges for both clinicians and managers [58].

References

1 Burnes B. *Managing Change*, 4th edn. FT/Prentice Hall, Harlow, 2004.
2 Walshe K, Boaden R. *Patient Safety: Research into Practice*. McGraw Hill/Open University Press, Maidenhead, 2006.
3 Walshe K. *Regulating Healthcare*. Open University Press, Maidenhead, 2003.
4 Miller E. *Systems of Organisation*. Tavistock, London, 1967.
5 Burns T, Stalker GM. *The Management of Innovation*. Tavistock, London, 1961.
6 Woodward J. *Industrial Organization: Theory and Practice*. Oxford University Press, London, 1965.
7 Beach SD. *Personnel*. Macmillan, London, 1980.
8 Berwick DM. *Escape Fire: Designs for the Future of Health Care*. Jossey-Bass, San Francisco, 2004.
9 Cummings TG, Worley CG. *Organization Development and Change*, 7th edn. South-Western College Publishing, Mason, OH, 2001.
10 Dawson P. *Organizational Change: A Processual Approach*. Paul Chapman Publishing, London, 1994.
11 Kanter RM, Stein BA, Jick TD. *The Challenge of Organizational Change*. Free Press, New York, 1992.
12 Pettigrew A, Ferlie E, McKee L. *Shaping Strategic Change*. Sage, London, 1992.
13 Stace D, Dunphy D. *Beyond the Boundaries: Leading and Re-Creating the Successful Enterprise*, 2nd edn. McGraw-Hill, Sydney, 2001.
14 Weick KE. Emergent change as a universal in organisations. *In*: Beer M, Nohria N, eds. *Breaking the Code of Change*. Harvard Business School Press, Boston, 2000: 223–41.
15 Wilson DC. *A Strategy of Change*. Routledge, London, 1992.
16 Back KW. This business of topology. *Journal of Social Issues* 1992; **48** (2): 51–66.
17 Allport GW. Foreword. *In*: Lewin G, Allport G, eds. *Resolving Social Conflict*. Harper and Row, London, 1948; pp. vii–xiv.
18 Bargal D, Gold M, Lewin M. The heritage of Kurt Lewin – introduction. *Journal of Social Issues* 1992; **48** (2): 3–13.
19 Lewin K. Frontiers in group dynamics. *In*: Cartwright D, ed. *Field Theory in Social Science*. Social Science Paperbacks, London, 1952: 188–237 (reprinted from *Human Relations*, 1947; **1** (1): 2–38).
20 Schein EH. Kurt Lewin's change theory in the field and in the classroom: notes towards a model of management learning. *Systems Practice* 1996; **9** (1): 27.
21 French W, Bell C. *Organization Development*, 6th edn. Prentice Hall, Upper Saddle River, NJ, 1999.
22 Dunphy DD, Stace DA. The strategic management of corporate change. *Human Relations* 1993; **46** (8): 905–18.
23 Kanter RM. *When Giants Learn to Dance: Mastering the Challenges of Strategy, Management, and Careers in the 1990s*. Unwin, London, 1989.
24 Peters T, Waterman RH. *In Search of Excellence: Lessons from America's Best-Run Companies*. Harper and Row, London, 1982.
25 Hayes J. *The Theory and Practice of Change Management*. Palgrave, Basingstoke, 2002.

26 Kanter RM. *The Change Masters*. Simon and Schuster, New York, 1983.

27 Hofstede G. Values and culture. *In*: Hofstede G, ed. *Culture's Consequences: International Differences in Work-Related Values*. Sage, Beverly Hills, CA, 1980: 13–53.

28 Scott T, Mannion R, Davies H, Marshall M. The quantitative measurement of organisational culture in health care: a review of the available instruments. *Health Services Researcher* 2003; **38**: 923–45.

29 Leape LL, Berwick DM. Safe health care: are we up to it? *British Medical Journal* 2000; **320**: 725–6.

30 Clarke S. The contemporary workforce: implications for organizational safety culture. *Personnel Review* 2003; **32** (1): 40–57.

31 Mearns K, Flin R, O'Connor P. Sharing 'worlds of risk': improving communication with crew resource management. *Journal of Risk Research* 2001; **4** (4): 377–92.

32 McCarthy D, Blumenthal D. Stories from the sharp end: case studies in safety improvement. *Milbank Quarterly* 2006; **84** (1): 165–200.

33 Kirk S, Marshall M, Claridge T, Esmail A, Parker D. Evaluating safety culture. *In*: Walshe K, Boaden R, eds. *Patient Safety: Research into Practice*. McGraw Hill/Open University Press, Maidenhead, 2006: 173–84.

34 Hatch MJ. *Organization Theory: Modern, Symbolic and Postmodern Perspectives*. Oxford University Press, Oxford, 1997.

35 Pettigrew AM, Whipp R. Understanding the environment. *In*: Mabey C, Mayon-White B, eds. *Managing Change*, 2nd edn. Open University Press/Paul Chapman Publishing, London, 1993: 5–19.

36 McDonald R, Waring J, Harrison S. Rules, safety and the narrativisation of identity: a hospital operating theatre case study. *Sociology of Health and Illness* 2006; **28** (2): 178–202.

37 Waring J. Adaptive regulation or governmentality: patient safety and the changing regulation of medicine. *Sociology of Health and Illness* 2007; **29** (2): 163–79.

38 Leape LL, Berwick DM. Five years after 'To Err is Human' – what have we learned? *Journal of the American Medical Association* 2005; **293** (19): 2384–90.

39 Khatri N, Baveja A, Boren SA, Mammo A. Medical errors and quality of care: from control to commitment. *California Management Review* 2006; **48** (3): 115–41.

40 Hale AR, Glendon A. *Individual Behaviour in the Control of Danger*. Elsevier Science, New York, 1987.

41 Parker D, Lawton R. Psychological approaches to patient safety. *In*: Walshe K, Boaden R, eds. *Patient Safety: Research into Practice*. McGraw Hill/Open University Press, Maidenhead 2006: 31–40.

42 Reason J. *Human Error*. Open University Press, Cambridge, 1990.

43 Reason J, Parker D, Lawton R. The varieties of rule-related behaviour. *Journal of Organisational and Occupational Psychology* 1998; **71**: 289–304.

44 Lawton R, Parker D. Individual differences in accident liability: a review and integrative approach. *Human Factors* 1998; **40**: 655–71.

45 West E. Sociological contributions to patient safety. *In*: Walshe K, Boaden R, eds. *Patient Safety: Research into Practice*. McGraw Hill/Open University Press, Maidenhead, 2006: 19–30.

46 Vaughan D. The dark side of organisations: mistake, misconduct and disaster. *Annual Review of Sociology* 1999; **25**: 271.

47 West E. Organisational sources of safety and danger: sociological contributions to the study of adverse events. *Quality and Safety in Health Care* 2000; **9** (2): 120–6.

48 Boaden R. The contribution of quality management to patient safety. *In*: Walshe K, Boaden R, eds. *Patient Safety: Research into Practice*. McGraw Hill/Open University Press, Maidenhead, 2006: 41–65.

49 Hackman JR, Wageman R. Total quality management: empirical, conceptual and practical issues. *Administrative Science Quarterly* 1995; **40** (2): 309–42.

50 Esmail A. Clinical perspectives on patient safety. *In*: Walshe K, Boaden R, eds. *Patient Safety: Research into Practice*. McGraw Hill/Open University Press, Maidenhead, 2006: 9–18.

51 Fox R. Training for uncertainty. *In*: Merton R, Reader G, Kendall P, eds. *The Student Physician: Introductory Studies in the Sociology of Medical Education*. Harvard University Press, Cambridge, MA, 1957: 207–41.

52 Gorovitz S, MacIntyre A. Toward a theory of medical fallibility. *Journal of Medicine and Philosophy* 1976; **1** (1): 51–71.

53 Tamuz M, Thomas EJ. Classifying and interpreting threats to patient safety in hospitals: insights from aviation. *Journal of Organizational Behavior* 2006; **27** (7): 919–40.

54 Hoff T, Jameson L, Hannan E, Flink E. A review of the literature examining linkages between organizational factors, medical errors and patient safety. *Medical Care Research and Review* 2002; **61**: 3–37.

55 Grol R, Baker R, Moss F, eds. *Quality Improvement Research: Understanding the Science of Change in Health Care*. BMJ Books, London, 2004.

56 Shapiro E. *Fad Surfing in the Boardroom*. Capstone Publishing, Oxford, 1996.

57 Lewis RQ, Fletcher M. Implementing a national strategy for patient safety: lessons from the National Health Service in England. *Quality and Safety in Health Care* 2005; **14** (2): 135–9.

58 Degeling P, Maxwell S, Kennedy J, Coyle B. Medicine, management, and modernisation: a 'danse macabre'? *British Medical Journal* 2003; **326** (7390): 649–52.

CHAPTER 6

How does the law recognise and deal with medical errors?

Alan F. Merry

About 2% of patients admitted to acute care hospitals suffer serious harm caused by medical errors. Medical errors come to the attention of the law through the complaints that arise from patients who are harmed in this way. However, only a minority of patients do complain, and many of these complaints are resolved locally through the processes administered by health care institutions. It follows that the vast majority of medical errors are in fact not dealt with (or recognised) by the law at all.

The legal response to medical errors and their consequences, when recognised, typically includes one or more of three elements: compensation, accountability and retribution. Each of these elements may feature to a greater or lesser extent in a variety of legal or regulatory mechanisms (Figure 6.1; Table 6.1).

Over the last 50 years there has been an international trend towards increased regulation of health care and legislation related to medical error has become very complex. Such legislation varies from country to country and from time to time, some jurisdictions operating under the common

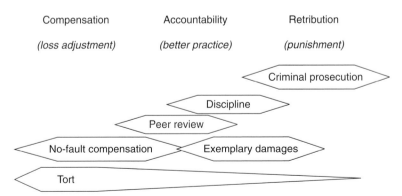

Figure 6.1 Dealing with accidental harm in health care: the elements of an appropriate response and some mechanisms by which these are usually provided (reproduced with permission from [16]).

Health Care Errors and Patient Safety. Edited by Brian Hurwitz and Aziz Sheikh.
© 2009 Blackwell Publishing, ISBN: 978-1-4051-4643-2.

Table 6.1 Some of the organisations and processes through which the law recognises and deals with medical errors.

- Internal institutional enquiries and processes (sometimes required by law, e.g. in relation to open disclosure)
- Offices safeguarding patients' rights (e.g. that of the Health and Disability Commissioner in New Zealand)
- Medical registration bodies (e.g. General Medical Council in the UK):
    Disciplinary processes
    Competency enquiries
- Civil courts:
    Actions for compensatory damages
    Actions for exemplary damages
- Coroner's courts:
    Inquests
- Criminal courts:
    Prosecutions for manslaughter

law (which depends primarily on precedence established by judgments in previous cases), while others deal with written legislative legal codes. Even when the law is codified, it has to be interpreted, and precedence in relation to identical legislation can be entirely different in different countries, or at different times. Since the 1996 report of Lord Woolf [1] there have been significant reforms to the way in which medical errors are handled in England and Wales. New Zealand and some Scandinavian countries have no-fault systems of compensating accidental injury (including injury arising from medical errors). In some countries, abortion and/or euthanasia are legal – a point which has little to do with medical errors but may have considerable relevance to the related issue of health care violations in countries where they are illegal. Legislation related to medical registration and discipline is often the major mechanism by which the law deals with medical errors and this too is characterised by considerable regional and temporal variation.

In practice, policy may be of greater practical importance than the law itself. For example, in the UK, the likelihood that a fatal medical error will result in prosecution for manslaughter may have increased in recent years (Figure 6.2) even though the relevant law has remained unchanged over this period. This probably reflects a change in prosecution policy [2].

It follows that any attempt to provide a comprehensive review of the ways in which medical error is recognised and dealt with by law would be prohibitively lengthy, so the focus here will be on the underlying principles and philosophical issues relevant to the legal response to errors and accidental harm in health care. I will distinguish between error, violation and sabotage, and explain the link between these concepts as understood by scientists and the legal concepts of negligence and recklessness. I will argue that error, as defined in this chapter, is not morally culpable, although it may at times require very careful enquiry to distinguish between error and violation as the

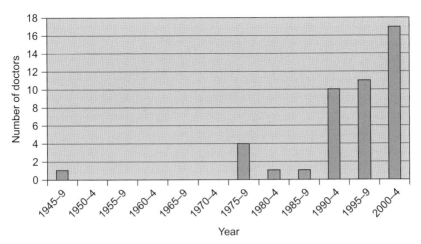

Figure 6.2 Number of doctors prosecuted for manslaughter in the UK in 5-year periods from 1945 to 2004 (data provided by R. E. Ferner and S. E. McDowell).

cause of an adverse event, and both may sometimes be involved. I will end with some suggestions for a better way in which the law might deal with errors and violations in health care.

The law, science, moral philosophy and medicine

The law is a man-made system of rules to govern the way people live together in society, and in the end it is made effective through punishment. From religious or deontological viewpoints, punishment may be seen as justified in its own right. A consequentialist justification for punishing those doctors who, through their medical errors, cause harm to patients might hold that this will deter other doctors from making the same mistakes in the future and thereby, on balance, will do more good than harm. Such an argument would be predicated on the notion that it is actually possible to deter error. In reality, an analysis based on the empirical and theoretical science of human cognition and behaviour demonstrates that this idea is unsustainable; it also demonstrates that to punish those in error is unjust.

Empirical scientific data on iatrogenic harm and medical error

Over the last decade it has become apparent that many patients are harmed by health care intended to help them. Harm of this type is often called 'iatrogenic' and the magnitude of this public health problem is now thought to rival that of traffic accidents. The scientific evidence quantifying this harm comes from various sources (Table 6.2). Probably the most compelling source has been a series of studies using trained researchers to screen

Table 6.2 Sources of information about things that go wrong in health care (modified from [16]).

Medical record review
Routine data collections (deaths, discharges, GP surveys)
Observational studies
Population surveys
Existing registers, reporting systems and audits for:
  morbidity and mortality
  adverse drug reactions
  equipment failure and hazards
Incident monitoring
Complaint investigations:
  hospital and state
  registration boards
  complaints commissioners
Medicolegal investigations
Root cause analyses (sentinel events)
Coronial investigations
Quality improvement and accreditation activities
Results of enquiries and investigations
Literature searches for common and rare events

medical records selected at random from acute care institutions for specified indicators of adverse events; records positive for these events are then subjected to more detailed expert review. These studies have shown that adverse events occur in about 10% of admissions to acute care institutions and that these contribute to permanent harm or death in about 2% of such admissions. After allowing for differences in the precise methods used in each study, the problem, it would appear, is of the same order of magnitude in the USA, UK, Australia, Denmark, New Zealand and Canada [3–8]. Many of these adverse events are due to medical error and are theoretically preventable.

Perhaps the most striking examples of preventable and tragic events arising from medical error are provided by the series of disasters involving the anti-cancer agent vincristine. Vincristine should only be administered intravenously, and is often given in combination with methotrexate administered intrathecally (that is, directly into the cerebrospinal fluid through a lumbar puncture). In Peterborough in 1990, and at Great Ormond Street Hospital some years later, junior doctors were asked to give these drugs with inadequate specific training and supervision, and ended up accidentally confusing the routes by which each drug was to be administered. Intrathecal vincristine leads inexorably to a painful death over a period of a week or two, and there does not seem to be any effective treatment. Many of the victims of these mistakes have been children. It is hard to imagine a more terrible situation for the child, or child's family. It is not surprising that the legal response to errors of this sort has been substantial. In both the Peterborough and the Great Ormond Street cases, the young doctors were charged with manslaughter [9].

Scientific theory: error, violation and intentional wrong doing

Error

There is a substantial body of empirical research on the nature of human error, and the cognitive processes by which errors occur have been extensively reviewed [10,11]. Given the constraints of space, a story may best illustrate several key points about human error, and about the way it is sometimes dealt with by the law.

On 9 June 1995, an Ansett New Zealand Dash 8 aircraft crashed in the foothills of the Tararua Ranges on its approach to Palmerston North Airport on a scheduled flight in bad weather [12]. Owing to a previously unidentified design flaw, there was difficulty in fully extending the undercarriage, and the pilot and co-pilot were distracted with doing this manually by means of a hydraulic pump, while continuing to descend, flying on instruments in cloud. The Ground Proximity Warning System should have alarmed 17 seconds ahead of impact, but malfunctioned, and only provided 4 seconds warning. This was inadequate under the circumstances, and in the ensuing collision between the aeroplane and a hillside four people died (a flight attendant and three passengers).

The police investigated the accident. Three years later they cleared the airline and the co-pilot of any criminal liability [13]. In January 1999, 5 years after the crash, they charged the pilot with manslaughter [14]. In June 2001, after a jury trial lasting 26 days and involving 22 witnesses, a thousand pages of evidence and a great deal of expense, he was found not guilty [15]. Understandably, the accident, the trial and the pilot (who was named) were all the subject of intense media publicity.

Several points are illustrated by this story.

1 Errors are not unique to health care: even in an industry with the reputation for a cultural and organisational commitment to safety, disastrous errors do occur, and blame-oriented responses often follow. Arguments about the appropriate legal response to medical errors should not be based primarily on the fact that these errors are made by doctors: the issues to be considered apply equally to other people involved in dangerous activities – in this case, pilots.

2 Errors are unintentional. In simple English, an error occurs 'when someone is trying to do the right thing, but actually does the wrong thing' [16]. In the present example, the pilots were fully engaged trying to sort out a difficulty with their aircraft's undercarriage, which seemed at the time to be the right thing to do. A more formal definition of error is 'the unintentional use of a wrong plan to achieve an aim, or failure to carry out a planned action as intended' [16].

3 Errors are not carelessness in the strict sense of the word 'care' – clearly these pilots would have cared a great deal about the risk of a crash.

4 Pilots sit at the front of the aeroplane and (unlike doctors) they are therefore usually the first to die when things go wrong. It is sometimes alleged that this is one of the reasons for the better safety record of the airline industry than of hospitals. However, the corollary of points 2 and 3 is that deterrence is useless in the prevention of errors. It is noteworthy that the manslaughter charges in relation to the vincristine tragedies in Peterborough and Great Ormond Street have been totally ineffectual in this regard: the same error has now occurred at least 15 times in the UK [17]. It is very unlikely that draconian punishment will reduce the incidence of medical errors.

5 Experts make errors; actually, all people make errors, but it is often (unrealistically) suggested that experts should get things right, and that errors are unacceptable from trained professionals. The errors made by experts may differ from those made by novices, but they still occur.

6 The consequences of an error tend to depend on more than one factor, and a great deal of luck is involved in this (the term 'moral luck' is often used). Typically, a sequence of events aligns to produce an outcome that might have been averted if any one of these events had not occurred. Underlying defects in the system or environment (known as latent factors – in this case failure in the undercarriage, failure in the warning equipment and the poor visibility are examples) each individually predisposes to error and their coincidence, to the disastrous consequences of an error when one occurs. This principle has been encapsulated by James Reason's 'Swiss cheese' model of accident causation [18] (see Figure 3.1, p.39).

7 The legal response to an error tends to depend on its outcome. In this case, the key error was that both pilots attended to the undercarriage at the same time; instead, one should have allocated his attention to flying the plane while the other dealt with the problem. If the pilots had done exactly the same thing, but circumstances (such as a different geographical setting) had dictated that no adverse event occurred, the error might never have been discovered. If it had been, the response would probably have been minor, and of an internal disciplinary nature. In the airline industry's alleged no-blame culture, the response might even have been constructive and educational rather than punitive. If the same set of circumstances had occurred, but the warning had sounded in time for the pilots to have averted the disaster, the error would no doubt have reached the wider public, and the response might have been more severe, but it is unlikely that criminal prosecution would have been involved. Many drug errors are made in health care, but only those which end up harming a patient tend to be punished. We tend to punish if there are consequences rather than because of any inherent culpability underlying an error (see Chapter 7).

8 The legal response to a serious accident is likely to be prolonged and expensive so it is important that it does promote future safety. In a criminal prosecution, the emphasis is placed on establishing the culpability or otherwise of an individual, and enquiry into the underlying causes of an event is quite often inhibited by the strict rules of the process. Tort is certainly a less blame-oriented alternative, but even in civil actions the focus tends to be on establishing the liability of an individual or organisation. Moreover, it is quite common for settlements to be made out of court, particularly in the case of egregious violations seen as difficult to defend (see below). A more investigative legal response might be more successful in identifying root causes and preventing the occurrence of similar problems in the future. There is an irony in a process likely to end the career of the particular professional who, through the accident, has no doubt learnt the relevant lessons and is very unlikely ever to make the same mistake again any more than the junior doctors who administered vincristine would make that type of drug error again.

Very similar points can be made about other medical errors. They are unintended and do not usually represent carelessness (although, as explained below, they may be associated with violations that do represent carelessness, a possibility that requires to be properly discounted); most practitioners care about their patients and they also care about their own professional reputations. Many errors go undetected, but even if detected the initial response today tends to be minimal or constructive, provided no one has been harmed. When harm does occur, law suits, discipline or criminal prosecution may well follow. The legal response tends to be proportionate to the *actual* consequences of the error, rather than to potential consequences or the moral culpability involved.

Violation

It is important to distinguish errors from violations. Many actions that cause patient harm and which are dealt with by the law as 'medical errors' are actually violations. Violations involve choice and are intentional. A simple English definition of violation is 'an act which knowingly incurs a risk' [16]. A more formal definition is this: 'a violation is a deliberate – but not necessarily reprehensible – deviation from safe operating procedures, standards or rules' [16]. Violations may predispose to errors. For example, drinking before driving makes error more likely. When investigating errors, associated violations are relevant to evaluating the degree of moral blame involved. It is not enough to argue that an error was completely unintentional if it was contributed to by an antecedent and morally culpable violation, which did involve intentional willingness to take risk, albeit no intention to cause harm. It could be argued that a violation was involved in the Dash 8 crash: the correct procedure in circumstances such as these is understood by pilots – one should concentrate on flying the aeroplane while the other attends to the problem. The key to differentiating violations from errors is the element of intentionality in relation to the breaking of the rule, and this seems to have been absent in this case. It can be very difficult to establish the mental processes behind a given event or action.

Except in cases of criminal intent (see Chapter 3) violation usually implies at least some disregard for safety, but not always: occasionally circumstances arise in which violation is unavoidable (Reason refers to these as 'systems double binds' [11]), or even in which it is appropriate to break a rule, because doing so is thought to create *less* risk on balance than following the rule. In other words, not all violations are equally culpable, and each needs to be considered on its merits, under the specific circumstances of the case. Assessing the moral culpability of a violation is made more complicated by the fact that rules may vary from time to time and place to place. For example, as mentioned above, in some jurisdictions abortion or euthanasia are serious violations (to say the least) but in other jurisdictions are within the rules governing provision of medical services.

Sabotage

Violation seldom implies intent to harm: the assumption of the person committing the violation is always that he or she will get away with it. James Reason calls intentional harm 'sabotage' [11] and this is clearly something quite different from either error or violation. In the context of health care, sabotage is morally culpable, and the legal response should reflect that culpability. For example, Harold Shipman murdered many of his patients and was sent to prison (see Chapter 3) [19]. Sabotage is only relevant to the present chapter because the high profile of such cases tends to colour the way in which society believes health care should be regulated, and therefore the way in which the law responds to medical error. This is misguided. The empirical data outlined above demonstrate that iatrogenic harm arising from medical error is a substantial public health problem, whereas genuinely evil doctors such as Shipman are rare, very difficult to identify and relatively straightforward to deal with once identified. Both problems matter, but to confuse unintentional iatrogenic harm with deliberate malice is counterproductive to managing either.

Variation in medical practice: a subtle form of medical error

One of the many inconsistencies in the way the law responds to medical error lies in its failure to recognise certain mistakes which are commonly made by doctors, and which arguably are at least as culpable and medically significant as events that do come to light.

John Wennberg has demonstrated variation in the provision of certain operations, far in excess of that which could be explained by differences between patients [20–22]. These differences seem to be attributable only to variations in approach by different doctors and different institutions, unsupported by evidence. The implication is that many patients fail to receive operations that are indicated, while others receive operations that they do not need. An unnecessary operation is a form of iatrogenic harm in itself, and the decision to undertake it must be either an error or a violation. Furthermore, if a technical error is made during such an operation, a strong argument can be made that the true root cause of this lies in the decision to operate in the first place. Unfortunately the law is very unlikely to elucidate this type of error, even though the potential for improving the overall quality of health care at this level is substantial.

Some implications of legal action against medical error

In general, law suits, disciplinary actions and even internal enquiries are very stressful for the doctors concerned, and so is the publicity that tends to accompany them. To some extent this is inevitable, but justice arguably requires that such stress should be proportionate to the moral culpability of the actions under review (accepting that inevitably this is in part an individual matter). In this context, there is a substantial difference between most other forms of legal response to medical accidents and a criminal prosecution for manslaughter. This can be appreciated if it is remembered that, of the legal processes typically evoked by medical error, only the latter involves the following:

- Being arrested and taken to a police station for charging.
- Having photographs and fingerprints taken by the police.
- Having to apply for bail.
- Restrictions on international travel.
- Being included on lists for court hearings that include other people charged with crimes like theft, assault and rape.
- The possibility of serving a prison sentence.

All of this is perfectly reasonable in cases of serious moral culpability, such as that of Harold Shipman, but much less reasonable in respect of unintentional medical error. The difference was made clear by the judge in one of the vincristine cases, who said: 'You are far from being bad men; you are good men who contrary to your normal behaviour on this one occasion were guilty of momentary recklessness' [23].

Some basic concepts relevant to the legal response to medical error

The law tends to work through legal rather than scientific concepts, and it is helpful to consider how these two frameworks interrelate, looking at some basic concepts.

1 *Duty of care*: The legal response to a medical error begins with the question: was there a duty of care? For doctors looking after patients the answer to this question is almost always in the affirmative, but there are circumstances in which some ambiguity may arise. For example, in the vincristine cases one might ask if a senior doctor associated with the case had a duty of care, and if so how well he or she discharged this duty. One might also ask this question about those responsible for administration within the institutions in which these disasters occurred.

2 *Standard of care*: The next question is whether the standard of care was adequate. The standard of care required in medical practice is almost always phrased in terms of reasonableness, and failures to meet this standard are generally referred to as negligence or recklessness.

3 *Negligence*: Negligence is usually defined by some variation on the theme of failing to have and to use reasonable knowledge, skill and care. This is sometimes called 'simple' or 'civil' negligence, and is the standard pertaining in the civil courts.

4 *What is reasonable?* A fundamental problem with the concept of 'reasonableness' in this context is that human error is never reasonable. How can it

be reasonable to give a patient the wrong drug, for example? The point generally considered is not whether an action or decision was reasonable, but whether it was one that might have been made by a reasonable person under the circumstances. Empirical data are highly relevant to this question. For example, data demonstrating that the vast majority of anaesthetists have given the wrong drug at some stage of their career [24] show that giving the wrong drug may be the sort of error any reasonable anaesthetist could on occasion make. On the other hand all the circumstances of the particular case should be considered. If an anaesthetist had chosen not to put labels on his or her syringes when preparing several of these for use in a case, this violation of a widely understood and accepted rule, antecedent to the error in question, might be construed as something a reasonable anaesthetist would never do.

In Bateman the judge said:

You should only convict a doctor of causing a death by negligence if you think he did something which no reasonably skilled doctor should have done. [25]

Further help can be obtained from the judge in Marshall v. Lindsey County Council, who said:

What is reasonable in a world not wholly composed of wise men and women must depend on what people presumed to be reasonable constantly do. [26]

The explanation, given by Lord Denning in his judgment in Whitehouse v. Jordan (an obstetric case) provides further assistance. He said that an error of judgment in a professional context did not amount to negligence. To test this, he said:

I would suggest that you ask the average competent and careful practitioner: 'Is this the sort of mistake that you yourself might have made?' If he says: 'Yes, even doing the best I could, it might have happened to me', then it is not negligent. [27]

However this passage was 'corrected' in the House of Lords by Lord Fraser, who suggested that what Lord Denning had meant to say was that an error of judgment was not necessarily negligent. Lord Fraser said:

The true position is that an error of judgment may, or may not, be negligent; it depends on the nature of the error. [28]

It may seem slightly ironic in the context of prosecuting a doctor for error, that an alleged mistake on the part of a senior judge should simply be corrected in this courteous manner, but this is how common law evolves; it is refined by subsequent (or higher) judges' reading and reformulation of judicial decisions and jurisprudential reasonings.

1 *Recklessness*: Recklessness is an attitude of mind regarding a violation and implies understanding that a substantial risk is incurred in taking (or

omitting) an action, but nevertheless choosing to take it. This is sometimes called 'subjective recklessness'. 'Objective recklessness' is a difficult concept which suggests that even if the person did not know he or she was taking a risk, the circumstances were such that any reasonable person would have appreciated the risk.

2 *The test for criminal charges*: It is generally held that something more than simple negligence should be required for a finding of criminal negligence. This is often called 'gross negligence'. Definitions of gross negligence tend to be circular, but emphasise that negligence should only be considered criminal if it involves seriously deficient behaviour. In practice, it can be very difficult to distinguish between gross negligence and recklessness, but, in England at least, it is clear that the test for negligent manslaughter is whether the breach of duty that led to the death of a patient involved gross negligence [29].

In New Zealand for many years it was held that simple negligence was sufficient for criminal prosecution, and a number of medical errors during the 1990s were the subject of manslaughter charges on this basis [30]. However, the Crimes Amendment Act of 1997 changed the requirement to one of a 'substantial departure' from reasonable knowledge, skill and care.

How the law works in practice

As already emphasised, the vast majority of medical errors are never recognised by the law. When they are, it might be thought that errors amount to negligence, and violations amount to recklessness. In fact, the linkage between these concepts is far from simple, and depends on the exact circumstances of each individual case. The key to obtaining a legal response to medical error that is scientifically and legally sound is well informed and articulated expert evidence.

In most parts of the world, the majority of errors that do reach the attention of the law are dealt with through litigation. In theory, the primary objective of an action in negligence is compensation. But in order to obtain compensation, the patient must prove negligence and that the negligence concerned caused the harm which is to be compensated. The latter element may be more difficult to prove than the former, because of uncertainties inherent in medical practice and the difficulty in proving causation in the case of particular individuals in a way that goes beyond more than 50% probability. Whatever the outcome in respect of compensation, the process also tends to punish the doctor through its impact on his or her reputation, through the stresses involved in the legal process and through the inevitable publicity associated with such cases. Ironically, patients often feel that they too have been punished, because the proceedings tend to be unpleasant and impersonal for all concerned (see Chapter 13). The vast majority of cases in some jurisdictions are settled out of court, and this tends to maximise the emphasis on compensation and reduce that on punishment. Ironically, the more egregious the case, the more likely it is to be settled in this way. Occasionally, courts impose exemplary damages with the express purpose of punishing a doctor or institution.

Overall, litigation is an inefficient and unreliable way of providing compensation for harm arising from medical error. It is often said that it is better than the alternatives, but the no-fault systems of compensation in New Zealand and Scandinavia seem to work to the satisfaction of these countries' populations. On the other hand, the threat of litigation may be of some value in increasing investment in safety. Conversely, it might produce perverse effects, such as increased insurance premiums for certain groups of doctors, which tend to be passed on to consumers in the form of an increase in the cost of health care.

Discipline through registration bodies such as the General Medical Council seems to have become more common in recent years, and focuses on accountability and punishment. Compensation is seldom provided through this route. The criminal courts are even more strongly oriented towards punishment; traditionally it has been very unusual for medical error to be dealt with as a crime, but the majority of the increased manslaughter prosecutions against doctors in England mentioned above (see Figure 6.2) have arisen out of errors [2]. In New Zealand, the similar rash of such prosecutions in the 1990s has given way (after a change in the Crimes Act) to a more enlightened focus on accountability, root cause analysis and improving the system, through the office of a Health and Disability Commissioner [31].

Should medical error be tolerated?

The fact that medical error often involves little or no moral culpability is an argument against a punitive legal response, but it is not an argument for tolerating medical errors or suggesting errors do not matter.

If it is accepted that many errors occur and produce harm largely through predisposing factors in the environment or system, then it seems obvious that punishing the doctors who make them without addressing these factors is unlikely to prevent a recurrence of the errors (and this has certainly been true in the case of the vincristine disasters). The fact that terrible harm has occurred to a patient may not in itself be a reason to punish someone, but it is, absolutely, a reason to take all reasonable steps to prevent such errors happening again. It is perverse in the extreme that few limits seem to be placed on the resources expended in the legal response to medical accidents once the courts are involved, but strict limits are applied to proactive investment into safety in health care. It is therefore critically important that the legal response to accidents in health care should promote safer practice.

The ideal legal response to medical errors that result in harm to patients

When a patient is harmed by a medical error the highest priority is timely and free provision of the health care needed to minimise that harm.

An acknowledgement of the fact that something has gone wrong, an empathic apology and an explanation are all essential, and should be given early and readily. This requirement has been called 'open disclosure', and is increasingly becoming enshrined in the policies of many institutions and in the legislation of many countries (see Chapter 7).

Appropriate compensation should be provided as of right, and should include the costs of any health care and rehabilitation and any loss of earning capacity arising from the accident. Ideally, compensation should not be linked to the need to prove fault (as it is in litigation). An appropriate analysis of why things went wrong and a concerted effort to correct any failings in the system and minimise the likelihood of a recurrence is essential.

The concept of a 'no-blame culture' is hard to sustain. Rather, the aim should be for a 'just culture' in which blame is restricted to those circumstances in which it is morally appropriate. In dealing with medical errors, for which by definition moral culpability is low, the primary objective of both the legal and the medical systems should be the promotion of safe and effective health care [10]. The focus should therefore be on those who do have the influence or authority to make changes and promote safety within the health care system. Prosecuting or suing practitioners who have no such influence or authority, such as junior doctors, simply sets the scene for the same errors to be made again.

References

1 Lord Woolf. *Access to Justice: Final Report to the Lord Chancellor on the Civil Justice System in England and Wales.* HMSO, London, 1996: 15.2.
2 Ferner RE, McDowell SE. Doctors charged with manslaughter in the course of medical practice, 1795–2005: a literature review. *Journal of the Royal Society of Medicine* 2006; **99** (6): 309–14.
3 Kohn LT, Corrigan JM, Donaldson MS, eds. *To Err Is Human: Building a Safer Health System.* National Academies Press, Washington, 1999.
4 Baker GR, Norton PG, Flintoft V et al. The Canadian Adverse Events Study: the incidence of adverse events among hospital patients in Canada. *Canadian Medical Association Journal* 2004; **170** (11): 1678–86.
5 Schioler T, Lipczak H, Pedersen BL et al. Incidence of adverse events in hospitals. A retrospective study of medical records. *Ugeskrift for Laeger* 2001; **163** (39): 5370–8.
6 Vincent C, Neale G, Woloshynowych M. Adverse events in British hospitals: preliminary retrospective record review. *British Medical Journal* 2001; **322**: 517–19.
7 Davis P, Lay-Yee R, Schug S et al. *Adverse Events in New Zealand Public Hospitals: Principal Findings from a National Survery.* Occasional paper. Ministry of Health, Wellington, 2001.
8 Runciman WB, Webb RK, Helps SC et al. A comparison of iatrogenic injury studies in Australia and the USA. II: Reviewer behaviour and quality of care. *International Journal for Quality in Health Care* 2000; **12** (5): 379–88.
9 Dyer C. Doctors cleared of manslaughter. *British Medical Journal* 1999; **318**: 148.
10 Merry AF, McCall Smith A. *Errors, Medicine and the Law.* Cambridge University Press, Cambridge, 2001.
11 Reason J. *Human Error.* Cambridge University Press, New York, 1990.
12 Swarbrick N. *Air Crashes.* 13 April 2007. Available at http://www.teara.govt.nz/EarthSeaAndSky/SeaAndAirTransport/AirCrashes/1/en.

13 Anon. Ansett cleared but heat stays on crash pilot. *New Zealand Herald* 1999.

14 Wall T. Five years later, pilot charged over fatal crash. *New Zealand Herald* 2000.

15 Anon. Dash 8 pilot found not guilty. *New Zealand Herald* 2001.

16 Runciman B, Merry A, Walton M. *Safety and Ethics in Healthcare: A Guide to Getting it Right.* Ashgate, Aldershot, 2007.

17 Dyer C. Doctor's manslaughter trial halted owing to defendant's health. *British Medical Journal* 2003; **327** (7407): 123.

18 Reason J. Human error: models and management. *British Medical Journal* 2000; **320**: 768–70.

19 Dyer C. Tighter control on GPs to follow doctor's murder convictions. *British Medical Journal* 2000; **320**: 331.

20 McPherson K, Wennberg JE, Hovind OB, Clifford P. Small-area variations in the use of common surgical procedures: an international comparison of New England, England, and Norway. *New England Journal of Medicine* 1982; **307** (21): 1310–14.

21 Wennberg J, Gittelsohn A. Small area variations in health care delivery. *Science* 1973; **182** (117): 1102–8.

22 Wennberg J, Gittelsohn A. Variations in medical care among small areas. *Scientific American* 1982; **246** (4): 120–34.

23 R v. Prentice (1993) 3 WLR 927.

24 Merry AF, Peck DJ. Anaesthetists, errors in drug administration and the law. *New Zealand Medical Journal* 1995; **108**: 185–7.

25 R v. Bateman (1925) All ER 45.

26 Marshall v. Lindsey County Council (1935) 1 KB 516.

27 Whitehouse v. Jordan (1980) 1 All ER 650.

28 Cheney FW, Posner KL, Lee LA, Caplan RA, Domino KB. Trends in anesthesia-related death and brain damage: a closed claims analysis. *Anesthesiology* 2006; **105** (6): 1081–6.

29 R v. Prentice, R v. Sullman, R v. Adomako, R v. Holloway (1994) QB 302.

30 Skegg PDG. Criminal prosecutions of negligent health professionals: the New Zealand experience. *Medical Law Review* 1998; **6**: 220–46.

31 Paterson R. Protecting patients' rights in New Zealand. *Medicine and Law* 2005; **24** (1): 51–60.

CHAPTER 7

The many advantages and some disadvantages of a no-blame culture regarding medical errors

Mavis Maclean

There is widespread dissatisfaction with the present system for compensating victims of medical injury. As there is no legal contract between doctor and patient in the National Health Service (NHS) the patient can only sue in tort for a wrong which has caused them harm. If the aims of a tort-based system are to compensate victims and deter future perpetrators, neither of these aims is being consistently achieved. Victims of medical mishap or injury can only receive financial compensation if they are able to identify an individual whose action caused their problem. This gives rise to two difficulties. Firstly it can be difficult to assess to what extent the problem is part of the underlying medical condition which brought the patient to seek treatment. Secondly it is becoming increasingly difficult to produce evidence linking the adverse incident to the action of an individual, given the complex nature of work carried out by medical professionals, and the development of team working where the actions of each individual are not always identifiable. Furthermore, it is unlikely that any evidence regarding intent will be found, as adverse incidents are by their nature accidental.

As a member of the Bristol Royal Infirmary Inquiry Panel, with research experience of compensation studies of road traffic and industrial accidents as well as accidents in the home [1] and in the course of medical care, I have long taken the view that compensation for illness and accident through the tort system is expensive, inefficient and unsatisfactory (see Chapter 6). But the evidence presented to the Bristol Inquiry, which was concerned with the mortality rate among children undergoing surgery for congenital heart conditions in the Bristol Royal Infirmary between 1984 and 1995, led me to the view that medical negligence is not only unsatisfactory in dealing with compensation and deterrence, but can actually make matters worse. The resulting culture of secrecy and blame makes it impossible to learn from previous

Health Care Errors and Patient Safety. Edited by Brian Hurwitz and Aziz Sheikh.
© 2009 Blackwell Publishing, ISBN: 978-1-4051-4643-2.

mistakes, which are our richest source of information in learning how to de better. The Inquiry [2] concluded that:

- The absence of a culture of safety and a culture of openness meant that concerns and incidents were not routinely or systematically discussed and addressed and thereby unsafe practices continued unchecked.
- The physical environment and working arrangements were as important to the safe care of patients as the technical skills of physicians.
- The absence of systems for monitoring the safety of clinical care at national or local level put the care of patients at risk.
- The absence of a systematic approach to learning from things that went wrong prevented effective remedial actions from being taken.

The key element in our view was the importance of accepting that not only accidents but also adverse events, or 'near misses' are frequent occurrences in any complex organisation, and inevitably so in the health service. The term is self-explanatory and comes from the excellent work done on safety in air travel [3]. The training and expertise of the medical professionals are, of course, essential for the provision of safe and effective care, but they are only part of the picture. Highly trained responsible people with the best of intentions will sometimes make mistakes. In addition, they work in a less than perfect environment. Equipment may be faulty, or premises less than ideal. In the Bristol case, the fact that surgeons and cardiologists were working in separate buildings some minutes walk apart (including a steep hill) contributed to less than optimal cooperative working. The difficulty of identifying the individual contribution to a mishap was described to us in the context of paediatric cardiac surgery at Great Ormond Street by Professor Marc de Laval where there may be up to 16 separate screens in theatre displaying information during surgery. This level of complexity makes it hard for any one individual to keep his eye on all the separate pieces of data, and although a major change in any reading would be noticed and responded to (e.g. a major change in blood pressure), it becomes hard to analyse the impact of a number of minor changes which taken together would indicate that a child was not doing well. It was these combinations of minor problems, where the information was analysed together, that in his view were more likely to lead to the loss of a child than a single major bleed or breathing difficulty.

We became convinced that the tort-based approach to medical mishap which seeks to find a responsible individual is no longer 'fit for purpose' in the modern medical context. In addition, by requiring a culprit to be found, and naming and shaming the professional concerned even though any money payment will be made by the appropriate union not the individual, the structure of the process provides an incentive to hide errors. This works against the development of medical audit and the possibility of learning not only from major incidents, but also from all the times when a procedure came close to disaster, as well as all those cases that could have gone better – which may well include most cases.

The government shared our interest in the systems approach, and in 2000 published *An Organisation with a Memory* [4] in which the expert group contrasted the individual-based approach to error as evidenced in the medical negligence approach with the systems approach, which assumes that humans are fallible and errors are inevitable.

When things go wrong whether in health care or another environment the response has often been an attempt to identify an individual or individuals who must carry the blame. The focus of incident analysis has tended to be on the events immediately surrounding an adverse event and in particular on the human acts or omissions immediately preceding the event itself … human error may sometimes be the factor that immediately precedes a serious failure but there are usually deeper systemic factors which if addressed would have prevented the error or acted as a safety net to mitigate its consequences … When an error occurs the important issue is not who made the error but how and why did the defences fail and what factors helped to create the conditions in which the errors occurred. [4]

In the Bristol report we stated unequivocally that clinical negligence litigation does not represent a systematic approach to accountability, far less to the proper analysis of error. Rather it is an entirely haphazard process. By institutionalising blame it breeds defensiveness. Errors cannot be treasured if, by acknowledging them, the health care system or the hospital may be sued.

We take the view that it will not be possible to achieve an environment of full open reporting within the NHS when outside it exists a litigation system the incentives of which press in the opposite direction … Within the NHS itself a policy of reporting sentinel events which is both open and non punitive should be pursued. By a non punitive policy we mean a policy which expressly indicates that the NHS prizes information and it will not punish those who report errors, even their own, except in circumstances of criminal behaviour. [2]

The government has been active in addressing the issues. The NHS Litigation Authority (NHSLA) has encouraged the admission of liability and the provision of explanations and apology to patients and relatives. This has already led to the earlier admission of liability, shorter cases and wider use of mediation. The NHSLA has also used a specialist panel of solicitors to good effect.

In addition the reforms to civil justice procedures instigated following Lord Woolf's report [5] have helped to promote a culture of settlement, and made cases quicker, cheaper and fairer to settle. Under these procedures a timetable is set out for the conduct of the case, and the court is asked to identify which matters it will be deciding upon at an early stage. The clinical negligence scheme was set up in 1995 to support NHS trusts in financing negligence enquiries, and offers discounted premiums for those who set up reporting systems to ensure compliance with their risk management standards. In 2001 the National Patient Safety Agency was set up which runs a mandatory reporting system for all mistakes, failures, errors and near-misses across the health service. And in 2001 the National Clinical Assessment Service was set up to support the NHS in dealing with medical professionals whose conduct gave rise to concern, so separating the regulatory function from the question of compensation. In the same year the National Clinical Assessment Authority was set up to support the NHS in dealing with local handling of cases and to carry our local clinical performance assessments.

No-fault schemes

The government has also been looking closely at no-fault schemes in Denmark, Sweden and particularly New Zealand where the no-fault scheme 'Making Amends' has been in operation since 1972. In New Zealand compensation is paid for personal injury as a result of an accident. So personal injury caused by medical error is included within the definition of personal injury. A *medical mishap* is defined as when the patient is given the correct treatment, properly given, but the patient has a complication which was both rare and severe. A *medical error* is defined as the failure of a registered health professional to observe a standard of care and skill reasonably expected in the circumstances. There is no recourse to common law action. Payments are made for medical treatment to victims, and also for loss of earnings (at 80% of previous salary) – the costs being met by a combination of general taxation, premiums charged to medical practitioners and levies on employers.

No-fault schemes are easy to administer but may prove costly if the rate of claim goes up. The Chief Medical Officer concluded that such a scheme would be unaffordable for the NHS [6]. Estimates suggest that even with a 25% reduction in the current rate of litigation, the cost would be between £1.6 billion and £4 billion, compared with £400 million spent on clinical negligence in 2001 [6]. A scheme has also been discussed that would have offered comprehensive compensation to neurologically compromised newborn infants, but this has been shelved. After rejecting both the status quo and the suggested moves towards a no-fault scheme, the Chief Medical Officer has now laid out the government scheme for investigations when things go wrong, remedial treatment when needed, and explanations and apologies for lack of financial compensation. The introduction of an NHS Redress Bill was announced in the Queen's Speech in 2005, and is now on the statute book of England and Wales [7]. The Bill requires trusts not only to offer financial compensation where appropriate, but also to help ensure that the claimant is being provided with a package of care to meet their needs.

There are, of course, some disadvantages to taking this path. The redress scheme makes hospitals investigate not only on response to a complaint but in response to adverse events. The time and resources required by the Act is likely to divert attention from other work. Furthermore, removing the risk that the loser in a case may have to pay the other side's costs may remove any disincentive to bringing claims which are not well founded, and so increase the level of legal activity. As it stands the 'Making Amends' scheme may make it easier to pursue small claims, while not offering any way to reduce the number of cases pursued through the conventional legal system.

However, it is important to go back to the views of those affected, the patients or victims and their families. Although the value of claims pursued over the last few years has increased dramatically from £31 million in 1974/5 to £446 million in 2001/2, these claims have a low success rate (only 24% of legally aided cases currently succeed) and research shows that the majority of those who have a complaint do not seek financial compensation as their primary goal but are driven to seek this when their requests for a clear explanation of what went wrong, and where appropriate an apology, is the primary request. Only when these more simple procedures are not followed do the claims for monetary compensation arise [8]. The British Medical Association has for many years been in favour of a no-fault scheme for compensation. The cynical response might be that of course they do not want to see their members in court. But they have put forward some strong arguments. They point out that the present tort-based system destroys the proper relationship between doctor and patient by introducing a confrontational element, and contributes to the current adversarial system which upholds the blame culture and prevents the heath professions being open about mistakes and learning from them.

On a personal note, as an academic used to fighting my corner in an individualistic, highly competitive professional world, my own experience of studying the no-blame culture was a revelation. To be free to admit to mistakes, and to share the experience of others who have been in a similar position is a thoroughly enabling experience, freeing the individual from the fear of failure and facilitating learning from the best of all sources, colleagues with parallel experiences. The concept of treasuring mistakes is a strange one, in that it sounds as if errors have an intrinsic value. This is hard to reconcile with a poor outcome for the patient. But no profession has a static knowledge base, and the contribution of acknowledged error to progress and development is real and extensive. There are issues to resolve about how to provide some form of confidentiality with respect to error-related information. But the Bristol Inquiry took the view that these problems were not insurmountable. There is little to lose, and a great deal to gain. Are we making progress? Professor Sir Ian Kennedy in his lecture 'Learning from Bristol; are we?', published by the Healthcare Commission in 2006, is optimistic about the culture changes within the NHS with respect to concerns for patient safety, though recognising that we have a long way to go.

References

1 Harris D, Hawkins K, Fenn P. *Compensation and Support for Illness and Injury*. Oxford University Press, Oxford, 1984.
2 Bristol Royal Infirmary. *Learning from Bristol. The Report of the Public Inquiry into Children's Heart Surgery at the Bristol Royal Infirmary 1984–1995*. CM 5207. HMSO, London, 2001: 352.
3 Vincent C, Neale G, Woloshynowych M. Adverse events in British hospitals: preliminary retrospective record review. *British Medical Journal* 2001; **322**: 517–19.

4 Department of Health. *An Organisation with a Memory*. Department of Health, London, 2000: 39.

5 Lord Woolf. *Access to Justice: Final Report to the Lord Chancellor on the Civil Justice System in England and Wales*. HMSO, London, 1996.

6 Deparment of Health. *Making Amends. A Consultation Paper Setting out Proposals for Reforming the Approach to Clinical Negligence in the NHS*. Department of Health, London, 2003: 112.

7 NHS Redress Act 2006. United Kingdom Parliament http://www.opsi.gov.uk/acts/acts2006/pdf/ukpga20060044en.pdf

8 Mulcahy L et al. *Mediating Medical Negligence Claims: An Option for the Future?* HMSO, London, 1999.

PART 2

Threats to patient safety

CHAPTER 8

Diagnostic errors: psychological theories and research implications

Olga Kostopoulou

The psychology of medical diagnosis has been studied for more than three decades [1]. Our knowledge of how clinicians reason and solve patient problems has greatly improved since the early studies of Elstein and colleagues [2], which remain pioneering in their methodology and findings.

There are two fairly distinct psychology approaches to the study of medical diagnosis. Cognitive psychology approaches medical diagnosis as a problem-solving activity, requiring a store of medical knowledge and reasoning processes with which to apply that knowledge to a given patient. The aim is to describe the knowledge representations involved and the processes by which they are activated during diagnosis, and use process measures to explain the diagnostic outcome. A common theme in this type of research is investigation of differences between groups of clinicians according to, for example, specialty or experience.

Structural approaches to the study of diagnosis, such as clinical judgment analysis, are essentially 'black box' or 'input–output' approaches, in that they do not describe reasoning processes but statistically model how the input (e.g. patient characteristics) determines the output (the decision, judgment or diagnosis). The statistical model, usually a regression model, of a single doctor identifies what information this doctor uses and how he/she weighs it to arrive at the decision. The model can be used to predict what this doctor would decide for other patients, whose characteristics are known and have been included as variables in the model. Structural approaches are idiographic, i.e. focus on single doctor decisions, but data can ultimately be aggregated at a group level, e.g. by specialty, experience or practice location [3].

This chapter will concentrate on cognitive psychology approaches to medical diagnosis and their contributions to the development of theory. In comparison to structural approaches, cognitive psychology approaches tend to use patient problems that are richer in information. They allow more flexibility in the range of methods that can be employed (e.g. standardised patients, think aloud techniques), and in the clinical information that can be presented to study participants. They allow clinicians to collect information as they

Health Care Errors and Patient Safety. Edited by Brian Hurwitz and Aziz Sheikh.
© 2009 Blackwell Publishing, ISBN: 978-1-4051-4643-2.

see fit. They are better suited to diagnosis, which often involves deciding between several alternatives – whilst structural approaches are suitable for studying judgments (e.g. estimates of likelihood) and decisions involving binary choice (heart disease vs no heart disease, patient A vs patient B, treatment vs no treatment).

A brief introduction to the various conceptualisations of diagnosis will be followed by their implications for explaining diagnostic error. Diagnostic error can result from deeply rooted tendencies in human reasoning, as well as the content and structure of the clinician's knowledge base. The hypothetico-deductive framework is adopted to present various types of diagnostic errors, not as the sole model for diagnosis but as an all-encompassing framework where the different conceptualisations of diagnosis can fit.

Psychological theories of diagnosis

A number of psychological theories and models have been proposed to explain how diagnosticians form mental representations of the problem to guide their information search and interpretation, and how knowledge is structured in long-term memory and called upon when required. They aim to predict the strategies that will be deployed in different types of diagnostic situations and the errors that are likely to arise during the process.

Diagnosis has been explained as the result of hypothetico-deductive reasoning – hypothesis generation and testing [2], 'pattern recognition' or matching of the presenting problem to a similar, previously encountered problem [4], abstraction from specific patient features to higher-order memory structures [5] or mapping patient cases to disease prototypes [6]. Experienced clinicians are likely to test hypotheses in difficult cases, whereas simpler, familiar cases are more quickly solved by rapid recognition of similar instances or prototype mapping. Novices, on the other hand, are expected to use their biomedical knowledge and employ causal reasoning to interpret symptoms and signs, due to their limited repertoire of patterns or due to poorly organised knowledge in memory making it difficult to access. According to Schmidt et al. [7], the development of diagnostic skill passes from the stage of slow and effortful reasoning with biomedical knowledge, to the application of clinical rules and prototype mapping, to pattern matching (recognition of past similar patients). The perceived difficulty of a patient case and the subsequent strategy employed will depend on the clinician's skill and experience [8]. With experience, clinicians become better at identifying the demands of the diagnostic problem at hand and move seamlessly between the different types of reasoning.

Hypothesis generation and associated errors

Hypothesis generation is the first step in the diagnostic process and it is critical for accurate diagnosis. Knowing what data to collect depends on the hypotheses generated [2] and has been linked to the level of expertise [9].

Clinicians and students at all levels of experience have been found to generate a small number of hypotheses early on in the process [2,10]. Barrows et al. [10] found that causes or hypotheses that are not generated initially are unlikely to be considered later (see Box 8.1 for an example). This can be linked to the difficulty of the human mind to restructure a problem once a solution strategy has been constructed, especially one that has worked well in similar problems in the past. This is known as 'cognitive set' [11].

Pattern recognition can also be thought of as hypothesis generation, where the recognised instance is the hypothesis entertained by the clinician that leads directly to action. Errors can result from clinicians confusing previous similar instances in visual diagnostic tasks (e.g. interpreting dermatology slides [12]) or not recognising novel situations as such. When novel situations are mistakenly perceived as familiar, diagnosticians will respond in ways that have worked in the past but are not currently appropriate, ignoring or explaining away counter-evidence. This is a common finding in both clinical and non-clinical diagnosis [13].

When there is partial feature matching, two or more competing hypotheses may be generated. Base rates, i.e. the incidence of diseases, seem to determine which hypotheses are considered [2]. Similarly, in other domains of diagnostic activity, recent research has shown that participants tend to generate hypotheses that are highly likely, and to ignore hypotheses that are implausible or unlikely [14]. It follows that a disease may not be seriously considered if its perceived likelihood is low. This might be of particular relevance in primary care, as, with experience, general practitioners' (GPs') perception of prevalence is expected to adapt to the characteristics of their patient population. On average and in comparison with hospital specialists, GPs encounter fewer serious diseases. This may lead them to not consider a condition that they perceive as unlikely.

A disease may also be considered because it is memorable, irrespective of its prevalence. This is likely to happen with serious conditions that have been misdiagnosed, leading to injury or death (e.g. meningococcal septicaemia in

---

Box 8.1: Example of a failure to generate the appropriate diagnostic hypothesis [15]

A patient, with a current diagnosis of depression and antidepressants taking, presents with fatigue and dry mouth. The doctor assumes that the presenting symptoms are due to the medication (known side effects) and the depression medication and spends the entire consultation testing the diagnosis of depression, which had initially been made by another doctor in the practice; the doctor decides to change the medication because it seems to be ineffective and is causing side effects. At no time does the doctor consider the alternative possibility of newly onset diabetes as a coexisting disease.

general practice), or with unusual cases that the clinician has encountered – which then become the subject of 'anecdotes' in the communication with and training of other clinicians [16]. Dawson and Arkes [17], also anecdotally, convincingly recount the case of an older clinician who was diagnosed with and operated for chronic appendicitis and who subsequently started diagnosing chronic appendicitis in many of his older patients presenting with new, non-specific abdominal pain, referring them for surgery. Recent evidence for the influence of 'availability bias' [18] on treatment decisions comes from Choudhry et al. [19]. The study found that doctors were less likely to prescribe warfarin to patients with atrial fibrillation after one of their patients had experienced a major adverse bleeding event associated with warfarin, than before such an occurrence. In diagnosis, the 'availability' of a diagnosis in memory, can lead to inappropriate diagnoses being triggered and pursued or to overestimating their prevalence.

In complex diagnostic situations, the correct hypothesis may not be generated initially. Generating inaccurate hypotheses or 'faulty triggering' [20], can result in an inability to account for the presenting clinical evidence [21] and the collection of irrelevant data. As more information is obtained and the clinical picture evolves, the initial hypothesis may need to be rejected and the problem reformulated. As mentioned earlier, fixation or 'cognitive set' [11] may prevent problem reformulation.

Hypothesis testing and associated errors

The outcome of the hypothesis generation process determines which hypotheses are tested. Hypotheses are tested by deducing what further symptoms should be present and then checking for their presence or absence [2]. This process can be subject to various biases that occur without awareness and are by-products of our cognitive system. The most notable bias in hypothesis testing is confirmation bias [22,23]. It can take various forms: for example, the clinician may start out with an initial hypothesis and search for evidence that supports it, discounting or explaining away evidence that points to an alternative diagnosis. Alternatively, the clinician may not try to disconfirm the preferred diagnosis or may not sufficiently revise confidence in the preferred diagnosis as new information is obtained ('conservatism' [24]). Another facet of confirmation bias is 'pseudo-diagnosticity' [25], whereby information is collected not because it is diagnostic (i.e. can help to differentiate between competing hypotheses) but because it is likely to be consistent with the favoured hypothesis. This can lead to inefficiency and cost by deferring additional laboratory tests thought to be of little diagnostic value, which can increase confidence but not necessarily accuracy [26].

Diagnostic decision making can be affected by the number of differential diagnoses considered. This is because the likelihood of the hypothesis under consideration (the focal hypothesis) is evaluated relative to other competing hypotheses. According to the support theory [27], the perceived likelihood of a hypothesis increases as its description becomes more detailed. Due to memory limitations, people compare the focal hypothesis against a set of alternatives described at a more general level. This leads to 'sub-additivity', i.e. underestimating the likelihood for the set of alternatives.

One of the studies of this phenomenon recruited 59 house officers at Stanford University [28]. Participants were divided into two groups and read the following description:

A well-known 22-year-old Hollywood actress presents to the emergency department with pain in the right lower quadrant of her abdomen of 12 hours' duration. Her last normal menstrual period was 4 weeks ago.

All participants were told that the patient had only one condition and the estimated probabilities should add to 100% (Table 8.1). Logically, 'none of the above' in the short list of differentials (group A) should be equally likely as ('appendicitis' + 'pyelonephritis' + 'pelvic inflammatory disease' + 'none of the above') in the long list of differentials (group B). In fact, its average estimated likelihood was significantly lower in group A. The study suggests that unpacking 'some other diagnosis' so that more alternatives are considered can alter likelihood estimates, by reminding doctors of diagnoses that they might have overlooked or by increasing the salience of diagnoses that they did consider but forgot or failed to pursue. The other noteworthy finding was that the average estimated likelihood of gastroenteritis, the leading diagnosis for group A, was significantly lower for group B. This suggests that if clinicians are prompted to consider other diagnoses, likelihood estimates for the focal diagnosis tend to decrease.

There is experimental evidence that consideration of different possibilities can improve probability judgments by increasing consideration for counterfactuals and counter-arguments [14]. Covey and Lovie [29] found that asking people to evaluate both the true positive rate and the false positive rate reduces inattention to false positives [30] but does not turn people into 'Bayesians' – most people still prefer to simplify the task by considering one

Table 8.1 Estimated probabilities of alternative diagnoses.

Group A estimated probabilities for:	Average estimates (%)	Group B estimated probabilities for:	Average estimates (%)
Gastroenteritis	31	Gastroenteritis	16
Ectopic pregnancy	19	Ectopic pregnancy	15
None of the above	50	Appendicitis	
		Pyelonephritis	
		Pelvic inflammatory disease	69
		None of the above	

hypothesis at a time. This focus of attention on a single possibility has been shown to inflate its estimated likelihood [28].

Knowledge base: content and structure

Knowledge content

Inappropriate hypotheses may be generated both because of insufficient biomedical knowledge and insufficient or inappropriate contextual knowledge. Experts have been found to make greater use of contextual information, whilst less experienced clinicians make greater use of biomedical knowledge because they cannot effectively use contextual information [31]. The widespread view in the psychology literature on clinical diagnostic reasoning is that experts make little use of biomedical knowledge if they can solve a case in less effortful ways. However, 'biomedical reasoning is an aid to diagnosis that is readily available to experts and is one which they will use effectively, if short-cut methods using contextual information are not available' [32, p. 220]. Faced with challenging problems in their specialty (nephrology), experts diagnosed much more accurately and provided more aetiological explanations based on basic science principles than residents in both internal and family medicine [33].

Knowledge structure: schemata and scripts

It is not only the knowledge content that can determine diagnostic accuracy but also its structure in memory. Theories of 'schemata' and 'scripts' attempt to explain how knowledge is organised in memory. Schemata are abstract representations of categories and contain generic knowledge about attributes, values and relations [34,35]. Scripts are 'event schemata' that account for people's stereotypical knowledge of often-encountered situations, e.g. going to a restaurant [36]. New events are encoded with respect to general scripts and subsequent recall is influenced by the script [37], helping us predict missing information or correct errors in information.

Feltovich and Barrows first coined the term 'illness script' [38, p. 138], thereby introducing the concept in the literature of medical reasoning. They hypothesised that a clinician understands a patient problem by constructing a story of how the problem came to be (the 'enabling conditions'), the major points of malfunction (the 'faults') and the associated consequences (the signs and symptoms). At every clinical encounter the clinician constructs a new script – a mental representation of the situation – through causal and associative reasoning. This enables hypothesis generation and testing. Illness scripts are therefore similar to 'story construction' as a way by which clinicians make sense of the presenting problem and choose a course of action [39,40].

Schmidt et al. [41] have also used the concept of scripts but with different meaning and implications. Scripts are abstract representations of diseases in memory (prototypes), activated almost unconsciously, against which each clinical encounter is compared. They do not require causal reasoning and contain relatively little knowledge about pathophysiological causes of symptoms and signs. They mostly contain clinically relevant information about the disease, its consequences and the context within which it develops, e.g. risk factors. Hypothesis generation and testing are seen as script activation and processing (assessment of fit between a script and a given clinical situation) [6].

Activation of disease prototypes can occur through abstraction from the patient's specific features to 'semantic qualifiers' [42]. For example, 'three times a month' becomes 'recurrent'. Increased use of semantic qualifiers has been correlated with greater diagnostic accuracy in both students and doctors [42]. However, a training programme to promote their use with second-year students was not successful, possibly due to the students' insufficient knowledge base [43].

Hamm's account of scripts utilizes both a semantic network and a production system [44]. Scripts are stored in memory as semantic networks of nodes. A node representing a disease is connected to other nodes (e.g. risk factors, symptoms and signs, treatments, past patients with that disease, etc.). When nodes representing features of the clinical situation become active (usually as a result of one or a handful of key features from the patient's presentation), activation spreads along the connections of the semantic network to associated script nodes. With experience (e.g. seeing many patients with the same disease presenting with a number of similar features), certain links between disease and symptoms become stronger and are activated more rapidly. At the same time, scripts have the form of condition–action rules ('if–then' rules), prescribing what to do but also allowing for new responses or solutions to be generated in novel situations through analogical reasoning and inductive learning [45].

Script theory is an attractive theory, consistent with evidence about the development of expertise in a number of domains. However, it lacks empirical support and does not enable precise predictions about the performance expected from clinicians at different levels of experience and for different types of diagnostic problems. As Hamm points out, it needs 'sharper definition before serious hypothesis testing can be done' [44, p. 335].

A synthesis of the literature

It is possible that clinicians use a mixture of strategies involving automatic activation of disease prototypes and their variations, memories of previous patient encounters, as well as more effortful causal reasoning. How they will reason and how effectively depends on the features of the case (familiarity, complexity, typicality), their previous experience with similar cases, the existence of relevant scripts in their memory and/or their knowledge of the underlying pathophysiology.

The observable products of hypothesis generation and testing are the gathering of clinical information in terms of history taking, physical examination, ordering of tests and sometimes referral to (other) specialists. The interpretation of clinical information is a more or less covert process that clinicians may externalise when providing explanations to patients or discussing the case with other clinicians. It has been suggested that information gathering is more problematic than information interpretation due to the difficulty in recognising what information has diagnostic value, and that if clinicians are provided with optimal diagnostic information, they will make optimal diagnostic decisions [46]. However, this was observed in a study that used hypothetical diseases ('disease A' and 'disease B') without context, which precluded the use of relevant clinical knowledge and 'scripts' to guide hypothesis generation and testing. It is therefore possible that the interpretation of information, either overinterpreting non-diagnostic information [2,47] or underweighing/misinterpreting critical information, can also determine the outcome of the diagnostic process (see Box 8.2 for examples). Other documented problems with information interpretation include failure to link evidence to appropriate hypotheses [48, 49], ignoring the disease prevalence when unexpected test information is obtained [30] and explaining away symptoms by wrongly attributing them to existing health problems [50, 51]. A recent selective review of the literature on clinical reasoning [54] suggests that inability to generate an appropriate mental representation can result in the random generation of hypotheses that are based on isolated findings in the case. Another well-known phenomenon is that of 'premature closure', i.e.

Box 8.2: Examples of clinicians underweighting critical information or overweighting non-critical information, when dealing with a patient presenting with chest pain [15]

Underweighting/misinterpreting critical information
GP assessing patient with chest pain: 'Now he says it goes down his right arm, which is unlikely to be angina unless he's got … his heart is the wrong way round. It tends to be your left arm. Now that could be a red herring, you've still got to be … it doesn't exclude it. It makes it less likely.'

Note: Right-sided radiation of chest pain has a likelihood ratio of 6.68 for acute coronary syndrome (ACS), whilst left-sided radiation of pain has a likelihood ratio of 1.22 [52]. Nevertheless, left-sided radiation is considered by many to be a typical feature of ACS.

Overweighting non-critical information
Another GP assessing the same patient: 'If he has no pain and he has pain only when he moves his arm, it's totally the musculoskeletal, but if he has pain right now in the chest, then it's totally different because he needs to get the ECG done or a blood test done to rule out acute coronary syndrome.' (The patient did not have pain during the consultation.) 'That's fine. So he's not needing to go to hospital now.'

Note: ACS does not necessarily present with chest pain [53].

abandoning data gathering too early and making a decision with insufficient or scant evidence [55,56].

The role of decision support systems in reducing diagnostic errors

The contribution of computerised decision support systems to the enhancement of clinical performance and quality of care is widely acknowledged in the areas of prescribing, test ordering, drug dosing and preventive care [57,58]. However, the role of diagnostic decision support remains unclear. Contentious issues include the way such programmes are constructed (Bayesian, logic, pattern recognition), how they derive information about individual patients (automatic retrieval from record vs clinician input), how they integrate in the clinical workflow, how they change the nature of the consultation, and how transparent they are to users – to name but a few. From de Dombal's early system that helped diagnose acute abdominal pain to 'Isabel', the diagnostic reminder system initially developed for paediatric conditions, a fundamental problem has been the lack of evidence as to which aspects of the diagnostic process need to be supported. Sometimes, clinicians may benefit from suggestions regarding differential diagnoses. Should these suggestions be offered early on in the consultation, or later on, when clinicians have more or less decided on a diagnosis but have failed to test some important possibilities? There may be times when clinicians will benefit more from suggestions as to how to test diagnostic hypotheses, e.g. what specific questions to ask the patient, what to look for in the physical examination or what investigations to order. Should the system leave it up to the clinician to recognise the need or should it provide prompts when important information about the patient is not recorded during the consultation? Finally, there may be situations where important information is obtained but not properly assessed. Should the system provide online advice about how information should be interpreted? We do not know the types of diagnostic situations where clinicians are likely to benefit the most from the above different types of support. Experimental studies based on psychological and learning theories should assess needs and likely impact before decision support is constructed.

Research implications

Diagnostic error is particularly important in settings where there is a large throughput in terms of patient contacts, disease presents early and is difficult to differentiate, and diagnosis has to be made without delay or availability of reliable diagnostic tools. This describes well the situation in primary care. Diagnostic error is the commonest cause of claims against GPs to medical defence societies [59]. Some of these errors are caused by system failures (e.g. incomplete records). Others are caused mainly by cognitive factors (e.g. the

GP giving too much weight to a normal mammogram or the GP diagnosing irritable bowel syndrome (IBS) in patients who turned out to have colon cancer, possibly due to relying on IBS prevalence). Investigation of patient claims happens months or years after the event. It is therefore difficult to identify the cognitive factors that were implicated as the relevant information is not necessarily recorded or is forgotten. Identifying the cognitive factors of errors is not the focus of such investigations. Furthermore, the details of patient claims are not freely available and open to scrutiny by researchers.

Is self-reporting by doctors a more fruitful approach in the identification and study of diagnostic errors? Most incident reporting studies in primary care receive very small numbers of diagnostic errors. For example, a US study [60] classified 3.9% of the reported errors as 'wrong or missed diagnosis'; in the UK, diagnostic error accounted for 2.6% of the reports in one study [61] and 0.5% of the reports in another [62]. An Australian study classified 14% of the reported errors as 'diagnostic', including diagnostic errors by pharmacists and hospital doctors [63]. An exception is an earlier Australian study [64] that found diagnostic error to be implicated in 34% of the reported incidents. Leaving aside the problems of different systems of error classification between these studies, reporting is likely to underestimate the extent of diagnostic error. There are several reasons why diagnostic errors might be under-reported:

1 There is a current research and policy emphasis on the system causes of error. Practitioners' self-reports may reflect this.

2 Admission of a diagnostic error can be embarassing and potentially harmful in terms of loss of patient and colleagues' trust, loss of self-confidence and potential litigation (see Chapters 6 and 7).

3 Practitioners tend to concentrate on errors that led to an adverse outcome[65–67]. A missed or delayed diagnosis that was subsequently detected and corrected may be considered as part of the normal diagnostic process.

4 Doctors may not be aware that they have made an error and even more so a diagnostic one. Feedback about the outcome of the diagnostic process is usually either absent or delayed. This is more the case in general practice than hospital specialties and can have implications for the improvement of GPs' diagnostic performance [68].

Record review may help to identify diagnostic errors but not their causes. The earlier discussion on theoretical approaches to diagnostic errors suggests that knowing what hypotheses are entertained during the diagnostic process and how information is interpreted is important for understanding why a diagnostic error occurred. Such information is unlikely to be found in patient claims, incident reports or patient records. Experimentation using realistic vignettes is more suitable to this end. The validity of vignettes as a measure of performance in diagnosis and management has been shown [69,70], but they need to be constructed so that they reflect real practice as much as possible (e.g. be interactive and sufficiently complex, impose time constraints and use evidence-based scoring criteria).

Psychological research has focused more on clinical reasoning and the development of diagnostic skill than diagnostic error per se. Nevertheless, one cannot study the latter without taking the former into account. Several methods have been employed to study clinical reasoning. For example, clinicians have been interviewed [71], have thought aloud whist reasoning about cases [72,73], and their management of standardized patients has been assessed [74]. They have made judgments over a large number of cases that have then been statistically modelled to identify which information has been influential [3,75]. Clinician information elicitation has been traced using hypothetical or real, computer- or paper-based case histories [2,76]. Clinicians have also been given scenarios as part of carefully controlled experiments designed to study particular heuristics or methods of reasoning [77–80]. Harries and Kostopoulou provide a review of the psychological approaches for measuring and modelling clinical reasoning and decision making [81].

Some research paradigms allow the information gathering process to be observed, whilst others present all information at once. In the 'immediate presentation' paradigm, vignettes are presented in full and experienced physicians with sufficient knowledge can exhibit 'forward reasoning' (no hypothesis testing) [82] because all the information is available to support this mode of reasoning. Some studies have presented case information in a series of sequentially revealed screens [73], keeping the sequence constant for all doctors. In 'active information search' (AIS) paradigms, clinicians can request any information in any sequence they see fit [2]. As a consequence, hypothesis testing takes place. AIS paradigms create a natural mode of reasoning, but do not indicate how information is interpreted and whether it is influential. Some studies have complemented AIS with thinking aloud [83] or questioning techniques [76]. However, in familiar diagnostic situations with experienced clinicians, verbalisation is likely to disrupt or not sufficiently capture the automatic mode of diagnosis (pattern recognition) [84].

Researchers of diagnostic reasoning and error should aim to use methods that:
• Are non-reactive, i.e. do not interfere with and change the nature of the diagnostic task.
• Allow a degree of experimental control in terms of, for example, the type, complexity, range and order of problems presented.
• Use representative diagnostic problems, i.e. problems that clinicians are likely to encounter in their everyday practice.
• Have reliable ways of measuring and scoring diagnosis and management.
• Use a 'gold standard' against which to measure diagnosis, e.g. diagnosis confirmed by definite test.

It is possible that some diagnostic difficulties are not resolvable within the current limits of knowledge and are inherent to the diagnostic situation. Kassirer and Kopelman [20] identified a category of 'no fault' errors, which refers to atypical or non-specific cases, extremely rare cases or rapidly evolving diseases, where clinicians would be likely to miss the diagnosis (e.g. very early presentations of meningococcal septicaemia). Studies of diagnostic reasoning and error should determine the bounds of acceptable professional judgment.

References

1 Norman G. Research in clinical reasoning: past history and current trends. *Medical Educuation* 2005; **39** (4): 418–27.

2 Elstein A, Shulman L, Sprafka S. *Medical Problem Solving: An Analysis of Clinical Reasoning*. Harvard University Press, Cambridge, MA, 1978.

3 Tape T, Heckerling P, Ornato J et al. Use of clinical judgment analysis to explain regional variations in physicians' accuracies in diagnosing pneumonia. *Medical Decision Making* 1991; **11** (2): 189–97.

4 Norman G, Brooks L. The non-analytical basis of clinical reasoning. *Advances in Health Science Education* 1997; **2** (2):173–84.

5 Grant J, Marsden P. The structure of memorized knowledge in students and clinicians: an explanation for diagnostic expertise. *Medical Education* 1987; **21**: 92–8.

6 Charlin B, Tardif J, Boshuizen H. Scripts and medical diagnostic knowledge: theory and applications for clinical reasoning instruction and research. *Academic Medicine* 2000; **75** (2): 182–90.

7 Schmidt H, Norman G, Boshuizen H. A cognitive perspective on medical expertise: theory and implications. *Academic Medicine* 1990; **65** (10): 611–21.

8 Elstein A. What goes around comes around: the return of the hypothetico-deductive strategy. *Teaching and Learning in Medicine* 1994; **6**:121–3.

9 Allen V, Arocha J, Patel V. Evaluating evidence against diagnostic hypotheses in clinical decision making by students, residents and physicians. *International Journal of Medical Informatics* 1998; **51** (2/3): 91–105.

10 Barrows H, Norman G, Neufeld V et al. The clinical reasoning of randomly selected physicians in general medical practice. *Clinical and Investigative Medicine* 1982; **5** (1): 49–55.

11 Luchins A. *Mechanization in Problem Solving. The Effect of Einstellung.* Psychological Monographs No. 54. 1942: 248.

12 Norman G, Rosenthal D, Brooks L et al. The development of expertise in dermatology. *Archives of Dermatology* 1989; **125** (8):1063–8.

13 Reason J. *Human Error.* Cambridge University Press, Cambridge, 1990.

14 Dougherty M, Gettys C, Thomas R. The role of mental simulation in judgments of likelihood. *Organizational Behavior and Human Decision Processes* 1997; **70**: 135–48.

15 Kostopoulan O, Oudhoff J, Nath R et al. Predictors of diagnostic accuracy and safe management in difficult diagnostic problems in family medicine. *Medical Decision Making* 2008; **28**: 668–80.

16 Alderson T, Bateman H. Doctors telling stories: the place of anecdote in GP registrar training. *Medical Teacher* 2002; **24** (6): 654–7.

17 Dawson N, Arkes H. Systematic errors in medical decision making: judgment limitations. *Journal of General Internal Medicine* 1987; **2** (2): 183–7.

18 Tversky A, Kahneman D. Judgment under uncertainty: heuristics and biases. *Science* 1974; **185**: 1124–31.

19 Choudhry N, Anderson G, Laupacis A et al. Impact of adverse events on prescribing warfarin in patients with atrial fibrillation: matched pair analysis. *British Medical Journal* 2006; **332**: 141–5.

20 Kassirer J, Kopelman R. Cognitive errors in diagnosis: instantiation, classification, and consequences. *American Journal of Medicine* 1989; **86** (4): 433–41.

21 Gruppen L, Palchik NS, Wolf F et al. Medical student use of history and physical information in diagnostic reasoning. *Arthritis Care and Research* 1993; **6** (2): 64–70.
22 Klayman J. Varieties of confirmation bias. *In*: Busemeyer J, Hastie R, Medin D, eds. *The Psychology of Learning and Motivation*, Vol. 32. Academic Press, San Diego, 1995: 385–418.
23 Nickerson R. Confirmation bias: a ubiquitous phenomenon in many guises. *Review of General Psychology* 1998; **2** (2): 175–220.
24 Edwards W. Conservatism in human information processing. *In*: Kleinmuntz B, ed. *Formal Representation in Human Judgment*. Wiley, New York, 1968: 17–52.
25 Kern L, Doherty M. 'Pseudodiagnosticity' in an idealized medical problem-solving environment. *Journal of Medical Education* 1982; **57**: 100–4.
26 Chapman G, Elstein A. Cognitive processes and biases in medical decision making. *In*: Chapman G, Sonnenberg F, eds. *Decision Making in Health Care: Theory, Psychology, and Applications*. Cambridge University Press, Cambridge, 2000: 183–210.
27 Tversky A, Koehler D. Support theory: a nonextensional representation of subjective probability. *Psychological Review* 1994; **101**: 547–67.
28 Redelmeier D, Koehler D, Liberman V et al. Probability judgment in medicine – discounting unspecified possibilities. *Medical Decision Making* 1995; **15** (3): 227–30.
29 Covey J, Lovie A. Information selection and utilization in hypothesis testing: a comparison of process-tracing and structural analysis techniques. *Organizational Behavior and Human Decision Processes* 1998; **75** (1): 56–74.
30 Eddy D. Probabilistic reasoning in clinical medicine: problems and opportunities. *In*: Kahneman D, Slovic P, Tversky A, eds. *Judgment Under Uncertainty: Heuristics and Biases*. Cambridge University Press, New York, 1982: 249–67.
31 Hobus P, Schmidt H, Boshuizen H et al. Contextual factors in the activation of first diagnostic hypotheses: expert-novice differences. *Medical Education* 1987; **21**: 471–6.
32 Gilhooly K, McGeorge P, Hunter J et al. Biomedical knowledge in diagnostic thinking: the case of electrocardiogram (ECG) interpretation. *European Journal of Cognitive Psychology* 1997; **9** (2): 199–223.
33 Norman G, Trott A, Brooks L et al. Cognitive differences in clinical reasoning related to postgraduate training. *Teaching and Learning in Medicine* 1994; **6**: 114–20.
34 Brewer W, Treyens J. Role of schemata in memory for places. *Cognitive Psychology* 1981; **13**: 207–30.
35 Rumelhart D. Schemata: The basic building blocks of cognition. *In*: Spiro R, Bruce B, Brewer W, eds. *Theoretical Issues in Reading Comprehension*. Lawrence Erlbaum Associates, Hillsdale, NJ, 1980.
36 Schank R, Abelson R. Scripts, plans, goals and understanding. Lawrence Erlbaum Associates, Hillsdale, NJ, 1977.
37 Bower G, Black J, Turner T. Scripts in memory for text. *Cognitive Psychology* 1979; **11**: 177–220.
38 Feltovich P, Barrows H. Issues of generality in medical problem solving. *In*: Schmidt H, De Volder M, eds. *Tutorials in Problem-Based Learning: A New Direction in Teaching the Health Professions*. Van Gorcum, Assen, Maastricht, 1984: 128–142.
39 Cox K. Stories as case knowledge: case knowledge as stories. *Medical Education* 2001; **35** (9): 862–6.
40 Charon R. Narrative and medicine. *New England Journal of Medicine* 2004; **350** (9): 862–4.
41 Schmidt H, Norman G, Boshuizen H. A cognitive perspective on medical expertise: theory and implication. *Academic Medicine* 1990; **65** (10): 611–21.
42 Bordage G, Lemieux M. Semantic structures and diagnostic thinking of experts and novices. *Academic Medicine* 1991; **66** (9): S70–S73.

43 Nendaz M, Bordage G. Promoting diagnostic problem representation. *Medical Education* 2002; **36** (8): 760–6.

44 Hamm R. Medical decision scripts: combining cognitive scripts and judgment strategies to account fully for medical decision making. *In:* Hardman D, Macchi L, eds. *Thinking: Psychological Perspectives on Reasoning, Judgment and Decision Making.* Wiley, Chichester, 2003: 315–45.

45 Anderson J. Skill acquisition: compilation of weak-method problem solutions. *Psychological Review* 1987; **94** (2): 192–210.

46 Gruppen L, Wolf F, Billi J. Information gathering and integration as sources of error in diagnostic decision-making. *Medical Decision Making* 1991; **11** (4): 233–9.

47 Friedman M, Connell K, Olthoff A et al. Medical student errors in making a diagnosis. *Academic Medicine* 1998; **73** (10): S19–S21.

48 Johnson P, Duran A, Hassebrock F et al. Expertise and error in diagnostic reasoning. *Cognitive Science* 1981; **5**: 235–83.

49 Kostopoulou O, Devereaux-Walsh C, Delaney BC. Missing celiac disease in family medicine: the importance of hypothesis generation. *Medical Decision Making.* In press.

50 Bhasale A. The wrong diagnosis: identifying causes of potentially adverse events in general practice using incident monitoring. *Family Practice* 1998; **15** (4): 308–18.

51 Kostopoulou O, Delaney BC, Munro CW. Diagnostic difficulty and error in primary care: a systematic review. *Family Practice.* In press.

52 Mant J, McManus R, Oakes R et al. Systematic review and modelling of the investigation of acute and chronic chest pain presenting in primary care. *Health Technology Assessment* 2004; **8** (2).

53 Fenton D, Baumann B, Stahmer S. Acute coronary syndrome. *eMedicine.* Available at http://www.emedicine.com/EMERG/topic31.htm (last updated 9 Jan. 2007; accessed 14 March 2007).

54 Bowen J. Educational strategies to promote clinical diagnostic reasoning. *New England Journal of Medicine* 2006; **355** (21): 2217–25.

55 Voytovich A, Rippey R, Suffredini A. Premature conclusions in diagnostic reasoning. *Journal of Medical Education* 1985; **60** (4): 302–7.

56 Dubeau C, Voytovich A, Rippey R. Premature conclusions in the diagnosis of iron-deficiency anemia: cause and effect. *Medical Decision Making* 1986; **6** (3): 169–73.

57 Mitchell E, Sullivan F. A descriptive feast but an evaluative famine: systematic review of published articles on primary care computing during 1980–97. *British Medical Journal* 2001; **322** (7281): 279–82.

58 Hunt DL, Haynes RB, Hanna SE et al. Effects of computer-based clinical decision support systems on physician performance and patient outcomes – a systematic review. *Journal of the American Medical Association* 1998; **280** (15): 1339–46.

59 Silk N. What went wrong in 1000 negligence claims. *Health Care Risk Report.* 2000.

60 Dovey S, Meyers D, Phillips RJ et al. A preliminary taxonomy of medical errors in family practice. *Quality and Safety in Health Care* 2002; **11** (3): 233–8.

61 Kostopoulou O, Delaney B. Confidential reporting of patient safety events in primary care: results from a multilevel classification of cognitive and system factors. *Quality and Safety in Health Care* 2007; **16** (2): 95–100.

62 Rubin G, George A, Chinn D et al. Errors in general practice: development of an error classification and pilot study of a method for detecting errors. *Quality and Safety in Health Care* 2003; **12** (6): 443–7.

63 Makeham M, Dovey S, County M et al. An international taxonomy for errors in general practice: a pilot study. *Medical Journal of Australia* 2002; **177** (2): 68–72.

64 Bhasale A, Miller G, Reid S et al. Analysing potential harm in Australian general practice: an incident-monitoring study. *Medical Journal of Australia* 1998; **169**: 73–6.

65 Taylor-Adams SE, Kirwan B. Human reliability data requirements. *International Journal of Quality and Reliability Management* 1995; **12** (1): 24–46.

66 Lawton R, Parker D. Barriers to incident reporting in a healthcare system. *Quality and Safety in Health Care* 2002; **11**: 15–18.

67 van der Schaaf T, Kanse L. Biases in incident reporting databases: an empirical study in the chemical process industry. *Safety Science* 2004; **42**: 57–67.

68 Ericsson K. Deliberate practice and the acquisition and maintenance of expert performance in medicine and related domains (invited address). *Academic Medicine* 2004; **79** (10): S70–S81.

69 Peabody JW, Luck J, Glassman P et al. Comparison of vignettes, standardized patients, and chart abstraction: a prospective validation study of 3 methods for measuring quality. *Journal of the American Medical Association* 2000; **283** (13): 1715–22.

70 Peabody J, Luck J, Glassman P et al. Measuring the quality of physician practice by using clinical vignettes: a prospective validation study. *Annals of Internal Medicine* 2004; **141** (10): 771–80.

71 DiCaccavo A, Reid F. Decisional conflict in general practice: strategies of patient management. *Social Science and Medicine* 1995; **41** (3): 347–53.

72 Denig P, Haaijer-Ruskamp F. Do physicians take cost into account when making prescribing decisions. *Pharmacoeconomics* 1995; **8** (4): 282–90.

73 Backlund L, Skånér Y, Montgomery H et al. Doctors' decision processes in a drug-prescription task: the validity of rating scales and think-aloud reports. *Organizational Behavior and Human Decision Processes* 2003; **91**: 108–17.

74 Beullens J, Rethans J, Goedhuys J et al. The use of standardized patients in research in general practice. *Family Practice* 1997; **14** (1): 58.

75 Harries C, Evans J, Dennis I et al. A clinical judgement analysis of prescribing decisions in general practice. *Le Travail Humain* 1996; **59** (1): 87–111.

76 Kostopoulou O, Wildman M. Sources of variability in uncertain medical decisions in the ICU: a process tracing study. *Quality and Safety in Health Care* 2004; **13** (4): 272–80.

77 Reyna V, Lloyd F. Physician decision making and cardiac risk: effects of knowledge, risk perception, risk tolerance, and fuzzy processing. *Journal of Experimental Psychology: Applied* 2006; **12** (3): 179–95.

78 McNeil B, Pauker S, Sox H et al. On the elicitation of preferences for alternative therapies. *New England Journal of Medicine* 1982; **306** (21): 1259–62.

79 Redelmeier D, Shafir E, Aujla P. The beguiling pursuit of more information. *Medical Decision Making* 2001; **21** (5): 376–81.

80 Redelmeier D, Shafir E. Medical decision making in situations that offer multiple alternatives. *Journal of the American Medical Association* 1995; **273**: 302–5.

81 Harries C, Kostopoulou O. Psychological approaches to measuring and modelling clinical decision-making. In: Bowling A, Ebrahim S, eds. *Handbook of Health Research Methods: Investigation, Measurement and Analysis*. Open University Press, Maidenhead, 2005: 331–61.

82 Patel V, Groen G. Knowledge-based solution strategies in medical reasoning. *Cognitive Science* 1986; **10**: 91–116.

83 Williamson J, Ranyard R, Cuthbert L. A conversation-based process tracing method for use with naturalistic decisions: an evaluation study. *British Journal of Psychology* 2000; **91**: 203–21.

84 Ericsson K, Simon H. *Protocol Analysis: Verbal Reports as Data*. MIT Press, Cambridge, MA, 1984.

CHAPTER 9

'Mince' or 'mice'? Clinical miscommunications and patient safety in a linguistically diverse community

Celia Roberts

I only know that these things mean something quite different to me from what they do to you.

Nora in *The Doll's House* by Henrik Ibsen, 1879

In any consultation there is always the possibility of misunderstanding. Indeed some sceptics would argue that we can never fully understand each other given that all communication is asymmetrical [1]. But on the whole we conduct ourselves on the assumption that we can come to a reasonable interpretation of what the other said. So, we take for granted that if misunderstandings surface, more communication will probably resolve the matter. In matters of patient safety in general practice, the quality of talk and the level of mutual understanding is crucial in appropriate diagnosis and coming to a shared agreement on what action to take.

Errors and misunderstandings remain euphemised in the medical world where a culture of striving for perfection still exists, despite a general acknowledgement that health care is a practice full of uncertainties. Health care professionals face daily dilemmas in communicating with patients. Either they assume they have understood, or made themselves understood, and ignore the goal of 'perfect' communication. Or, in striving to minimise uncertainty and ensure there are no misunderstandings, they are drawn into an increasingly imperfect world. The act of seeking clarification produces its own communication problems, since the communicative resources used that created difficulties in the first place are the ones re-used to resolve them.

Recent research on misunderstandings suggests that mismatched or 'unvoiced agendas' can frequently lead to errors in how patients act on advice and treatment [2,3]. And it is commonplace to assume that medical jargon is the source of much misunderstanding for patients. However, there is

Health Care Errors and Patient Safety. Edited by Brian Hurwitz and Aziz Sheikh.
© 2009 Blackwell Publishing, ISBN: 978-1-4051-4643-2.

much more to misunderstanding than unfamiliar jargon or different agendas, important though these are.

Misunderstandings are on a continuum from complete non-understandings to an illusion of understanding which may be maintained over the whole interaction and only surface and be resolved later or never at all. Some of these implicit misunderstandings are misalignments that stem from different perspectives between doctors and patients and these are often most evident in remote consultations such as telephone medicine [4]. Apart from simple 'slips of the ear', misunderstandings are mutually constructed by all participants in an encounter so cannot be separated off from how people also have to maintain 'conversational involvement' [5]. So misunderstandings are a joint production and are not distinct from how conversation is maintained. A simple but potentially hazardous example is when 'yes' can either mean 'that's correct' or 'I'm listening to you (even if I'm not sure I have understood)'.

While there is a potential for problems of understanding in any consultation, the linguistic and cultural diversity of patient populations in most cities and large towns in much of the western world, the Middle East, Asia, parts of Africa and Latin America creates new challenges for medical encounters. These globalised cities are a mix of long-term residents from traditional sending countries, asylum seekers and refugees and new economic migrants. For example in London, over 300 languages are spoken [6]. The challenges of multilingual health care environments have an impact on policy and practice at many levels. Most responses coalesce around two themes. The first focuses on culturally specific health beliefs and assumes that if doctors know enough about different attitudes and responses to illness experiences [7] then they will be able to act appropriately. The second response is to tackle the 'language barrier' and argue for more interpreters or to assume that there is a reasonable matching of linguistic minority patients and doctors, for example for the South Asian communities in many urban areas of the UK.

There are several problems with these two responses, which stem from the assumption that language and culture are separate and are to be treated separately. The tendency to discuss 'culture' in terms of static, culturally specific health beliefs separate from language is now widely critiqued in both the medical and the sociolinguistic literature [8–10]. Despite some evidence of different health beliefs, research shows that western models of medicine predominate [11]. A more culturally hermeneutic model, in which several meaning systems are seen in play together offers an alternative more in tune with 21st century communities [12]. Illness narratives may combine folk and religious notions, brought along from early socialisation, with popular beliefs and institutional knowledge absorbed from residence in a new country. But even if it was possible to understand these meaning systems in some abstract or general way for every ethno-linguistic group in the patient population, it does not account for the dynamic way in which these systems inter-relate over time or how they are manifested in particular encounters.

Another problem is the way the 'language barrier' is conceived and seen as separate from sociocultural values about the self and power relations. The issue of English language ability has been treated as an either/or matter: you either speak English or you do not [13]. Yet patients who do not speak a local or standard variety of English may be anywhere on a continuum of ability in terms of their accuracy, fluency, structuring of explanations and presentation of symptoms [14,15]. Many minority ethnic patients who were born abroad have learnt and used a variety of English in their country of origin or previous countries of residence. They may be considered expert users of English abroad and assume that there will be no problems of communication in the UK. However, as discussed below, miscommunication can easily occur. 'Expert' is a relative term.

Perhaps because of this continuum of ability, the available literature on language problems is conflicting. Some research is emphatic about the problems [8,16] while other research downplays them [17]. It is assumed that it is easy to decide when a patient needs an interpreter (or not), and the fact that interpreter-mediated consultations can produce their own problems is rarely systematically addressed. In addition, some patients prefer to communicate directly with their doctor [18,19]. A dramatic example of how, even with interpreters, errors can be made is shown in Byrne and Long's classic study [20]. Some way into the consultation, it transpired that the small group of minority ethnic workers were consulting about a patient who was not physically present in the surgery.

Misunderstandings in interaction

Neither the 'health beliefs' nor the 'language barrier' literature deals in detail with the interactional ways in which misunderstandings and the potential for error can arise in a consultation. Detailed discourse analysis puts a microscope on interaction [21] and reveals some of the teeming life within it. Specifically, it illuminates the different levels of misunderstanding that can occur, how these can interact together and how they may be resolved or not.

The rest of this chapter examines how misunderstandings occur when patients and doctors have to manage the consultation in English, wherever they are on the continuum of ability. It is based on a study of general practice in South London [15] in which 232 video recordings were analysed.* The first example (Box 9.1) is typical of patients with enough English to come to the surgery without an interpreter but still with many difficulties in processing apparently straightforward enquiries. Here, a young Portuguese-speaking hotel worker has hurt her leg while at work.

This example illustrates the multicausal nature of misunderstandings. Although the patient's immediate safety and well-being were not at risk, since

*Patients with Limited English and Doctors in General Practice: Educational Issues (2001/3): the PLEDGE project was funded by the Sir Siegmund Warburg Foundation. Two hundred and thirty-two video recordings were made with 19 different doctors in Lambeth, South London.

Box 9.1: Accident at work

1	D	(Turns to patient)
2	P	yes er accident yesterday
3	D	ah what was accident
4	P	yeah no er
5	D	what happened
6	P	accident at hotel
7	D	ah you work in the hotel
8	P	yes
9	D	**what is your job C**
10	P	**erm yesterday at 4 o'clock yeah and alarm alarm the uh the er fire**
11	D	oh
12	P	the doors
13	D	ah
14	P	and er close
15	D	right
16	P	and in there oof
17	D	which er
18	P	in the hotel in the sixth floor
19	D	**right do you work in the hotel**
20	**P**	**today <u>no:</u>**
21	D	yesterday
22	P	yeah
23	**D**	**which hotel**
24	P	er dolphin square dolphin
25	D	dolphin
26	P	square
27	D	oh dolphin square hotel
28	P	yeah
29	D	**so: this happened while you were working while you were working**
30	P	**huh oh today <u>no</u>**
31	D	**no yesterday you were working**
32	P	**erm yeah**
33	D	**what's your job what do you do**
34	P	**erm 9 o'clock**
35	D	**no what <u>is</u> your job what (.) is (.) your job**
36	P	**oh job e::rm**
37	D	cleaner or
38	P	cleaner yeah and er clean the chambermaid
39	D	ah chambermaid
40	P	yeah sorry
41	D	no problem

See Appendix 9.1 for the transcription system used. D: doctor; P: patient.

her physical injury was clear to see, it shows how quickly wrong inferences on both sides can lead to protracted clarification sequences. Lines 9 and 10 and 33–36 show that the processing of an apparently simple question about her job is problematic. Then, at line 19 the doctor seeks to confirm that she is an employee, and a confusion arises over whether this is a habitual action (she works at the hotel) or a completed action (she worked there today) (line 20). Again at lines 29–31 there is a similar misunderstanding over how time is grammaticalised in English, with the doctor trying to establish that the accident (a completed action) happened while she was working (the past continuous verb form). While the patient wants to deal with the 'here and now' of her injury, the doctor's agenda, and so control of topic, concerns the fact that this was an industrial accident and requires bureaucratic procedures. So, the basic processing of words, how time is conceptualised in English and lack of institutional knowledge combine together to produce this misunderstanding.

The example in Box 9.1 shows that misunderstandings and potential errors are joint productions. The patient's limited English and lack of knowledge about institutional procedures combines with the lack of clear signposting from the doctor about his agenda – that he needs details about her employer and her job – and with his failure to realise that time, duration and the habitual nature of activities are concepts subtly encoded in the verb system in English. While the conditions for misunderstandings to arise are produced by patient and doctor, as in this case, for the purposes of analytical clarity, the focus will first be on misunderstandings initially caused by patients and then on those primarily caused by doctors.

Misunderstandings caused by patients

The language ability of patients who do not have English as their expert language is often judged in some undifferentiated way as 'poor' English or a question of accent, but the potential for misunderstanding arises through many different channels of talk. On the one hand there are narrowly linguistic and paralinguistic features and on the other broader aspects of self-presentation and interactional management. But, as indicated above, it is often a cluster of features together that cause problems of understanding. The more linguistic features are, pronunciation and word stress, intonation and speech delivery, and grammar and vocabulary. Misunderstandings with pronunciation are often resolved because the context narrows down interpretive possibilities but often this is not the case. For example, an elderly Arabic speaker when describing nose bleeds talks of /bluk/ and in the context it could be either 'blood' or 'black'.

In the consultation shown in Box 9.2 with an Albanian patient there is confusion between /mit/ and 'meat', /mince/ and 'mice', and /cow/ and 'coal'. She tries to explain to the doctor what she thinks is causing the rash on her neck and arms. Both sides work hard to understand the other but on three

---

Box 9.2: Skin rash

1	P	I think from /mit/ because
2	D	milk
3	P	/mit/
4	D	mit what is mit
5	P	/mit/ ((laughs)) I don't know /mit/ erm
6	D	er
7	P	/mince/ I think
8	D	mice
9	P	yeah
10	D	like rat
11	P	yeah
12	D	you have mice at home
13	P	what do you- /mince/ no but meat you know to eat erm I can't say in English
14	D	can you draw it
15	P	no I don't know how to /write/ this er
16	D	is it a food
17	P	eah food food I think from er from /cow/ you know
18	D	from
19	P	/cow/
20	D	coal?
21	P	no no /cow/
22	D	cow from cow
23	P	yes
24	D	ah beef
25	P	beef yeah
26	D	ah beef ah

---

occasions, the different ways of pronouncing vowels: the short and long 'i' sound (mit/meat), the short 'i' sound and the /ai/ sound (mince/mice) and the different sounds of 'o' as in /au/ and /ou/ (cow/coal) lead to quite a protracted clarificatory sequence. This includes a further misunderstanding at lines 14 and 15 when the doctor tries to repair the confusion by asking the patient to draw what she thinks is the cause of the rash. What is important here is that twice the patient, in order to keep the conversation going, agrees with the doctor's wrong inference (lines 9 and 11). This receipt token ('yes' or 'yeah') as the conversation analysts call it, is particularly frequent when one speaker is struggling to communicate in a second or foreign language. If the doctor had taken these two confirmations at face value, the possible diagnosis and advice to the patient would have been quite different.

Differences in word stress can also cause as many misunderstandings as pronunciation. This is particularly the case in patients' English which is influenced by syllable-timed languages such as French, many West African languages and Caribbean Creoles. This means that each syllable occurs at regular intervals rather than in local or standard English where only each *stressed* syllable occurs at regular intervals. For example, a patient from the Gambia speaks about bathing in <u>Dettol</u>, stressing each syllable equally and the GP does not immediately understand the reference.

With patients who speak fluent English but in a way that is influenced by their expert language and styles of communicating from their early years, the illusion of understanding is more frequent and misunderstandings may not be resolved. Differences in intonation and other features of speech delivery are often the hidden causes of misunderstanding and since they are fleeting signals processed below the level of consciousness, they are hard to identify or take account of.

The tunes, rhythm and stress in speech help to chunk information into units, distinguish what is important, make the contrast between given and new information and to establish speaker perspective. These are all important features of communicative style and differences in style make it difficult to process the other's meaning. One frequent cause of misunderstanding is the difference between the way in which standard/local speakers of English and other speakers of English show emphasis and contrast, to make a point or a correction. In local/standard English this is routinely done through contrastive stress, e.g. 'Did you go this week?' 'No, <u>last</u> week'. In the next example (Box 9.3), there is an ambiguity which is not resolved because the

---

Box 9.3: Dog bite

1	D	what kind of dog was that (.) it was somebody's (.) =dog=
2	P	=yes= somebody's
3	D	it was a stray dog
4	P	no no it was somebody's dog
5	D	right
6	P	yes I:: made an enquiry they said that- **they they told me**
7		**the dog go to the vet regular**
8	D	<u>right</u> okay
9	P	**but that's <u>what</u> they said**
10	D	right (.) <u>right</u> right so did you know the owner or =did=
11	P	=I= know the owner==
12	D	= =oh fair enough (.) so
13	P	**erm:: ((laughs)) (but)**
14	D	did you see any doctor then
15	P	no

patient's use of contrastive stress is different from the doctor's. The patient's English has many characteristics of Nigerian English.

The patient was bitten by a dog when on holiday in Nigeria and the doctor explores the circumstances with a view to deciding whether a rabies immunisation is necessary (lines 1 and 3). Told the dog reportedly sees a vet regularly (lines 6–7), and the patient knows its owner (line 11), the GP appears satisfied the evidence is authoritative – he says 'oh fair enough so' (line 12). He may also interpret the way the patient latches swiftly onto his question about knowing the owner (at line 11, indicated by =) as an indicator of the patient's knowledge about the dog's background, whereas for the patient this may simply be part of his conventional style of communicating. Later in the consultation he suggests to the patient that an immunisation is not indicated. However, during the early stage of history taking shown above, the patient implies that he is not convinced that the dog is free from rabies ('they told me the dog go to the vet regular but that's what they said'; lines 6, 7 and 9). In British English, contrastive stress to convey this suspicion would emphasise the *verbs* 'told' and 'said': 'they told me the dog goes to the vet regular, but that's what they said' (implication: and not what they actually *do*). Instead, the patient's intonation system focuses on the *agent* (the acquaintance, 'they'), and the *content* of the agent's utterance – the 'what'. The patient also hints at his sceptical perspective by using the word 'but' twice and at line 13, by the use of a hesitation marker and laughter. Yet the difference between the participants' intonation systems means the hint is not consolidated categorically and the matter remains unresolved.

Just as in Box 9.1 where the misunderstandings were multicausal, we see here that conveying a clear message also relies on a number of features of speech delivery. Words alone do not convey intention. Where different intonation systems meet, ambiguities may result and, as in this case, the patient's safety might have been at risk. There were many similar examples in the data when patients and doctors tried to sort out what pills patients were currently taking; again, differences in contrastive stress made it difficult to disambiguate the references to the assortment of pills prescribed and (not) taken.

The broader aspects of self-presentation and interactional management are commented on by general practitioners but less to do with their potential for misunderstandings, oversights and possible errors. These features of talk and interaction tend to create more unresolved misunderstandings as patients and GPs talk past each other without quite knowing why. Lengthy explanations and stories by patients may be hard to follow and do not fit with doctors' expectations of how the consultation generally is run. Long linear phases may result where the doctor glazes over and gives minimal responses. Or, conversely, the doctor makes possibly incorrect or inappropriate inferences from little or insufficiently understood patient information and narratives, which may not subsequently be interrogated or refuted by patients.

Styles of self-presentation and interaction are part of the socialisation process that starts at an early age. For example, knowing how much to reveal about yourself, learning how to tailor requests to instructional norms or how and when to take a turn in conversation are all aspects of sociocultural knowledge learnt through 'networks of relations' [22] over time. While there is a long tradition of studying how illness experiences differ cross-culturally, with certain national groups reporting more gastrointestinal symptoms, the French more mood changes and the Filipinos cardiovascular symptoms [7], the London study found that the clearest differences were in communicative styles [23].

These differences in styles were categorised in four ways. The first two concern self-presentation: low self-display and different ways of structuring information. The second two relate to the interaction: topic overload and recycling, and overlapping/interrupting talk.

The different ways in which patients present self and symptoms have consequences for how doctors take a history and make a diagnosis and how potential errors in misdiagnosis can arise. While local speakers of English tend to follow a pattern of symptom description, context and evaluative stance, other patients tend to focus on only one of these three or reveal very little of their symptoms, context or stance [24]. Some patients hand over a letter or empty bottles or give a brief opening statement such as 'I pain here too much' and wait for the doctor to question and infer. Similarly, the structuring of the narrative may be very different with patients providing extensive contextual background when the doctor expects to hear the main reason for the visit at the beginning.

In the example given in Box 9.4, a Bangladeshi patient opens his story by talking about work and his worrying symptoms to set the context for his

---

Box 9.4: Social security 1

1	D	have a seat (2.5) right
2	P	{see} I'm coming ask er – for er I used to work{ing} part-time
3		(0.5)
4	D	yes
5	P	and er at the moment I couldn't work since last week because I feel very <u>weak</u>
6		(. .) and I was loo- er losing <u>blood</u>
7	D	losing blood= =
8	P	= =yeah and er the toilet was {quite a} long time and I going in to hospital for
9		erm (1.0) er fifteen of this month {[this is= ((hands letter to doctor))
10	D	=thank you
11	P	=the letter]} which tells also [doctor M---]
12	D	[why] ah I see so you've been referred to have a test
14	P	and further testing and er it doesn't get any better

request for a letter. When the doctor does not respond after line 3, the patient then gives more context about the reason why he is working part time. Because of the way he structures his self-report, both at utterance level and at the more general level, the doctor and patient rapidly become mired in the background detail of the case. He has some worrying symptoms which, together with his concern about obtaining social security revealed later, produce conditions for anxiety. Neither side can find a way of clarifying the main reason for his visit, since the very language resources they use only serve to create more uncertainty. It is only after 3 minutes into the consultation that the patient mentions social security and it is a further 9 minutes before the doctor signs the form relating to his request. However, after 11 minutes of the consultation have passed the patient is still uncertain about whether he has the right document for social security (Box 9.5).

In lines 1–9, the patient is reiterating what social security want. This seems to be a reprise of the earlier pattern, where he establishes at length the context before getting to the main point. The doctor, however, at line 10 interprets this as an implied criticism and starts a sequence about the adequacy of the form she has signed for him. They appear to reach an agreement at line 16 but the patient is still concerned. He appears to want an individualised letter while the doctor is following institutional procedure. The consultation ends without a satisfactory resolution for the patient.

This style of structuring information so that the context or comment come first and the main topic later is widely used in South and East Asian languages but the GP on viewing the video said that she was quite uncertain as to where the consultation was going. The consultation takes 12 minutes but the patient does not appear to be reassured either about his physical condition or about his financial worries.

Misunderstandings caused by doctors

The extensive communications literature tends to focus on medical jargon as the chief culprit in misunderstandings caused by doctors, with aspects of speech delivery as an also-ran. The London study [15], however, showed that many problems arose in less recognised areas. Again, as with the misunderstandings initially caused by patients, these can be divided into two broad categories: linguistic features related to how, in particular, concepts of time and causality are grammaticalised, and sub-medical, everyday vocabulary and metaphor, on the one hand, and sociocultural assumptions and interactional management, on the other.

As Box 9.1 shows, linguistic difficulties experienced by patients are in part to do with doctors' lack of awareness of what aspects of language are difficult to process. In particular aspects of patient history, duration, precise onset of symptoms and so on are difficult for patients with limited English. For example, the metaphor of space in 'How long have you had … ?' is the most common question about time and can immediately cause problems. Indeed metaphors are

---

Box 9.5: Social security 2

1	P	so what's happened they go (.) I was (.) you know (.) little ? job because
2		of my illness but they want they want to know the proof of the doctor
3	D	the full
4	P	they need you know the proof of the doctor you see the letter from a
5		doctor
6	D	right
7	P	you know job seek allowance people
8	D	right
9	P	you see you know this letter from your doctor that you are sick
10	D	right (.) I thought that that would do
11	P	yes
12	D	will that not do that should be it
13	P	yeah
14	D	that's enough
15	P	that's enough yeah
16	D	yeah yeah that's what we normally do
17	P	that's what I explained to them but they don't believe me you see they say we
18		need a letter from your doctor
19	D	we- well they they can write to me if they want a letter (.) you know
20	P	yeah
21	D	that that should be enough
22	P	yeah
23	D	that- that's a a letter I'll give you (.) here you are
24	P	if you if you give me= =
25	D	= =that's me (gives a card with her name and address on it) um
26	P	if you I can = (show them) you can anything more
27	D	=and you can if there's anything that they want= =
28	P	= =you tell the you write a letter to my doctor
29	D	they can write to me and I will inform them okay (.) but they shouldn't
30		need a private letter as well
31	P	thank you very much
32	D	OK

everywhere [25] and are often not perceived as such since they are so ingrained in our talk, and are how we see the world [26]. Often, when doctors are trying hard to be patient-centred and face-saving, there are 'bursts of metaphor' which either present an increased chance of misunderstanding or, as in the example in Box 9.6, a chance for both patient, who in this case is a local English speaker, and doctor to align to each other's metaphors. The doctor is trying to reassure the patient that going to the counsellor will be helpful and not daunting.

The sociocultural assumption of patient-centredness and shared decision making, paradoxically, can create some of the most profound misunderstandings and ambiguities. This is for several reasons. Firstly, these assumptions are not necessarily shared between doctor and patient and this overarching difference can affect any attempts to involve patients more. Secondly, there are several strategies (often encouraged by communication textbooks [27]) to be more patient-centred by explaining more and talking more about the process of communication.

In the London study [15], one of the clearest patterns occurring between doctors and patients for whom English was not their expert language was patient interruption of a doctor explanation, usually done to present a new topic. This tended to produce a more traditional consultation than an involving, sharing one and meant that many patients left the consultation without the explanations, advice and reassurance that contribute to the safe healing

---

Box 9.6: Depression

1	D	it's not easy because don't forget there's quite a lot of soul baring times and you might be quite difficult but I think you need to go through tha+t stage I I I think gone are the days where you could just
2	P	it's where to start with her now
3	D	doesn't matter doesn't matter don't don't even think about that the the thing about counselling is that it doesn't matter what you do what you say where you start because they will guide you
4	P	right
5	D	so you don't have to plan a speech you know you don't need to say well what do I start the session on
6	P	mm
7	D	just let it go just let it flow
8	P	okay
9	D	so it's not anything you need to premeditate

[phone call]

| 10 | D | don't run out |
| 11 | P | ((laughs)) |

Underlined words in this box are metaphors.

process. Patient-centredness is often modelled by showing doctors talking more about communication. This metacommunication is intended to give space to patients and involve them in the doctor's decision-making process. However, when talk itself is the problem, more talk and the abstract nature of metacommunication, removes the topic from the 'here and now' and adds an additional communicative burden.

A third reason relates to the attempts to be respectful and face-saving to patients as part of the patient-centred model. Doctors seem very aware of the need to save face and be more indirect when dealing with potentially embarrassing and difficult moments. Similarly humour and social chat is quite routinely used to mitigate a mild rebuke or probe for possible problems. This indirectness is conveyed through language features, intonation and interactional markers. The less both sides share a style of communication and underlying sociocultural assumptions about the nature of the consultation, the more likely this indirectness will cause misunderstandings. In the example in Box 9.7, the doctor's attempt to elicit the patient's concerns and expectations lead to an unresolved sequence.

Box 9.7: Baby with diarrhoea

1	D	so how much i- how often is she breast feeding
2	P	little bit= =
3	D	= =little bit (.) right so you're virtually stopped (.) **so what sort of questions have you got in your mind for me today** (.) what do you want me to do (..) =today=
4	P	no: =she say= eh: the lady she say if you want to contacting doctor eh: you want eh: talk him
5	D	yeah= =
6	P	= =I say yes I am happy with e- with you
7	D	right ok
8	P	because definitely when I am coming with you when I go back I
9		will go back happy
10	D	((laughs)) (I) hope so
11	P	because I will look to see you and your doctor k… I like it
12	D	good= =
13	P	= =when when I come in will come in the you know ((tut)) when I go
14		back my home I'm happy
15	D	right
16	P	((laughs))
17	D	**so you want me to (.) check her over**
18	P	yeah =[ ]=
19	D	=I'll examine her= yes

At line 3, the doctor switches from checking how the baby is fed to a patient-centred metacommunicative question: 'So what sort of questions have you got in your mind for me today?' This attempt to elicit the patient's concerns and expectations is difficult on many levels. It assumes that the patient, from Somalia, is familiar and comfortable with strategies for patient-centredness. The talk about talk is also abstract and hard to process. In addition, perhaps because the doctor herself finds these elicitations slightly awkward, the question is expressed as a metaphor (the metaphor of the mind as a container). Eventually, the doctor answers the question herself at line 17 and the moment passes when any other patient worries might be displayed.

These problems caused by doctors do not refer to situations where the doctors themselves may be less linguistically expert than their patients. The data from which these examples are drawn show experienced doctors who, even if they have trained overseas, have practised in the UK over a long period and are comfortable in English. The issue of the communication skills of a minority of overseas doctors has been of concern to the General Medical Council and the National Clinical Assessment Service. And although there was no evidence of talk that was unintelligible or of basic difficulties in understanding the style of local British patients, there was evidence of interactional differences, misunderstandings and unresolved agendas. Some overseas-trained GPs seemed relatively uncomfortable with using talk as a patient-centred eliciting and therapeutic tool. Patients' topics were often closed down early so that the doctor's agenda could be pursued and there was less mutuality and mitigation when diagnosing, explaining and deciding on an action plan.

In the consultation from which the following example is taken, there were unresolved agendas that related to the patient's concerns: she was worried about her heart and the doctor only discussed her breathing; she was concerned about the amount of fluid that had to be drained off around her wound and received no explicit response; she sought reassurance about how she could self-help after her operation and he failed to acknowledge the patient's 'moral self'; and rather than discussing her antibiotic use, he ignored her remarks and used the computer record to check her prescription. Finally, he failed to align to her jokey, self-deprecating tone and the rather strained social relations throughout which may account for many of the ambiguities that remain. This misalignment is illustrated an extract from the case (Box 9.8). The patient's remark 'God looks after me' is presented as a 'throw away' remark in a low falling tone, closing off that phase of the consultation with a light evaluative comment. But the doctor does not 'read' the intonational cue and interprets it as a significant statement about religious beliefs. Her response to his question is accompanied by a laugh and a rather strangely worded claim 'I like me church' which seems to indicate embarrassment. There are several such uncomfortable moments which may serve to create conditions that inhibit open communication and negotiation.

Box 9.8: Check-up after an operation

1	P	was lucky (.) God looks after me a lot (lo) (1.5)
2	D	do you go the church
3	P	oh yes I like (me church) ((laughing))

Conclusion

Although misunderstandings and the problem of unvoiced agendas can occur in any consultation, our London based research study found that they occur much more frequently and are more protracted when doctor and patient do not share the same language background. The very means of attempting to solve miscommunication, the different linguistic/cultural resources each side uses, may have caused it in the first place. GPs and patients find themselves in a 'looking glass world' in which questions and their responses seem bizarre to the one on the other side of the desk. In contexts where mutual understanding is a struggle and both sides may leave the consultation asking themselves 'what happened there?', the potential for missed opportunities in diagnosing, treatment and shared agreement on action is always present.

Missed opportunities and wrong inferences can result from apparently small and fleeting features of language difference. Yet many of such differences can have large interactional consequences in terms of the quality of the consultation and, as the examples illustrate, potential consequences for patient's well being and safety. General exhortations to listen and respect patients do not grapple with the detailed ways in which both sides have to negotiate meaning together. A more informed understanding of how differences feed into the interpretive processes on each side is a starting point. Together with this awareness raising, is the need for a more expert approach to 'talk' and how problems of talk can be prevented, managed and repaired when doctor and patient do not share a common first language.† In an increasingly globalised world, multilingual encounters will entail more focus on the language and communicative style of patients and doctors if the uncertainties, ambiguities and potential errors in consultations are not to increase.

Appendix 9.1: Transcription conventions

=word=	overlapping talk
word= =	latching (one speaker following another with no pause)
(.)	micro-pause, less than 1 second
(2.0)	estimated length of pause of 1 second or more, to nearest 0.5 of a second

---

† A DVD *Doing the Lambeth Talk* based on the PLEDGE research and produced by King's College London is an example of an awareness raising intervention.

wor:d	segmental lengthening
wor-	truncation
[ ]	inaudible speech
[word]	unclear speech
((laughs))	non-lexical occurrence
{[word]}	talk overlayed by non-lexical occurrence
word	stressed syllable
/wod/	indicates non standard pronunciation
(lo)	falling tone

References

1 Taylor T. *Mutual Misunderstanding: Scepticism and the Theorizing of Language and Interpretation*. Routledge, London, 1992.

2 Britten N, Stevenson F, Barry C, Barber N, Bradley C. Misunderstandings in prescribing decisions in general practice: qualitative study. *British Medical Journal* 2000; **320**: 484–8.

3 Barry C, Bradley C, Britten N, Stevenson F, Barber N. Patients' unvoiced agendas in general practice consultations: qualitative study. *British Medical Journal* 2001; **321**: 1246–50.

4 Drew P. Misalignments in 'after-hours' calls to a British GP's practice: a study in telephone medicine. In: Heritage J, Maynard D, eds. *Communication in Medical Care: Interaction between Primary Care Physicians and Patients*. Cambridge University Press, Cambridge, 2006: 416–44.

5 Gumperz J. *Discourse Strategies*. Cambridge University Press, Cambridge, 1982.

6 Baker P, Eversley J, eds. *Multilingual Capital: The Languages of London's School Children and the Relevance to Economic, Social and Educational Policies*. Corporation of London, London, 2000.

7 Helman C. *Culture, Health and Illness*. Sage, London, 1985.

8 Ahmad W. Making black people sick; 'race' ideology and health research. In: Ahmad W, ed. *'Race' and Health in Contemporary Britain*. Open University Press, Buckingham, 1993: 11–33.

9 Stubbs P. 'Ethnically sensitive' or anti-racist? Models for health research and delivery. In: Ahmad W, ed. *'Race' and Health in Contemporary Britain*. Open University Press, Buckingham, 1993: 34–47.

10 Gumperz J. On interactional sociolinguistic method. In: Sarangi S, Roberts C, eds. *Talk, Work and Institutional Order*. Mouton de Gruyter, Berlin, 1999: 452–71.

11 Bhopal R. Asians' knowledge and behaviour on preventative health issues: smoking, alcohol, heart disease, pregnancy, rickets, malaria prophylaxis and surma. *Community Medicine* 1986; **8**: 315–21.

12 Good BJ, Good MD. The meaning of symptoms: a cultural hermeneutic model for clinical practice. In: Eisenberg L, Kleinman A, eds. *The Relevance of Social Science for Medicine*. Reidel, Dordrecht, 1981: 165–96.

13 Health Education Authority. *Social Focus on Ethnic Minorities*. Health Education Authority, London, 1992.

14 Ali N. Fluency in the consulting room. *British Journal of General Practice* 2003; **53**, 514–15.

15 Roberts C, Moss B, Wass V, Sarangi S, Jones R. *Patients with Limited English and Doctors in General Practice: Education Issues. Final Report Submitted to the Sir Siegmund Warburg Voluntary Settlement*. King's College London, London, 2003.

16 Donaldson L. Health and social status of elderly Asians: a community survey. *British Medical Journal* 1986; **293**: 1079–82.

17 Rashid A, Jagger C. Attitudes to and perceived use of health care services among Asian and non-Asian patients in Leicester. *British Journal of General Practice* 1992; **42**: 197–201.

18 Green G, Lee M, Eldridge K, Bradby H. *Mental Health of Chinese Women in Britain*. Final report to the ESRC, No. R0002223822. 2002.

19 Smaje C. *Health, 'Race' and Ethnicity: Making Sense of the Evidence*. Kings Fund Institute, London, 1995.

20 Byrne PS, Long BEL. *Doctors Talking to Patients*. Royal College of General Practioners, Exeter, 1976.

21 Roberts C, Sarangi S. Theme-oriented discourse analysis of medical encounters. *Medical Education* 2005; **39**: 632–40.

22 Gumperz JJ. The linguistic and cultural relativity of inference. *In*: Gumperz J, Levinson S, eds. *Rethinking Lingusitic Relativity*. Cambridge University Press, Cambridge, 1996: 374–406.

23 Roberts C, Moss B, Wass V, Sarangi S, Jones R. Misunderstandings: a qualitative study of primary care consultations in multilingual settings, and educational implications. *Medical Education* 2005; **39**: 465–75.

24 Roberts C, Sarangi S, Moss B. Presentation of self and symptom in primary care consultations involving patients from non-English speaking backgrounds. *Communication and Medicine* 2004; **1** (2): 159–69.

25 Skelton JR, Wearn AM, Hobbs FDR. A concordance-based study of metaphoric expressions used by GPs and patients in consultation. *British Journal of General Practice* 2002; **52**: 114–18.

26 Lakoff G, Johnson M. *Metaphors We Live By*. University of Chicago Press, Chicago, 1980.

27 Silverman J, Kurtz S, Draper J. *Skills for Communicating with Patients*. Radcliffe Medical Press, Oxford, 1999.

CHAPTER 10

Clinical transitions: implications for patient safety

Alan Forster

This chapter examines the safety of 'health care transitions'. During their treatments, patients often undergo changes in their physical location (such as when they get discharged from hospital) or in their providers (e.g. hospital-ised patients experience a change of staff nightly, when an on-call physician, who is not their regular doctor, becomes responsible for their care). These changes or transitions are required to ensure that most appropriate care is available in the most appropriate setting 24 hours a day. Whilst necessary, health care transitions can pose considerable risks to patient safety if they are not performed properly. In particular, risk of harm is heightened during tran-sitions due to ineffective transmission of information.

There are several types of transitions in health care (Box 10.1). They occur when patients are admitted to, or discharged from, a health care facility; when patients are transferred between services within a facility; or when responsibility for patient care is 'signed over' between health care providers. There are obvious differences between the different types of transitions – such as the type of transport that occurs. There are also several similarities – such as the need to ensure adequate information sharing. The specific processes of care that are generic to all transitions are termed 'transitional care', and have been defined formally as the *set of actions* designed to ensure *coordination and continuity of health care* as patients transfer between different locations or dif-ferent levels of care in the same location [1].

Box 10.1: Types of transitions in health care

- Admission to hospital
- Transfer between services within a health care facility
- 'Sign over', when on-call physicians take responsibility or nursing shift changes
- Transfer between facilities
- Discharge home from hospital

Health Care Errors and Patient Safety. Edited by Brian Hurwitz and Aziz Sheikh.
© 2009 Blackwell Publishing, ISBN: 978-1-4051-4643-2.

There is a need for health care providers to better appreciate the impact of transitional care on health care outcomes. Increasing specialisation of health services coupled with limited health care resources has led to more transitions during the provision of care. For example, a single patient with a single problem such as breast cancer may see three different health care teams for treatment: surgical, radiotherapeutic and oncological. Further, as co-morbidity is increasingly the norm in ageing inpatient populations there may be several other distinct teams involved in the care of a woman with breast cancer. For example, in a recent cohort study of breast cancer patients, almost half had at least one co-morbidity predictive of an increased likelihood of dying, with 9% suffering from ischaemic heart disease and 12% having diabetes mellitus [2]. Thus, breast cancer patients may undergo many transitions between different specialists responsible for different aspects of their care and between different locations including inpatient and outpatient settings. Box 10.2 outlines some of the transitions possible for a hypothetical breast cancer patient admitted to hospital for an acute myocardial infarction.

There are concerns that increasing specialisation has lead to fragmentation of care, which in turn has lead to suboptimal patient outcomes [3]. Many processes of care must be coordinated when a transition occurs. If there is inadequate treatment planning by the transferring health care providers, insufficient capacity to provide care by the receiving providers, or poor communication between both sets of providers, then in many instances health services may need to be replicated and patient well-being may suffer.

This chapter will discuss the following types of transitions: admission to hospital, transfer between two inpatient services, discharge from hospital, and sign out of patient responsibility between providers. I will start each section with a clinical example. Then, I will describe evidence suggesting that each transition type poses a risk to patient safety. I will then highlight any interventions that have been shown to reduce risks related to the transitions, and will conclude each subsection with a prediction regarding how this transition could be improved in the future.

Box 10.2: Examples of transitions for a hypothetical woman with breast cancer and coronary artery disease admitted following a myocardial infarction

• *Admission to hospital*: admission to hospital after experiencing a myocardial infarction
• *Transfer between services within a health care facility*: step down from the coronary care unit to the regular ward
• *Transfer between facilities*: transfer from the regional cardiac center to the local community hospital
• *Discharge home from hospital*: discharge home directly from the hospital

Adverse events due to transition to hospital

Clinical example

A 62-year-old woman with a history of congestive heart failure and multiple previous hospitalisations for pulmonary oedema is admitted to hospital for a bowel resection. Prior to admission, she was taking furosemide 80 mg twice per day in order to maintain an appropriate fluid balance. At admission to hospital, the treating physician inadvertently omitted her diuretic. On post-operative day 6 (after her intravenous (IV) fluids were discontinued and she had resumed a diet), the patient developed severe dyspnoea associated with an arterial oxygen saturation of 85%. This was subsequently diagnosed as acute pulmonary oedema which responded promptly to diuresis medication.

Extent of the problem and its cause

The clinical example describes a woman for whom there was an inadvertent discrepancy in her pre-hospital medications and her intra-hospital medications. Given her high dose of furosemide and previous admissions for pulmonary oedema, it was likely that she would be particularly sensitive to perturbations in volume status. It is likely that omission of her furosemide was a contributing factor in the development of the pulmonary oedema. Other competing explanations, such as an excessive IV rate and postoperative fluid mobilisation are less likely to be the cause at this late stage after the operation.

Less is known about adverse events occurring as a result of the transition to hospital than is known about adverse events following other transitions, such as those occurring post-discharge. It is likely that adverse events at this time are less common given that at admission there is an increase in monitoring, as opposed to the decrease that occurs when patients leave hospital. While the monitoring aspect seems less important at hospital admission, there are data suggesting that prescribing errors frequently occur when patients enter hospitals. In certain circumstances, these errors can lead to harm, as they did in the clinical example.

A recently published systematic review identified that medication errors were exceedingly common at hospital admission [4]. The 22 studies included in the review had a number of different methodologies, which limited the ability to perform a formal meta-analysis. However, using the most conservative definition of error in the review (in which errors due to discrepancies in non-prescription drugs were excluded), there is likely to be at least one error in medication during the hospital admission process in 10% to 65% of cases. This range jumps to between 34% and 95% if one also considers a history of past medication allergies or adverse drug reactions as contraindications to ordering medications upon admission. The error estimates varied significantly in this review due to methodological differences in the included studies (some studies included only errors of omission while others also included errors of commission, and errors in dosing and frequency).

Although this range of medication errors is distressingly high, it is important to note that many errors have no potential to cause patient harm. Cornish et al. rated such errors in terms of their potential to cause serious harm and found that, fortunately, only 6% of errors were judged to carry such risk [5] (Table 10.1). Comparing the different types of errors, errors of commission were most commonly associated with the potential to cause harm. Fortunately, these error types were the least frequent. Overall, the types of errors occurring at admission include: errors of omission (46%), discrepancies in dose (25%), discrepant frequencies in medication taking (17%) and errors of commission (11%). Another study of patients transferred from nursing homes to hospital has found similar results [6].

There are few data to suggest other types of errors or adverse events experienced by patients at their admission to hospital. Another type of error

Table 10.1 Types of unintended medication order discrepancies (from Tam et al. [4], by permission of the publisher. © 2005 Canadian Medical Association).

Type of error	Example	Relative frequency	Proportion of errors having the potential to cause serious harm
Omission	A patient admitted because of recurrent presyncope was taking digoxin 0.125 mg daily before admission to hospital. The digoxin therapy was not recorded in the medication history	46%	5%
Comission	A stroke patient with aphasia was admitted to hospital. The family provided the medication vials from home, and these medications were ordered, including propafenone. After recovering from his aphasia, the patient stated that his cardiologist had advised him to stop the propafenone therapy several months ago	11%	25%
Incorrect frequency	A patient admitted for diabetes management was taking amlodipine 5 mg twice daily. The treating physician ordered amlodipine 5 mg daily	17%	4%
Incorrect dose	A patient admitted because of a gastrointestinal bleed was taking metoprolol 12.5 mg twice daily before admission to hospital, but the medication history and medication orders indicated metoprolol 50 mg twice daily	25%	0%

could relate to the inability of hospital-based physicians to access information describing community-based care. In one series of 1002 emergency department visits, physicians did not have access to necessary and existing information in 32% of cases [7]. While this proportion is extremely high, it is unknown how often this lack of information leads to harm.

In conclusion, when patients enter hospital it is likely that their admitting physician will make an error when ordering their home medications. Many of these errors will not cause harm but a small fraction of them could. While this latter point is reassuring, it is not entirely comforting as the high error rate appears to point to carelessness on the part of the admitting physicians. While this might be true, there are other potential explanations. Patients come into hospitals with complex problems that are often in a state of flux. In addition, patients are often on a large number of medications for the management of chronic health problems. In fact, many of these medications may be for prevention of potential health problems as opposed to management of symptoms, for example lipid-lowering agents. Thus, the high error rate may in part reflect the physician's prioritisation of the new acute problem over the management of chronic health problems.

Interventions

Based on our knowledge of the types of problems at admission, the most obvious solutions are based on preventing medication errors. With respect to medication errors, the process of 'medication reconciliation' is promoted as a method for doing so [8,9]. This involves a careful review of the patient's pre-hospital medication history, as well as the indications for those treatments. It then ensures that any hospital orders *reflect* these past treatments as well as the current problem. The medication orders do not necessarily need to be exactly the same as those taken prior to admission given that the new condition may result in a change. However, medication reconciliation is supposed to avoid any inadvertent medication errors. While this process seems to be a component of the standard process physicians perform taking a history from the patient, it differs in its use of an explicit process usually by someone other than the treating physician. While there are, as yet, no trials demonstrating the effectiveness of this approach on reducing in-hospital adverse events, a number of organisations (such as the influential Institute for Healthcare Improvement (see www.ihi.org/ihi) and the World Health Organization Collaborating Center on Patient Safety Solutions (see http://www.who.int/patientsafety/en/) and accrediting bodies now mandate that medication reconciliation is performed. The costs and logistics of implementing this intervention are not trivial (which makes its undemonstrated status in evidence terms all the more important), as it can take 20–30 minutes to complete medication reconciliation for a single patient at admission. Thus, hospitals are likely to have to dedicate significant resources to this task if they hope to achieve it.

The future

Health systems urgently need electronic health records spanning the entire continuum of care. The physician in hospital needs the most up-to-date outpatient prescription information at the time of admission. Perhaps more importantly, the physician needs access to the community provider's notes and treatment plans, and the results of any tests. It will be almost impossible to reduce error rates at a reasonable cost without access to such information.

Adverse events due to transitions between hospital services

Clinical example

A 60-year-old man is admitted to the intensive care unit (ICU) with sepsis secondary to a urinary tract infection. In the ICU, the patient receives a chest X-ray to assess central venous line placement. The ICU physician reviews the X-ray immediately and determines the line placement does not require adjustment. A week later, the ICU clerical staff receives the final radiology report for the X-ray indicating a 1 cm solitary pulmonary nodule with recommendations for a computed tomography (CT) scan of the chest. The patient had already been discharged home, his condition having improved rapidly. The ICU had filed the report and did not notify the physicians who took over his care on the medical ward or the patient's family doctor that an important X-ray report was pending. The patient returned to the same hospital 14 months later with an inoperable non-small cell lung cancer.

Extent of the problem and its cause

In the above case, a cancer that was likely curable by pneumonectomy transformed into a fatal disease due to an error. The ICU physician cared most about the immediate reason for performing the X-ray, that is, whether a central venous catheter was adequately placed for inotrope administration. This physician failed to take note of the solitary pulmonary nodule, probably because he was so focused on the line placement. No physician saw the final report of the X-ray, which recommended a CT scan, as there was no formal protocol to sign off such reports. All the physicians were unaware of the abnormality and incorrectly assumed that other physicians received the final report.

There are few data describing the prevalence of adverse events experienced by patients when they undergo a transfer between services. The example highlights one potential error that can occur – the failure to follow up test results that return after patient transfer. Other problems can include inappropriate transfers and medication errors. Finally, mishaps such as equipment problems can occur during the transfer of a potentially unstable patient.

A failure to communicate anticipated results by the transferring physician has the potential to lead to serious problems. Roy and colleagues provide the most comprehensive study on the issue of pending test results following a transition [10]. His group evaluated a cohort of 2644 medical patients in a Boston teaching hospital at the time they were discharged from hospital.

Forty-one per cent of patients had test results pending at the time of transfer. Of these tests, 9.4% were deemed to be potentially actionable – a test result was 'actionable' if it could have changed the management of the patient by requiring a new treatment or diagnostic test (or repeated testing), modification or discontinuation of a treatment or diagnostic testing, scheduling of an earlier follow-up appointment, or referral of the patient to another physician or specialist. For patients with such tests, the investigators then informed their physician of the test results. These physicians reported that for a third of the tests they did not even know a test had been performed. Inpatient physicians were more likely to be aware of test performance than the patient's primary care physician (75% of inpatient physicians were aware vs 54% of primary care physicians; $P=0.02$). In addition, only 62% of physicians had the results, even though the test had been completed. Again, inpatient physicians were more likely to have the result than those in primary care (70% vs 46%). The new information reported to the physicians by the investigators prompted urgent changes in treatment plans for 13% of patients with actionable lab results.

Another potential cause of adverse events following the transition of a patient between services within an institution is inappropriate transfers. Usually such transfers occur because the transferring service is no longer required, as when care intensity is stepped down and patients are transferred from the ICU to the regular ward. Alternatively they can occur when the receiving service has a specialised role within the institution, for example when a stroke patient is transferred to a rehabilitation service in anticipation of discharge. These transitions can be inappropriate if patients are not clinically stable at the time of discharge or if the receiving service has inadequate capacity to care for the patient.

Several investigators have demonstrated an association between night-time transfers out of the ICU and increased mortality. Research conducted in Australia, Canada and the UK has shown that the risk of in-hospital death increases by 33–70% for night-time versus daytime ICU transfers, after adjusting for factors also associated with death [11–16]. The hypothesis posed by these investigators is that patients discharged from the ICU at night are transferred prematurely as a result of a need to admit another critically ill patient. Supporting the argument that overnight bed pressures are causing this problem is a perception that 43% of night-time discharges were considered premature versus 5% of daytime discharges [15].

In-hospital transfers can also be inappropriate if the receiving service does not have the capacity to care for a patient. For example, when patients are in the ICU the usual nurse to patient ratio is typically 1:1 or at most 1:2. When patients are transferred to the hospital ward this ratio increases to between 1:4 and 1:10. If a patient requires more intensive monitoring than can be provided by a nurse who is simultaneously caring for 3–9 other patients then the patient may suffer as a result. This problem occurs because patients' need for intensity of monitoring and staff input often changes gradually but transitions usually involve quantum steps in the intensities with which these inputs can be provided. A similar issue arises when a patient requires special equipment or skills that are not standard on the receiving ward. For example, if continuous cardiac monitoring is required and the ward does not have telemetry beds then, unknown to ward staff, the patient could experience arrhythmias. Similarly, if the patient needs tracheostomy care but the nurses on the ward are unfamiliar with such devices, then life-threatening airway problems may ensue.

A third area of concern related to intra-hospital transitions are medication errors. Pronovost and colleagues demonstrated that for patients transferred from the ICU significant proportions of patients experience such a problem [17]. Similar to the situation at admission, despite the large numbers of errors occurring, resultant actual harm was unfortunately not measured.

A fourth problem related to intra-hospital transitions is mishap due to equipment problems during transfer into and out of ICUs. Several studies demonstrate that equipment failures occur during 33–45% of transfers undertaken [18–22]. Examples of these equipment failures include: the loss of battery power for such devices as cardiac monitors, IV pumps and portable ventilators; disconnection of central lines, arterial lines or ventilator tubing during transfers; inadvertent patient extubation; tanks containing supplemental oxygen running empty; hypothermia due to ambient air exposure; and, prolonged delays for various reasons.

Interventions

There are few proven interventions to reduce adverse events during the transition between hospital services. Medication reconciliation methods as described by Pronovost et al. [17] hold some promise, although feasibility issues will be challenging – as it is for medication reconciliation at hospital admission. However, as there are no randomised trials of this intervention, its effectiveness in terms of reducing errors is unknown. Therefore, the degree of effort made to reduce these mistakes needs to be balanced carefully with other initiatives.

Problems such as night-time ICU discharges and failure to communicate pending test information appear to have an impact on patient mortality. Therefore, if one were setting priorities for interventions, then it might be more appropriate to tackle the issue of premature discharges in some way. At the same time, the causes of these other problems may be more difficult to solve given existing resources in most health systems.

The future

To improve intra-hospital transitions, better communication methods are needed. Transferring physicians need to communicate specific issues known to be the cause of errors at the time of transfer. These include: the medication regimen, pending test results and the clinical stability of the patient at the time of discharge. It is likely that electronic health records can facilitate this communication. However, improved communication can occur in the absence of such a technology, as long as specific issues are dealt with in verbal or written forms. Conversely, the availability of electronic health records does not ensure that such communication will take place. Gandhi outlines a framework for this in communicating pending test results [23] (Figure 10.1). Other authors have recommended the use of standard communication methods to be used during transitions. For example, the Institute for Healthcare Improvement advocates a shared mental model in communication during transfers known as 'situation background assessment and recommendation' (SBAR) [24]. This standard communication technique is designed to ensure that recommendations on important issues are acknowledged by both parties involved in the transition. Regardless of whether an explicit communication method is used, the transferring and receiving teams must take note of important issues explicitly.

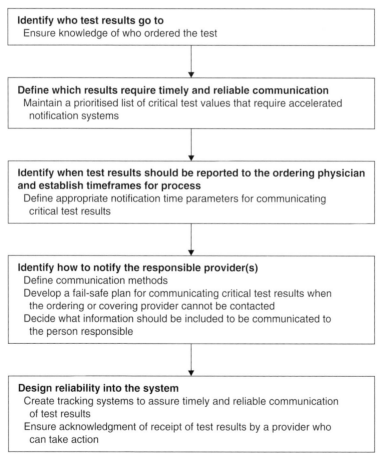

Figure 10.1 A framework for communicating critical test results (from Ghandi [23], reprinted with permission).

Finally, during intra-hospital transitions physicians must also be certain that the receiving service has the technical capacity and human resources required to provide adequate care. As staffing levels may vary during the course of a day or week, it may be necessary to prohibit transfers at certain periods. If such transfers are repeatedly necessary due to bed pressures, then hospitals need to enhance capacity in the ICU or in the step-down service.

Adverse events due to transition from hospital

Clinical example

A 75-year-old man with chronic atrial fibrillation on warfarin prophylaxis is admitted to hospital with pneumonia. The patient had been taking 1 mg of warfarin for many years with a relatively stable international normalised ratio (INR) and no prior episodes of bleeding or embolic phenomenon. At admission his INR was 2.5. After a 3-day hospitalisation, the patient was discharged home on oral antibiotics. During his hospital stay, his physicians did not adjust his warfarin dose and did not reassess his INR. Following discharge, the patient was to remain on his antibiotics for another 11 days. There were no instructions to have his INR tested. He returned to the emergency department 6 days after discharge with a painful knee subsequently identified as a haemarthrosis due to an INR of 6.2.

Extent of the problem and its cause

Adverse events occurring in the immediate post-hospitalisation period, like the one illustrated in the case, are common and clinically important. This patient was on a low dose of warfarin suggesting that he is sensitive to its effects and that he could have a relatively narrow tolerance to dosing modifications. He is discharged home on a class of medications well known to potentiate the effect of warfarin [25]. INR perturbation in patients recently hospitalised with medical illness is well established [26–28].

In several respects, the case highlights a typical post-discharge adverse event: the patient is elderly and has complex health issues that require multiple medications, some of which are inherently risky and need to be monitored closely. There are multiple providers (one in the hospital and one in the community) looking after the patient, with uncertain delineation of responsibilities. Specifically, who was responsible for ensuring the patient's INR was followed in the days immediately following discharge?

Two studies of hospitalised medical patients have found that one in five patients experience an adverse event during the first month after discharge [29,30]. A third of post-discharge adverse events lead to an emergency department visit, a readmission to hospital or a death (Figure 10.2). Post-discharge adverse events are most commonly adverse drug events but include also nosocomial infections, diagnostic errors, procedural complications and management errors (Figure 10.3). Although some of these problems develop after discharge, many may first have developed in hospital, becoming manifest

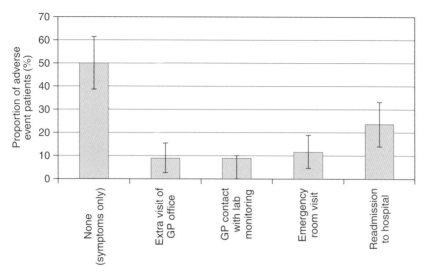

Figure 10.2 The association of different health services with adverse events (from Forster et al. [29], reprinted with permission).

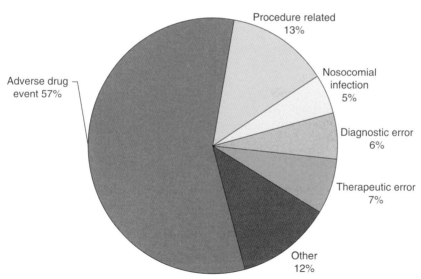

Figure 10.3 Types of adverse events affecting medical patients following hospital discharge; 78 adverse events were classified according to their type [29].

only after discharge [29,30]. Although this research focused specifically on medical patients, the same types of problems are similarly prevalent in surgical patients in whom postoperative wound infections are more important, affecting up to 10% of patients [31].

Adverse drug events account for almost three-quarters of post-discharge adverse events [27]. Given that medication use is ubiquitous it is important to identify factors associated with adverse drug events. For example, specific drugs increase the risk of adverse drug events, including the use of anticoagulants, antibiotics, analgesic agents (including narcotics), corticosteroids and hypoglycaemic agents. Furthermore, the more medications prescribed at discharge the higher the risk of post-discharge adverse drug event. Also, post-discharge adverse events are caused almost exclusively by medications that are newly prescribed at the time of discharge or by those in which dosage has been changed. Finally, patients who remember being taught about the side effects of their medications are almost half as likely to experience an adverse event [27]. Therefore, interventions to improve medication safety should involve education, targeting high-risk medications that are recently changed or started.

A large proportion of post-discharge adverse events are preventable or ameliorable. In the aforementioned studies almost two-thirds could have been avoided or their severity significantly reduced if simple measures had been implemented. These measures can be categorised as follows: interventions to improve patient education about the treatment plan, including medication side effects; interventions to improve the communication with primary care providers; and interventions to improve the monitoring of patients following hospitalisation. All of the preventable or ameliorable adverse events could have been influenced if one or more of these intervention types were implemented [29,30].

Other research suggests that poor inter-physician communication is related to poor patient outcomes following hospital discharge. In a prospective cohort study, van Walraven and colleagues showed that discharge summaries describing the hospital care are often not available to physicians at the time they see patients following hospital discharge [32]. While physicians generated a discharge summary for over three-quarters of the patients, the document was only available for 15% of the post-discharge visits. The discrepancy in these two frequencies is due to delay in receiving the document arising from the hospital transcription service and regular postal service, as well as the fact that patients see many physicians post discharge while the discharge summary is typically sent only to the primary care doctor. Although a copy resides within the hospital record, other treating physicians may have trouble accessing the document. The study showed that the availability of the discharge document at the time of the doctor visit was shown to have a clinically important effect in reducing post-discharge emergency department visits and hospital readmissions.

The same research group also showed that poor continuity of care is related to poor outcomes post discharge. They used administrative data and a retrospective cohort design to study all patients hospitalised in the province of Ontario, Canada. After adjusting for important co-variates, patients who were seen in the post-discharge period by their hospital physician were significantly less likely to experience urgent readmission or to die [33].

In summary, post-discharge adverse events are common. The majority are preventable or ameliorable. Analyses of preventable and ameliorable adverse events, as well as epidemiological studies of particular risk factors, show that communication and continuity of care are important predictors with respect to poor post-hospital outcomes. In addition, prevention of complications related to drug therapies should be targeted as a majority of post-discharge adverse events are related to their use.

Interventions

There are several promising interventions that have been shown to reduce the risk of poor patient outcomes following hospital discharge. These interventions are generally multifaceted and include the use of specially trained personnel performing novel tasks specifically designed to improve post-discharge care.

Coleman et al. has had considerable success with the use of an advanced practice nurse who functions as a so-called 'transition coach' [1,34]. Table 10.2 describes the interventions performed by the transition coach. This individual works with the patient before they are discharged to help improve understanding of their underlying health condition and treatments. In addition, the transition coach helps to prepare a health care diary or 'patient health record', which outlines the patient's health problems, the medications prescribed, follow-up plans and emergency contact numbers. The patient takes this diary with him or her to any post-discharge visit. Following discharge, the transition coach telephones the patient several times to determine whether there are any medication-related questions or new health problems and the coach even performs a home visit to continue teaching and performing assessments of the patient's condition and medication use.

In a large integrated delivery system in Colorado, Coleman's group demonstrated that this intervention significantly reduced readmission rates and hospital costs for complex internal medicine patients. They randomised over 700 medical patients to receive the transition coach intervention versus standard care, and found over 30% relative reductions in readmission rates at 30, 90 and 180 days following hospital discharge and a 20% reduction in hospital costs [34].

A similar, but somewhat less intensive, intervention is a pharmacist-based intervention described by Schnipper et al. [35]. In this study, a hospital-based pharmacist performs medication reconciliation for internal medicine patients at the beginning of a patient's hospital encounter. Medication reconciliation is a process of ensuring that there are no unintended order discrepancies between the medication regimens in two different locations. The pharmacist then provides specific teaching about medications and medication use in preparation for discharge from hospital. Following discharge, the pharmacist telephones the patient to review medication-related questions and problems.

In a randomised, controlled trial design Schnipper's group demonstrated that there was an improvement in patient outcomes associated with this

Table 10.2 Transition coach tasks as designed by Coleman et al. [34], with permission. ©2006 American Medical Association.

| Stage of intervention | Four pillars | | | |
	Medication self-management	patient-centred record	Follow up	Red flags
Goal	Patient is knowledgeable about medication and has medication management system	Patient understands and uses PHR to facilitate communication and to ensure continuity of care plan across providers and settings; patient manages PHR	Patient schedules and completes follow-up visit with primary care provider or specialist and is prepared to be an active participant in interactions	Patient is knowledgeable about indications that condition is worsening and how to respond
Hospital visit	Discuss importance of knowing medications and having a system in place to ensure adherence to regimen	Explain PHR	Recommend primary care provider follow-up visit	Discuss symptoms and drug reactions
Home visit	Reconcile pre-hospitalisation and post-hospitalisation medication lists	Review and update PHR	Emphasise importance of follow-up visit and need to provide primary care provider with recent hospitalisation information	Assess condition
	Identify and correct discrepancies	Review discharge summary	Practice and role-play questions for primary care provider	Discuss symptoms and adverse effects of medications
		Encourage patient to update and share PHR with primary care provider or specialist at follow-up visits		
Follow-up telephone calls	Answer remaining medication questions	Remind patient to share PHR with primary care provider or specialist	Provide advocacy in getting appointment, if necessary	Reinforce when primary care provider should be telephoned
		Discuss outcome of visit with primary care provider or specialist		

PHR, personal health record.

intervention [35]. Preventable adverse events occurred in 1% of patients randomised to the intervention versus 11% in the control group ($P < 0.01$). Unfortunately, there was no effect of the intervention on return visits to the emergency department or hospital. The small number of serious adverse events which prompted an emergency department visit probably explains the discrepant results.

Dudas et al. [36] also used components of the pharmacist intervention described above. His group simply had a pharmacist contact internal medicine patients by telephone several days following their discharge to ask them a few simple questions regarding their medications and condition. In a randomised trial at an American university hospital, this group showed that return visits to the emergency department occurred significantly less often in patients receiving the intervention versus those receiving standard care (10% vs 24%; $P < 0.05$) [36].

While the preceding interventions have demonstrated a beneficial effect, not all studies of similar interventions concur. A Cochrane review of a 'discharge planning' intervention did not demonstrate a beneficial effect on some health care outcomes [37]. It is important to note that this study did not evaluate patient safety outcomes. In addition, the interventions were very different as they did not focus on medication safety per se, but rather focused on the social aspects of the patient's health. A more recent randomised trial evaluating the impact of an advanced practice nurse intervention, which was similar to but not as intensive as Coleman's intervention, on patient safety outcomes did not show any benefit [38]. An important difference between these studies and the successful interventions described above was the intensity of the post-discharge monitoring and follow up. This suggests that the hospital service discharging a patient must take some responsibility for ensuring monitoring for a period after the patient returns home.

The future

Improving post-discharge safety requires efforts to improve patient self-efficacy, interprovider communication and patient monitoring. The promising findings described above addressed these issues to a greater or lesser degree. Before recommendations for widespread implementation can be made, the promising results found in these studies need to be confirmed by studies performed in other health systems, in multiple hospitals and other patient populations. In addition, the interventions described above are quite labour intensive. They need to be made as efficient as possible if there is any hope of performing them consistently for all patients, given the limited resources available to most health systems.

Automating some tasks may help. For example, van Walraven demonstrated that automating discharge summary generation and distribution is superior to a manual process [39]. This work relied on abstracting data from hospital data systems, a capability that many hospitals will soon have as their information systems improve. A modification of this approach is to export the medication orders from the pharmacy information system to generate a paper prescription.

Automating some of the post-discharge telephone monitoring using interactive voice response systems may also be of some benefit, principally by improving efficiency of calls [40]. The goal of automation is to ensure that these important tasks of communication and monitoring get done while freeing up time for providers to focus on the important tasks of implementing and overseeing treatments as well as on helping patients to better understand their health problems and treatments.

Adverse events due to transitions between providers

Clinical example

At 3:00 pm, a patient with a background history of left ventricular dysfunction and congestive heart failure is admitted to hospital with severe dehydration due to a gastrointestinal illness. The patient initially receives appropriately intensive rehydration treatment with intravenous crystalloid. At 5:00 pm, the treating house officer reassesses the patient and determines the patient still to be hypovolaemic. She recommends an IV infusion at a continual rate. At 6:00 pm, the treating house officer performs 'handover' to the on-call physician and asks him to check the patient's volume status and electrolytes at 10:00 pm. The on-call physician does not see the patient at 10:00 pm as he is overwhelmed with other duties at that time and is unaware of the critical need to check on the patient. At 2:00 am that night, the on-call physician receives a call from the nurse as the patient is in severe respiratory distress. On assessment, the patient was found to be grossly fluid overloaded and severely hypokalaemic.

Extent of the problem and its cause

The example highlights the challenge of ensuring appropriate 'handover' or 'sign out' of responsibilities between providers. The patient's status was tenuous at 5:00 pm. Despite a need for fluids, there was little margin for error given her known left ventricular dysfunction. Despite an attempt to ensure appropriate assessment of the problem, the patient developed problems because the on-call physician did not see the patient at the appropriate time. The on-call physician was aware the patient needed to be seen but because he did not appreciate the critical need to assess the patient, deferred it until a later time. If seen earlier, the crisis occurring at 2:00 am may have been averted.

The need to share tasks amongst providers is a result of the requirement to provide 24-hour per day coverage to patients. Existing communication systems are possibly inadequate and can potentially lead to problems by not ensuring effective transmission of information. Potentially exacerbating this issue are recent concerns related to the relationship between extended work hours and decreasing physician performance [41]. These concerns have led to changes in regulations for work hours. While this may have the benefit of ensuring rested health care providers, there may be an undesirable impact on overall safety due to the failure adequately to 'sign over' responsibilities. The new work hour legislation in Europe and North America means that cross coverage will be more common and in turn makes the problems related to handover even more pressing to solve.

Although there are a number of papers purporting a relationship between ineffective sign over and patient safety, there are few data systematically evaluating the relationship between sign over and adverse events. In addition, one of the most important papers evaluating this particular issue tackled the problem indirectly, by evaluating the impact of cross-coverage in a Boston teaching hospital rather than studying sign over per se [42]. In this particular hospital, after-hours coverage was occasionally assigned to cross-covering house staff (i.e. house staff not assigned to the team to which the patient was admitted). The investigators note that cross-covering house staff may not have the same knowledge of patients as house staff covering their own patients. In a multivariate analysis adjusting for confounding factors, the investigators found that when patients received cross-coverage they had a six-fold increase in the odds of experiencing a preventable adverse event [38].

There are a number of other studies that assess the adequacy of communication during handovers [43–45]. Frequently omitted content during sign out includes information on medications, active problems and pending tests. Frequent failure-prone communication processes included no face-to-face communication and illegible or unclear notes. Another of these studies highlights certain cognitive biases that might predispose physicians to be poorly understood. Other studies evaluated barriers to effective communication. These include language barriers, inadequate time, poor physical setting, the medium of communication and the social setting.

Interventions

There are no randomised trials evaluating interventions that reduce the risk of adverse events caused by poor sign over. However, there are two studies of computerised sign-out interventions that show that this may be an effective intervention [46,47]. These studies are described in the subsequent paragraphs.

Petersen et al. evaluated a computerised sign-out programme at the Brigham and Women's Hospital in Boston using a before–after design [47]. They found that the implementation of a computerised sign-out system decreased the odds ratio for a patient suffering a preventable adverse event during cross-coverage. Van Eaton and colleagues evaluated the implementation of a computerised sign-out system for a surgical service. In a cross-over randomised trial, they evaluated the impact of the sign-out system on several process of care measures [46,48]. They found that their system decreased the number of patients missed on rounds, increased the time spent seeing patients and decreased the total amount of time spent on rounds. While the study did not specifically address patient outcomes, the simple fact that fewer patients were forgotten during rounds suggests that over time the system will have an impact on patient safety.

The future

Improving handover of patient responsibilities requires technical solutions to ensure access to patient information by cross-covering physicians. The early data on computerised systems to facilitate handover suggest that such solutions hold promise for improving patient safety. The systems have the benefit of ensuring access to complete information in a relevant format [48]. For example, the data in the sign-out form can be structured to contain relevant fields: current active problems, medications and pending tests.

Conclusion

The different transitions I have discussed carry with them different risks of adverse events. Transitions from hospital to home are associated with a one in five chance of adverse events and many of these outcomes are clinically important. The other transitions I have discussed – transitions to hospital, transitions within hospitals and transitions between providers – appear to be associated with a lower risk of harm. However, there are relatively few studies evaluating them from the perspective of adverse events. Furthermore, the consequences of such adverse events may be as significant or even more so, especially when considering transfers out of the ICU. While the risk of harm may differ by transition type, many of the contributing factors for adverse events seem to be the same.

Transitional care includes several common processes which need to be attended to, irrespective of the type of transition taking place. In the preceding sections, I have highlighted different aspects of transitions that need to be addressed when a patient is transferred. *Effective communication of the treatment plan* is fundamentally important to all transfers. The treatment plan must include the current active problems, the current medication regimen and the pending test results. Given that poor communication is a weakness that impacts on all transitions, it makes sense for hospitals and health systems to address this issue as a top priority. *Ensuring that the providers who will be receiving the patient have adequate capacity* to care for them is as necessary. Finally, *preparing the patient so that he/she is ready for the transfer* is important. For patients discharged home, preparation includes educating them about the discharge plan and follow-up issues. For patients undergoing an intra-hospital transfer, preparation includes ensuring that the patient is in a suitable condition to undergo transfer at that time.

References

1 Coleman EA, Boult C, American Geriatrics Society Health Care Systems Committee. Improving the quality of transitional care for persons with complex care needs. *Journal of the American Geriatrics Society* 2003; **51** (4): 556–7.
2 Tammemagi CM, Nerenz D, Neslund-Dudas C, Feldkamp C, Nathanson D. Comorbidity and survival disparities among black and white patients with breast cancer. *Journal of the American Medical Association* 2005; **294** (14):1765–72.

3 Coleman EA, Berenson RA. Lost in transition: challenges and opportunities for improving the quality of transitional care. *Annals of Internal Medicine* 2004; **141** (7): 533–6.

4 Tam VC, Knowles SR, Cornish PL, Fine N, Marchesano R, Etchells EE. Frequency, type and clinical importance of medication history errors at admission to hospital: a systematic review (review). *Canadian Medical Association Journal* 2005; **173** (5): 510–15.

5 Cornish PL, Knowles SR, Marchesano R et al. Unintended medication discrepancies at the time of hospital admission. *Archives of Internal Medicine* 2005; **165** (4): 424–9.

6 Boockvar K, Fishman E, Kyriacou CK, Monias A, Gavi S, Cortes T. Adverse events due to discontinuations in drug use and dose changes in patients transferred between acute and long-term care facilities. *Archives of Internal Medicine* 2004; **164** (5): 545–50.

7 Stiell A, Forster AJ, Stiell IG, van Walraven C. Prevalence of information gaps in the emergency department and the effect on patient outcomes. *Canadian Medical Association Journal* 2003; **169** (10): 1023–8.

8 Santell JP. Reconciliation failures lead to medication errors. *Joint Commission Journal on Quality and Patient Safety* 2006; **32** (4): 225–9.

9 Barnsteiner JH. Medication reconciliation: transfer of medication information across settings-keeping it free from error (review). *Journal of Infusion Nursing* 2005; **28** (suppl 2): 31–6.

10 Roy CL, Poon EG, Karson AS et al. Patient safety concerns arising from test results that return after hospital discharge. *Annals of Internal Medicine* 2005; **143** (2): 121–8.

11 Wunsch H, Mapstone J, Brady T et al. Hospital mortality associated with day and time of admission to intensive care units (see comment). *Intensive Care Medicine* 2004; **30** (5): 895–901.

12 Beck DH, McQuillan P, Smith GB. Waiting for the break of dawn? The effects of discharge time, discharge TISS scores and discharge facility on hospital mortality after intensive care. *Intensive Care Medicine* 2002; **28** (9): 1287–93.

13 Duke GJ, Green JV, Briedis JH. Night-shift discharge from intensive care unit increases the mortality-risk of ICU survivors. *Anaesthesia and Intensive Care* 2004; **32** (5): 697–701.

14 Uusaro A, Kari A, Ruokonen E. The effects of ICU admission and discharge times on mortality in Finland. *Intensive Care Medicine* 2003; **29** (12): 2144–8.

15 Goldfrad C, Rowan K. Consequences of discharges from intensive care at night (see comment). *Lancet* 2000; **355** (9210): 1138–42.

16 Tobin AE, Santamaria JD. After-hours discharges from intensive care are associated with increased mortality. *Medical Journal of Australia* 2006; **184** (7): 334–7.

17 Pronovost P, Weast B, Schwarz M et al. Medication reconciliation: a practical tool to reduce the risk of medication errors. *Journal of Critical Care* 2003; **18** (4): 201–5.

18 Beckmann U, Gillies DM, Berenholtz SM et al. Incidents relating to the intra-hospital transfer of critically ill patients. An analysis of the reports submitted to the Australian Incident Monitoring Study in Intensive Care (see comment). *Intensive Care Medicine* 2004; **30** (8): 1579–85.

19 Gillman L, Leslie G, Williams T et al. Adverse events experienced while transferring the critically ill patient from the emergency department to the intensive care unit. *Emergency Medicine Journal* 2006; **23** (11): 858–61.

20 Wallen E, Venkataraman ST, Grosso MJ et al. Intrahospital transport of critically ill pediatric patients. *Critical Care Medicine* 1995; **23** (9): 1588–95.

21 Lovell MA, Mudaliar MY, Klineberg PL. Intrahospital transport of critically ill patients: complications and difficulties (see comment). *Anaesthesia and Intensive Care* 2001; **29** (4): 400–5.

22 Smith I, Fleming S, Cernaianu A. Mishaps during transport from the intensive care unit. *Critical Care Medicine* 1990; **18** (3): 278–81.

23 Gandhi TK. Fumbled handoffs: one dropped ball after another. *Annals of Internal Medicine* 2005; **142** (5): 352–8.

24 Haig KM, Sutton S, Whittington J. SBAR: a shared mental model for improving communication between clinicians. *Joint Commission Journal on Quality and Patient Safety* 2006; **32** (3): 167–75.

25 Wells PS, Holbrook AM, Crowther NR, Hirsh J. Interactions of warfarin with drugs and food. *Annals of Internal Medicine* 1994; **121** (9): 676–83.

26 van Walraven C, Austin PC, Oake N, Wells P, Mamdani M, Forster AJ. The effect of hospitalization on oral anticoagulation control: a population-based study. *Thrombosis Research* 2007; **119** (6): 705–14.

27 Forster AJ, Murff HJ, Peterson JF, Gandhi TK, Bates DW. Adverse drug events occurring following hospital discharge. *Journal of General Internal Medicine* 2005; **20** (4): 317–23.

28 Hylek EM, Chang YC, Skates SJ, Hughes RA, Singer DE. Prospective study of the outcomes of ambulatory patients with excessive warfarin anticoagulation. *Archives of Internal Medicine* 2000; **160** (11): 1612–17.

29 Forster AJ, Murff HJ, Peterson JF, Gandhi TK, Bates DW. The incidence and severity of adverse events affecting patients after discharge from the hospital (see comment). *Annals of Internal Medicine* 2003; **138** (3): 161–7.

30 Forster AJ, Clark HD, Menard A et al. Adverse events affecting medical patients following discharge from hospital. *Canadian Medical Association Journal* 2004; **170** (3): 345–9.

31 Delgado-Rodriguez M, Gomez-Ortega A, Sillero-Arenas M, Llorca J. Epidemiology of surgical-site infections diagnosed after hospital discharge: a prospective cohort study. *Infection Control and Hospital Epidemiology* 2001; **22** (1): 24–30.

32 van Walraven C, Seth R, Austin PC, Laupacis A. Effect of discharge summary availability during post-discharge visits on hospital readmission. *Journal of General Internal Medicine* 2002; **17** (3): 186–92.

33 van Walraven C, Mamdani M, Fang J, Austin PC. Continuity of care and patient outcomes after hospital discharge. *Journal of General Internal Medicine* 2004; **19** (6): 624–31.

34 Coleman EA, Parry C, Chalmers S, Min Sj. The care transitions intervention: results of a randomized controlled trial. *Archives of Internal Medicine* 2006; **166** (17): 1822–8.

35 Schnipper JL, Kirwin JL, Cotugno MC et al. Role of pharmacist counseling in preventing adverse drug events after hospitalization. *Archives of Internal Medicine* 2006; **166** (5): 565–71.

36 Dudas V, Bookwalter T, Kerr KM, Pantilat SZ. The impact of follow-up telephone calls to patients after hospitalization. *Disease-A-Month* 2002; **48** (4): 239–48.

37 Parkes J, Shepperd S. Discharge planning from hospital to home (review). *Cochrane Database of Systematic Reviews* 2000; **4**: CD000313 (update in *Cochrane Database of Systematic Reviews* 2004; **1**: CD000313; PMID: 14973952).

38 Forster AJ, Clark HD, Menard A et al. Effect of a nurse team coordinator on outcomes for hospitalized medicine patients. *American Journal of Medicine* 2005; **118** (10): 1148–53.

39 van Walraven C, Laupacis A, Seth R, Wells G. Dictated versus database-generated discharge summaries: a randomized clinical trial (see comments). *Canadian Medical Association Journal* 1999; **160** (3): 319–26.

40 Forster AJ, van Walraven C. Using an interactive voice response system to improve patient safety following hospital discharge. *Journal of Evaluation in Clinical Practice* 2007; **13**: 346–51.

41 Fletcher KE, Davis SQ, Underwood W, Mangrulkar RS, McMahon LF, Jr, Saint S. Systematic review: effects of resident work hours on patient safety. *Annals of Internal Medicine* 2004; **141** (11): 851–7.

42 Petersen LA, O'Neil AC, Cook EF, Lee TH. Does housestaff discontinuity of care increase the risk for preventable adverse events? *Annals of Internal Medicine* 1994; **121** (11): 866–72.

43 Solet DJ, Norvell JM, Rutan GH, Frankel RM. Lost in translation: challenges and opportunities in physician-to-physician communication during patient handoffs. *Academic Medicine* 2005; **80** (12): 1094–9.

44 Beach C, Croskerry P, Shapiro M, Center for Safety in Emergency Care. Profiles in patient safety: emergency care transitions (see comment). *Academic Emergency Medicine* 2003; **10** (4): 364–7.

45 Sabir N, Yentis SM, Holdcroft A. A national survey of obstetric anaesthetic handovers. *Anaesthesia* 2006; **61** (4): 376–80.

46 Van Eaton EG, Horvath KD, Lober WB et al. A randomized, controlled trial evaluating the impact of a computerized rounding and sign-out system on continuity of care and resident work hours. *Journal of the American College of Surgeons* 2005; **200** (4): 538–45.

47 Petersen LA, Orav EJ, Teich JM et al. Using a computerized sign-out program to improve continuity of inpatient care and prevent adverse events. *Joint Commission Journal on Quality Improvement* 1998; **24** (2): 77–87.

48 Van Eaton EG, Horvath KD, Lober WB et al. Organizing the transfer of patient care information: the development of a computerized resident sign-out system (see comment). *Surgery* 2004; **136** (1): 5–13.

CHAPTER 11

Medicines management

Rachel L. Howard, Anthony J. Avery

Drug-related morbidities (DRMs) are associated with a substantial proportion of patient morbidity in primary care. Some of the most serious DRMs result in hospital admissions. Estimates vary, but a meta-analysis of 68 studies worldwide found a mean of 4.9% (95% confidence interval (CI) = 0.1%) of hospital admissions were drug-related [1], whilst a systematic review of 15 studies in industrialised countries found a median of 7.1% (interquartile range (IQR) = 5.7, 16.2) [2]. Drug-related admissions were four times as common in older patients compared to younger patients [1].

Although not all DRMs can be avoided, a substantial proportion will be associated with errors in medicine management, which can cascade into preventable or ameliorable DRMs [3]. The outcome of preventable drug-related morbidities (PDRMs) can vary in severity from minor adverse events which can be resolved with minimal treatment, to more severe adverse events requiring hospital admission and causing death. Around two-thirds of all drug related hospital admissions are considered to be preventable [2]. A survey of 661 patients in US primary care found that 3% (20/661) experienced PDRMs and nearly 8% (51/661) ameliorable DRMs over a 3-month period [4]. A large US cohort study (over 30 000 person-years), found a rate of 13.8 PDRMs per 1000 person-years [5]. A systematic review of 13 studies worldwide found a median of 3.7% (range 1.4–15.4) of admissions to be drug related and preventable [6]. These preventable PDRMs represent a significant burden to patients and health care systems.

Importantly, improvements in medicines management that reduce the numbers of medication errors are likely also to reduce the incidence of PDRMs. This would benefit patients by reducing avoidable illness and health care systems by reducing the cost of care. Estimates of the cost of treating PDRMs vary between countries, presumably due to differences in cost of health care and methods used to estimate costs [7]. Beijer et al. estimate the cost of preventable drug-related hospital admissions in the Netherlands to be between £110 million and £256 million per annum, whilst estimates of the annual cost of drug-related admissions in the UK range from £380 million to £466 million [1]. Whichever estimate is used, it is clear that DRM

Health Care Errors and Patient Safety. Edited by Brian Hurwitz and Aziz Sheikh.
© 2009 Blackwell Publishing, ISBN: 978-1-4051-4643-2.

represents an important, and potentially avoidable, burden on health care resources.

Studies of medication errors have highlighted problems at multiple stages of the medicines management process with errors associated with PDRM most commonly occurring at the prescribing, monitoring and patient administration stages [5,6]. Previous reviews of methods to improve medicines management have highlighted a number of strategies to combat these medication errors [10–12] (Box 11.1). Since the publication of these reviews, further evidence for the effectiveness of these interventions has become available and this chapter focuses on recent studies of interventions to improve primary care medicines management. Where appropriate we have also drawn upon studies conducted in secondary care, particularly where evidence from primary care is lacking.

Prescribing decision

The first step in delivering a medicine to a patient is the prescribing decision. This decision should be based on the consideration of various factors including the condition being treated, existing and past conditions, concurrent medication and previous allergies or intolerance to medication. In order to make a safe prescribing decision, this complex array of information has to

---

Box 11.1: Strategies to improve medicines management identified in previous reviews

• Developing a systems-based approach to errors (rather than a blame approach) [11]
• Educating health professionals about medical errors and risks associated with specific drugs [11]
• Computerised prescriber order entry [10,11]
• Computerised decision support to assist in selecting appropriate drugs, avoiding contraindicated drugs and highlighting monitoring requirements (based on agreed protocols) [12]
• Bar code dispensing of medication to reduce dispensing errors [10,11]
• Automated dispensing by robots [10]
• Medication reviews performed by pharmacists or training for other health care professionals to improve the quality of these reviews [12]
• Computerised support for repeat prescribing and ensuring appropriate intervals between medication reviews [12]
• Shared decision making to improve patient adherence and increase patient knowledge of their medication [12]
• Expanding the role of clinical pharmacists [11]
• Computerised adverse drug event detection [10]

be assimilated and interpreted during a short appointment (often 10 minutes or less in primary care). It is not surprising, therefore, that errors occur at this stage in the medicines management process.

There are a range of ways in which the safety of prescribing decisions could be improved and in this section we focus on decision support and education of prescribers.

Decision support

Paper- or computer-based decision support systems can include disease- or drug-specific guidelines. They are usually based on a mixture of evidence from the literature and expert opinion, which aim to guide prescribers towards the most appropriate medication [13].

A systematic review of trials of clinical decision support systems has identified a number of features that enhance their chances of success [14] (Box 11.2). Kawamoto et al.'s review found that 94% (30/32) of systems that incorporated all four of these features were successful in improving clinical care compared with only 46% (18/39) of systems which had none of these features. The authors identified a further three factors associated with success (Box 11.2).

Walton et al.'s systematic review of 15 studies of computerised drug dosage advice provided in hospital settings found that these systems reduced the time to therapeutic control, the incidence of toxic drug levels and adverse drug reactions, and the length of hospital stay [15]. Garg et al.'s review of 100 studies published up to September 2004 found that computerised clinical decision support systems incorporating reminders and disease management or drug dosing systems consistently improved practitioner performance but had no consistent impact on patient outcomes [16]. However, such systems are not universally effective. Eccles et al. found that a computerised decision

---

Box 11.2: Factors associated with the success of clinical decision support systems [14]

Four factors associated with success:
- Automatic provision of decision support
- Providing decision support at the time and location of decision making
- Providing a recommendation rather than just an assessment
- Using a computer to generate the decision support

Three further factors that enhance the chances of success:
- Requiring clinicians to document a reason for not following recommendations
- Providing periodic feedback on compliance with system recommendations
- Providing decision support results to patients and physicians

---

Box 11.3: Potential solutions to problems with computerised decision support [20]

- Making it difficult to override hazard alerts and ensuring reasons for overriding alerts are entered
- Providing a clear display of alerts
- Highlighting drugs with similar names
- Coding clinical conditions to enable the system to generate relevant alerts
- Providing alerts for extreme or clinically relevant test results

---

support system for asthma and angina patients had no impact on the process of care, consultation rates or patient reported outcomes [17]. Further investigation found that minimal usage of the software during the study was a likely explanation for the lack of effect.

Although computerised decision support has been shown to be effective in certain circumstances, recognised problems include drug interaction alerts not appearing when they should, and unnecessary alerts, which increase the likelihood of important alerts being overridden [18]. A questionnaire survey of 236 UK general practitioners found that 28% admitted to frequently or very frequently overriding alerts without properly checking them, 19% sometimes overrode alerts because they were too busy to check them, and 22% were frequently annoyed by alerts [19]. An expert panel has developed potential solutions to these problems [20] (Box 11.3), but these solutions have yet to be widely adopted.

Education
In addition to decision support, educational interventions have also been shown to impact on behaviour at the decision-making stage. A complex intervention, which included educational outreach [21], was more successful at increasing the prescribing of thiazide diuretics as first-line treatment for hypertension in Norway than passive guideline dissemination (relative risk 1.94 (95% CI = 1.49–2.49)), but had no impact on other quality outcome measures [22]. Importantly, the cost savings from the change in prescribing would cover the cost of the intervention within 2 years [23]. O'Brien et al.'s systematic review of the effect of educational outreach on professional practice and health care outcomes has also highlighted the benefits of educational outreach at the decision-making stage of the medicines management process [24].

In addition to educational outreach, education of general practitioners for safe prescribing can be included in vocational training schemes, and is part of training courses for supplementary and independent non-medical prescribers in the UK. Also, all prescribers should engage in continuing professional development (CPD) to ensure that they remain up to date. Such training

---

Box 11.4: The top ten drugs most commonly associated with preventable drug-related hospital admissions [6]

- Antiplatelets (including aspirin when used as an antiplatelet)
- Diuretics
- Non-steroidal anti-inflammatory drugs
- Anticoagulants
- Opioid analgesics
- Beta-blockers
- Drugs affecting the renin–angiotensin system, e.g. angiotensin-converting enzyme inhibitors
- Drugs used in diabetes, e.g. insulin and sulphonylureas
- Positive inotropes, e.g. digoxin
- Corticosteroids

---

could focus on those drug groups most frequently associated with preventable drug-related admissions to hospital [6] (Box 11.4). Increasing prescribers' awareness of the risks associated with these drugs is likely to improve their management of patients taking them, thereby reducing the risk of PDRMs.

Prescribers can target their CPD to topics relevant to these patient groups by undertaking relevant audits. For instance, prescribers could audit the use of non-steroidal anti-inflammatory drugs (NSAIDs) in patients aged 75 or over (a patient group recognised to be at high risk of adverse events) [25]. If at-risk patients were identified, this could stimulate a training session highlighting the risks of prescribing NSAIDs to this patient group and identify alternative treatment options. CPD can also be stimulated through significant event auditing. Significant events can be identified in everyday practice, for instance if a patient has had a drug-related admission to hospital. Significant event audits involve one person presenting the details of the case to the rest of their team or practice. This stimulates discussion about how the significant event arose, and helps to identify a series of actions including addressing educational needs and changes to practice (see Chapter 14). Performing significant event audits can be difficult for health care professionals because it can require them to admit that a patient's care has been suboptimal and to think reflexively about their clinical practice [26]. Despite this, significant event analysis is generally viewed positively by general practitioners for its educational value [27], although little is known about its effectiveness in reducing medication errors.

Generating and signing prescriptions

Once the prescribing decision has been made, a prescription must be generated and signed. Prescriptions can be handwritten, printed or electronically transmitted. Problems can arise when illegible handwriting results in the dispenser selecting the wrong medication and/or dose. An obvious solution is electronic prescribing (known as computerised physician order entry (CPOE) in the USA). Prescriptions generated through this method are either printed or electronically transmitted and therefore legibility is less of an issue (although problems can occur when printed prescriptions are very faint). There are, however, potential problems with electronic prescribing. Medications are often selected from alphabetical drop down lists, increasing the possibility of accidentally selecting the wrong medication [18]. In addition, failure to cancel medications which are no longer required can lead to inappropriate prescriptions continuing to be issued [28]. Although electronic prescribing has been widely used for many years in UK primary care, there has been little research into its efficacy in reducing errors. There is some evidence, however, from CPOE programmes implemented in hospital settings [29–31]. Two studies collected data from voluntary error reports before and after CPOE implementation [30,31]. This method of data collection is inherently biased because personnel are more likely to be vigilant (and therefore more likely to report errors) following a system change – therefore any improvement in safety may be underestimated. Spencer et al. compared errors before and after the introduction of a CPOE system on two medical units in a US teaching hospital. The CPOE system prevented duplications, alerted to allergies (where allergy information was entered) and generated standardised printed prescriptions but was not linked electronically to the pharmacy. An overall increase in error reporting was found after the implementation of CPOE. There was a significant increase in reported errors associated with pharmacy preparation (some due to transcription errors), but a non-significant reduction in prescribing errors [30].

Upperman et al. compared errors before and after CPOE introduction to a paediatric hospital [31]. The CPOE system included full electronic records, prescribing warnings, electronic transmission of prescriptions to a pharmacy, and cross-linking to an on-line formulary. Adverse drug events that resulted in harm were reduced from 0.005 per 1000 doses before CPOE to 0.003 per 1000 doses after CPOE [31]. This equated to preventing one adverse drug event (harmful and non-harmful) every 64 patient-days. Although this does not sound like a significant impact, it is equivalent to preventing approximately one error every 2 days on a 30-bed ward.

Closer examination of the types of errors seen in these two studies shows that electronic transmission of prescriptions eliminated transcription errors [31], whereas manual transmission of prescriptions to the pharmacy increased dispensing errors [30]. The increase in dispensing errors described by Spencer et al. stemmed from the system of sending a new prescription to the pharmacy when a dose was changed. There was no mechanism for cancelling earlier prescriptions which had been issued to the pharmacy and this resulted in duplicate medications and inappropriate dose increases [30]. In addition, although Upperman et al. eliminated transcription errors by electronic transmission of prescriptions, a new error was instigated: selecting the wrong drug from a drop down list [31].

Nebeker et al. studied the incidence of PDRM in 937 patients admitted to a highly computerised hospital in the USA [29]. The computerised medical record contained all medications, medical notes and test results, but not images and flow sheets used by anaesthetists and nurses. The system did not include decision support for drug selection, dosing or monitoring. Adverse drug events resulting in harm were identified using prospective chart review of 937 admissions [29]. Twenty-seven per cent of the 483 clinically significant adverse drug events (129/483) detected in this study were associated with 172 errors. Only 35 of these were errors in the execution of tasks (as opposed to errors in decision making). Sixty-one per cent of these (21/35) were associated with ordering and the remainder with dispensing (1%), administration (13%) and monitoring (25%). The low number of adverse drug events associated with errors in task execution supports the benefits of CPOE in reducing harmful errors. However, without sophisticated decision support, errors in decision making will not be prevented.

Information provision and patient counselling

Adequate provision of information is essential if patients are safely to administer their medication and respond appropriately to drug-related problems. There is no agreement on what information should be given to patients, but common sense would suggest the following: name of medicine, why it is taken, how much to take, when to take, how to take, important and/or common side effects to be aware of, and how to respond if these arise. Sources of information can include verbal counselling by prescribers and pharmacists, medication labels, information leaflets, books and (increasingly) the internet.

Adequate counselling regarding medication is thought to impact on both patient adherence and numbers of adverse drug events. Levels of patient counselling vary from simple information provision to patient-centred interventions that focus on shared decision making and patient empowerment. It is widely believed that patient-centred care will improve patient outcomes although there is little evidence to support this [32].

Self-management education programmes in chronic disease have the potential to increase patient empowerment and improve patient outcomes. Warsi et al. reviewed 71 studies of self-management education programmes and found varying effects on disease control [33]. Significant improvements were found in the control of diabetes, blood pressure and asthma, but self-management programmes had no effect on arthritis. Face-to-face education between patients and health care personnel was associated with improved outcomes.

Beney et al.'s systematic review found that patient-oriented interventions by pharmacists improved patient adherence to medication [34]. These interventions were multifaceted, however, involving prescription reviews as well as patient counselling. The cause of the improved adherence is therefore unclear. Bluml et al. found that follow-up visits with a pharmacist, which included patient counselling as well as disease monitoring, resulted in high levels of patient adherence to cholesterol-lowering therapy over a 2-year period (94% of patients continued to take their medication at 2 years and patients were considered to be adherent at 90% of their follow-up visits) [35]. Lowe et al. reported a positive impact from clinical pharmacists visiting patients at home to provide patient counselling, assess patients' ability to take their medication, and rationalise medication regimens [36]. This intervention resulted in a 12% increase in doses of medication taken compared to the control group (80% in control and 91% in intervention).

But simply increasing patient adherence may not result in positive outcomes. Holland et al. found an increase in hospital admissions and home visits by GPs in response to a pharmacist intervention that included patient counselling and assessment of ability to self-medicate [37]. One possible reason for this adverse outcome was thought to be increased patient adherence to medication.

Dispensing medication

Accurate dispensing is essential to the safe provision of medication. This requires accurate selection of the medicine, accurate labelling and distribution to the right patient. Spencer et al.'s evaluation of errors associated with a CPOE system highlights the risk of transcription errors when prescription details are manually entered onto a pharmacy computer system [30]. Where prescriptions are handwritten, this risk is further exacerbated by illegible handwriting, whilst printed prescriptions may be too faint to be legible. Misreading prescriptions is one of the most common causes of dispensing errors [38]. Electronic transfer of prescriptions has the potential to eliminate the risk of transcription errors [31]. Problems also occur at the point of selecting medication, however, as a result of confusion between similar drug names. Awareness of this risk is increased by a list of names likely to cause confusion [39]. In addition, bar codes can increase the speed and accuracy of dispensing [40].

Irrespective of technological advances such as bar coding, a second check on the accuracy of dispensing will remain important. Wherever possible, this check should be made by a second person. At present, however, this is not always possible in community pharmacy. In these cases, it is important to have a time delay between dispensing a medication and checking the final prescription. The final check can be relatively straightforward when original packs are dispensed. However, some patients require multicompartment compliance aids (MCAs) where tablets are removed from their original packaging and mixed together in small compartments. This increases the risk of missing dispensing errors. Nunney and Raynor found that 50% of pharmacists had concerns about their ability to check MCAs [41].

Dispensing should not, however, simply be a supply process. In addition to supplying the medication, the pharmacist has an opportunity to check on the appropriateness of the prescription, identify drug-related problems, help patients resolve these problems and act as a source of information for patients. Studies of pharmacist interventions have, however, had mixed results. The majority of interventions relate to missing information on prescriptions or supply problems 67% (131/196), a smaller proportion to clinical issues 33% (65/196), with a few requiring contact with the prescriber 26% (50/196) [42]. Pharmacies with lower dispensing volumes identify more prescribing problems (four-fold difference in reporting rates between high- and low-volume pharmacies) [42]. Encouraging community pharmacists to provide extended pharmaceutical care services increases the percentage of problems identified. Pharmacists providing a repeat dispensing service identified potential problems in 12% (196/1614) of patients [43], whilst pharmacists questioning patients about drug-related problems following discharge to home identified drug-related problems in 64% (277/435) of patients [44].

Patient administration

The importance of safe and accurate provision of medicines to patients becomes clear when patients begin to administer their medication. At this point patients choose whether or not to take the medication, how to administer it and how to manage any problems which may arise as a result of their decisions with limited or no support from others. In order for people to make informed decisions at this stage, they need to have adequate information available to them. Patients' decisions may not align with the actions desired by the prescriber; this may be because they have received insufficient information or have priorities that differ from those of the prescriber. In addition, patients may experience practical difficulties when administering their medication. Some of these difficulties may be associated with the frequency of administration (once or twice daily regimens are better adhered to than more frequent ones) [45]. Therefore, simplified regimens are recommended [46]. Other problems can arise through difficulty opening medicine containers and impaired vision [47] so it is important to assess patients' ability to open containers and to supply administration aids as necessary. A range of suitable aids is available including non-clicklock lids, lids with wings, devices to help pierce blister packs, tablet cutters, and MCAs. MCAs may not be without their difficulties and there is, as yet, no clear evidence that they improve adherence or patient outcomes. Patients who use MCAs usually have lower levels of knowledge about their medication, and (as described above) it can be more difficult accurately to dispense medication into MCAs [41].

A systematic review has focused on strategies to improve patient adherence to medication, including complex interventions that may be difficult to transfer into everyday practice [46]. The authors suggest that making every effort possible to recall non-attenders and keep them in care is likely to be most effective, although there is little evidence to support this view [46]. Hanlon et al. found that interventions by clinical pharmacists which included patient counselling, home visits and medication reviews improved patient adherence to medication [48].

Monitoring medication

All medications have the potential to cause side effects and therefore require some form of monitoring. Inadequate monitoring is commonly associated with preventable adverse drug events [49]. Monitoring can range from a clinical check (assessing efficacy and adverse effects) to blood tests and other investigations. With some high-risk medications such as methotrexate and warfarin, there are guidelines in place as to the frequency of monitoring required. However, for the majority of medications there are no strict guidelines and little evidence to support the frequency of monitoring [50]. One reason why patients may not be adequately monitored is the difficulty of keeping track of who needs monitoring, when and by whom. Problems can also arise as a result of prescribers' lack of awareness of the need for monitoring, what to monitor for and what action to take if abnormal results are identified. Nebeker et al. found that 33% (57/172) of errors associated with adverse drug reactions related to the failure to start or complete adequate monitoring for common reactions [29]. Clinical computer systems can be programmed to provide reminders for patients requiring monitoring. In addition, they can be linked to pathology laboratory computer systems, facilitating the automatic transfer of test results. Raebel et al. found that alerting pharmacists to missing baseline monitoring (by linking first dispensings of drugs to the absence of laboratory test results) was successful in increasing baseline monitoring of new medications compared to usual care (79.1% vs 70% of patients receiving baseline monitoring) for some (but not all) medications [51]. Importantly, 7% (68/1010) of tests obtained through the intervention were abnormal, and in 91% (62/68) of cases prescribers followed pharmacist recommendations regarding repeat tests, dose adjustments or changes to medication regimens. Clinical computer systems can be adapted to alert prescribers to the need for baseline and long-term monitoring at the point of prescribing rather than after dispensing. Computer systems can also be programmed to alert prescribers to extreme or clinically relevant results, although, at present, such a facility is not routinely available in the UK [20].

An alternative strategy is to educate prescribers about the importance of monitoring, what to monitor and when. Thomas et al. found that brief educational reminders and feedback on levels of monitoring were effective at reducing levels of inappropriate test requests [52]. It seems likely that similar strategies could be used to increase appropriate monitoring.

Repeat prescribing

Patients on long-term medication require repeat prescriptions. Ideally, the process of issuing repeat prescriptions represents an opportunity to reassess the appropriateness of medication, look for drug interactions and assess ongoing requirements for medication. This assessment does not always take place, but there are some strategies which can help improve the safety of the repeat prescribing process.

Primary care computer systems in the UK can be used to differentiate between those prescriptions which are for one-off use (acute) and those which are for long-term use (repeat). Repeat prescriptions are usually authorised for a limited period of time or number of issues (depending on the computer system used). When the time limit is reached, prescriptions should be reviewed before making a further authorisation of repeats. Current recommendations in England suggest a maximum interval between reviews of 12 months, and 6 months for patients aged over 75 years if they are taking four or more medications [25]. Clinical computer systems can be programmed to alert prescribers (or the person issuing the prescription) to the need for a review and to under- or overuse of medication [20].

Not all long-term prescriptions are suitable for the repeat prescribing process. Those medications that require frequent monitoring, such as methotrexate, are usually more safely managed as acute prescriptions that patients request depending on the frequency of monitoring. This helps to ensure that blood test results are checked before a prescription is issued, and that these prescriptions are not mixed up in the pile of repeat prescriptions and that the prescriber is responsible for reviewing them prior to signing [53].

Recently, in the United Kingdom, community pharmacists have been required to offer repeat dispensing services. Under this system, prescriptions are authorised for a finite period of time. At the end of each repeat prescription the patient should attend the surgery for a review. In the meantime, patients attend their community pharmacist for further supplies, bypassing the need for the patient to obtain further prescriptions from their doctor. Research conducted on this system prior to its implementation found that more compliance problems were identified with the community pharmacist repeat prescription service than with the usual GP surgery-managed service [43].

As described above, when a repeat prescription comes to the end of its authorisation, a medication review should be performed to identify possible prescription problems and to assess the need for continuing the medication. Medication reviews can be conducted by a variety of health care professionals including doctors, pharmacists and nurses (depending on their qualifications). The type of prescription problem identified varies depending on the professional conducting the review [54]. After training nurses and doctors in how to perform medication reviews, Krska et al. found a significant increase in the numbers of problems identified [54]. Before training, doctors missed an average of 1.75 problems per patient. After training they missed 0.8 problems per patient. This increase in problem identification was also associated with an increase in changes to medication. Nurses were more likely to identify monitoring requirements and discrepancies in medication use with the medication record than doctors, but doctors were more able to identify clinical issues such as inappropriate indications, doses and formulations, drug interactions and untreated indications. Importantly, these medication reviews were conducted with the patient present. This offers an ideal opportunity to identify adverse effects and compliance problems, and to assess knowledge gaps about medication.

There is an increasing body of evidence relating to clinical pharmacists performing medication reviews in a community setting [55,56] and the acceptability of these reviews to GPs [57]. The outcomes of pharmacist-led medication reviews are variable [37,56], although a recent systematic review found an overall reduction in hospital admissions as a result of pharmacists' interventions [58].

In addition to patient-centred medication reviews, audits of the prescribing of high-risk drugs (see Box 11.4) can be used to identify patients at an increased risk of PDRM. This approach is being tested in the PINCER trial [59] – a cluster randomised trial which uses a series of computer-based queries to search primary care clinical computer systems to identify patients at an increased risk of morbidity from nine drug groups. In the trial, intervention practices are randomised to receive clinical pharmacist support for up to 12 weeks to help resolve problems with individual patients and to develop new medicine management systems to help avoid problems in the future. Control practices receive details of the patients identified by the computer search, but no support in resolving these problems. At present it is not known whether this intervention will be successful in reducing the incidence of potentially hazardous prescribing in primary care, but the results of the study are eagerly awaited.

Conclusion

This review of systems to help improve medicines management at various stages of the medicines use process has identified a number of strategies that may be helpful. There is a growing body of literature to support the use of computer systems in improving medicines management, although there remains a need to expand this evidence base, especially in the primary care setting. Existing studies of computer systems also present a cautionary tale. Computer systems are not a panacea for preventing medication errors. They can successfully tackle some types of errors, but in doing so risk creating new forms of errors. The implementation of new strategies to reduce medication errors needs to be carefully assessed to identify (and mitigate against) any new errors which they may predispose to.

At present, few studies are able to show an impact from the many interventions described on adverse drug effects or hospitalisation. It seems likely that, for a significant impact to be seen, move than one intervention will be required at multiple stages in the medication use process. This is supported by a computer simulation study that applied the outcomes from a number of different information technology-based interventions to data from 6966 hospital-based medication orders and found that significant reductions in events were seen only when all five interventions were combined [60].

References

1 Beijer HJM, de Blaey CJ. Hospitalisations caused by adverse drug reactions (ADR): a meta-analysis of observational studies. *Pharmacy World and Science* 2002; **24**: 46–54.
2 Winterstein AG, Sauer BC, Hepler CD, Poole C. Preventable drug-related hospital admissions. *Annals of Pharmacotherapy* 2002; **36**: 1238–48.
3 Howard RL. *The underlying causes of preventable drug-related admissions to hospital.* PhD thesis, University of Nottingham, Nottingham, 2006.
4 Gandhi TK, Weingart SN, Borus J, et al. Adverse drug events in ambulatory care. *New England Journal of Medicine* 2003; **348**: 1556–64.
5 Gurwitz JH, Field TS, Harrold LR, et al. Incidence and preventability of adverse drug events among older persons in the ambulatory setting. *Journal of the American Medical Association* 2003; **289**: 1107–16.
6 Howard RL, Avery AJ, Slavenburg S, et al. Which drugs cause preventable admissions to hospital? A systematic review. *British Journal of Clinical Pharmacology* 2007; **63**: 136–47.
7 Rodriguez-Monguio R, Otero MJ, Rovira J. Assessing the economic impact of adverse drug effects. *Pharmacoeconomics* 2003; **21**: 623–50.
8 Wiffen P, Gill M, Edwards J, Moore A. Adverse drug reactions in hospital patients. *Bandolier Extra* 2002: 1–15.
9 Pirmohamed M, James S, Meakin S, et al. Adverse drug reactions as cause of admission to hospital: prospective analysis of 18 820 patients. *British Medical Journal* 2004; **329**: 15–19.
10 Bates DW. Using information technology to reduce rates of medication errors in hospitals. *British Medical Journal* 2000; **320**: 788–91.
11 McCarter TG, Centafont R, Daly FN, Koricha T, Leander JZ. Reducing medication errors. A regional approach for hospitals. *Drug Safety* 2003; **26**: 937–50.
12 Avery AJ, Sheikh A, Hurwitz B, et al. Safer medicines management in primary care. *British Journal of General Practice* 2002; **52** (Suppl): S17–S22.
13 National Institute for Health and Clinical Excellence. *Reviewing and Grading the Evidence.* National Institute for Health and Clinical Excellence, London, 2006.
14 Kawamoto K, Houlihan CA, Balas EA, Lobach DF. Improving clinical practice using clinical decision support systems: a systematic review of trials to identify features critical to success. *British Medical Journal* 2005; **330**: 765–8.
15 Walton RT, Harvey E, Dovey S, Freemantle N. Computerised advice on drug dosage to improve prescribing practice. *Cochrane Database of Systematic Reviews* 2001; **1**: CD002894 (DOI: 10.1002/14651858.CD002894).
16 Garg AX, Adhikari NKJ, McDonald H, et al. Effects of computerized clinical decision support systems on practitioner performance and patient outcomes. *Journal of the American Medical Association* 2005; **293**: 1223–38.
17 Eccles M, McColl E, Steen N, et al. Effect of computerised evidence based guidelines on management of asthma and angina in adults in primary care: cluster randomised controlled trial. *British Medical Journal* 2002; **325**: 941–4.

18 Avery AJ, Savelyich BS, Teasdale S. Improving the safety features of general practice computer systems. *Informatics in Primary Care* 2003; **11**: 203–6.
19 Magnus D, Rodgers S, Avery AJ. GPs' views on computerized drug interaction alerts. *Journal of Clinical Pharmacy and Therapeutics* 2002; **27**: 377–82.
20 Avery AJ, Savelyich BS, Sheikh A, et al. Identifying and establishing consensus on the most important safety features of GP computer systems: e-Delphi study. *Informatics in Primary Care* 2005; **13**: 3–12.
21 Soumerai SB, Avorn J. Principles of educational outreach ('academic detailing') to improve clinical decision making. *Journal of the American Medical Association* 1990; **263**: 549–56.
22 Fretheim A, Oxman AD, Velsrud K, et al. Rational prescribing in primary care (RaPP): a cluster randomized trial of a tailored intervention. *PLoS Medicine* 2006; **3** (6).
23 Fretheim A, Aaserud M, Oxman AD. Rational prescribing in primary care (RaPP): economic evaluation of an intervention to improve professional practice. *PLoS Med* 2006; **3** (6).
24. O'Brien MA, Oxman AD, Davis DA, et al. Educational outreach visits: effects on professional practice and health care outcomes. *Cochrane Database of Systematic Reviews* 1997; **4**: CD000409 (DOI: 10.1002/14651858.CD000409).
25 Department of Health. *Medicines for Older People: Implementing Medicines-related Aspects of the NSF for Older People*. Department of Health, London, 2001.
26 Iedema RAM, Jorm C, Long D, et al. Turning the medical gaze in upon itself: root cause analysis and the investigation of clinical error. *Social Science and Medicine* 2006; **62**: 1605–15.
27 Bowie P, McKay J, Dalgetty E, Lough M. A qualitative study of why general practitioners may participate in significant event analysis and educational peer assessment. *Quality and Safety in Health Care* 2005; **14**: 185–9.
28 Chen YF, Avery AJ, Neil KE, et al. Incidence and possible causes of prescribing potentially hazardous/contraindicated drug combinations in general practice. *Drug Safety* 2005; **28**: 67–80.
29 Nebeker JR, Hoffman JM, Weir CR, Bennett CL, Hurdle JF. High rates of adverse drug events in a highly computerized hospital. *Archives of Internal Medicine* 2005; **165**: 1111–16.
30 Spencer DC, Leininger A, Daniels R, Granko RP, Coeytaux RR. Effect of a computerized prescriber-order-entry system on reported medication errors. *American Journal of Health-System Pharmacy* 2005; **62**: 416–19.
31 Upperman JS, Staley P, Friend K, et al. The impact of hospital wide computerized physician order entry on medical errors in a pediatric hospital. *Journal of Pediatric Surgery* 2005; **40**: 57–9.
32 Mead N, Bower P. Patient-centred consultations and outcomes in primary care: a review of the literature. *Patient Education and Counseling* 2002; **48**: 51–61.
33 Warsi A, Wang PS, LaValley MP, Avorn J, Solomon DH. Self-management education programs in chronic disease. *Archives of Internal Medicine* 2004; **164**: 1641–9.
34 Beney J, Bero LA, Bond C. Expanding the roles of outpatient pharmacists: effects on health services utilisation, costs, and patient outcomes. *Cochrane Database of Systematic Reviews* 2000; **2**: CD000336 (DOI: 10.1002/14651858.CD000336).
35 Bluml BM, McKenney JM, Cziraky MJ. Pharmaceutical care services and results in project ImPACT: hyperlipidaemia. *Journal of the American Pharmaceutical Association* 2000; **40**: 157–65.
36 Lowe CJ, Raynor DK, Purvis J, Farrin A, Husdon J. Effects of a medicines review and education programme for older people in general practice. *British Journal of Clinical Pharmacoloy* 2000; **50**: 172–5.

37 Holland R, Lenaghan E, Harvey I, et al. Does home based medication review keep older people out of hospital? The HOMER randomised controlled trial. *British Medical Journal* 2005; **330**: 293–5.

38 Ashcroft DM, Quinlan P, Blenkinsopp A. Prospective study of the incidence, nature and causes of dispensing errors in community pharmacies. *Pharmacoepidemiology and Drug Safety* 2005; **14**: 327–32.

39 USP Center for the Advancement of Patient Safety. *Use Caution – Avoid Confusion*. 2001. Available at http://www.usp.org/pdf/EN/patientSafety/qr792004-04-01.pdf (accessed 19 July 2006).

40 Kaushal R, Bates DW. Information technology and medication safety: what is the benefit? *Quality and Safety in Health Care* 2002; **11**: 261–5.

41 Nunney JM, Raynor DKT. How are multi-compartment compliance aids used in primary care? *Pharmaceutical Journal* 2001; **267**: 784–9.

42 Chen YF, Neil KE, Avery AJ, Dewey ME, Johnson C. Prescribing errors and other problems reported by community pharmacists. *Therapeutics and Clinical Risk Management* 2005; **1**: 333–42.

43 Bond C, Matheson C, Williams S, Williams P, Donnan P. Repeat prescribing: a role for community pharmacists in controlling and monitoring repeat prescriptions. *British Journal of General Practice* 2000; **50**: 271–5.

44 Paulino EI, Bouvy ML, Gastelurrutia MA, Guerreiro M, Buurma H. Drug related problems identified by European community pharmacist in patients discharged from hospital. *Pharmacy World and Science* 2004; **26**: 353–60.

45 Claxton AJ, Cramer J, Pierce C. A systematic review of the associations between dose regimens and medication compliance. *Clinical Therapeutics* 2001; **23**: 1296–310.

46 Haynes RB, Yao X, Degani A, et al. Interventions to enhance medication adherence. *Cochrane Database of Systematic Reviews* 2005; Issue 4: CD000011 (DOI: 10.1002/14651858. CD000011.pub2).

47 Beckman A, Bernsten C, Parker M, Thorslund M, Fastbom J. The difficulty of opening medicine containers in old age: a population-based study. *Pharmacy World and Science* 2005; **27**: 393–8.

48 Hanlon JT, Lindblad CI, Gray SL. Can clinical pharmacy services have a positive impact on drug-related problems and health outcomes in community-based older adults. *American Journal of Geriatric Pharmacotherapy* 2004; **2**: 3–13.

49 Howard RL, Avery AJ, Howard PD, Partridge M. Investigation into the reasons for preventable drug related admissions to a medical admissions unit: observational study. *Quality and Safety in Health Care* 2003; **12**: 280–5.

50 Coleman JJ, Ferner RE, Evans SJW. Monitoring for adverse drug reactions. *British Journal of Clinical Pharmacology* 2006; **61**: 371–8.

51 Raebel MA, Lyons EA, Chester EA, et al. Improving laboratory monitoring at initiation of drug therapy in ambulatory care. A randomized trial. *Archives of Internal Medicine* 2005; **165**: 2395–401.

52 Thomas RE, Croal BL, Ramsay C, Eccles M, Grimshaw J. Effect of enhanced feedback and brief educational reminder messages on laboratory test requesting in primary care: a cluster randomised trial. *Lancet* 2006; **367**: 1990–6.

53 National Patient Safety Agency. *Towards the Safer Use of Oral Methotrexate*. National Patient Safety Agency, London, 2004.

54 Krska J, Ross SM, Watts M. Medication reviews provided by general medical practitioners (GPs) and nurses: an evaluation of their quality. *International Journal of Pharmacy Practice* 2005; **13**: 77–84.

55 Zermansky AG, Petty DR, Raynor DK, et al. Clinical medication review by a pharmacist of patients on repeat prescriptions in general practice: a randomised controlled trial. *Health Technology Assessment* 2002; **6** (20).

56 Holland R, Smith R, Harvey I. Where now for pharmacist led medication review? *Journal of Epidemiology and Community Health* 2006; **60**: 92–3.

57 MacRae F, Lowrie R, MacLaren A, Barbour RS, Norrie J. Pharmacist-led medication review clinics in general practice: the views of Greater Glasgow GPs. *International Journal of Pharmacy Practice* 2003; **11**: 199–208.

58 Royal S, Smeaton L, Avery AJ, Hurwitz B, Sheikh A. Interventions in primary care to reduce medication related adverse events and hospital admissions: systematic review and meta-analysis. *Quality and Safety in Health Care* 2006; **15**: 23–31.

59 PINCER Trial. *PINCER Trial: Reducing Rates of Clinically Important Errors in Medicines Management in General Practice.* 2006. Available at www.pincertrial.org (accessed 12 March 2007).

60 Anderson JG, Jay SJ, Anderson M, Hunt TJ. Evaluating the capability of information technology to prevent adverse drug events: a computer simulation approach. *Journal of the American Medical Informatics Association* 2002; **9**: 479–90.

CHAPTER 12

The patient's role in preventing errors and promoting safety

Jo Ellins, Angela Coulter

In 2001, the UK Department of Health published a major report into patient safety, *An Organisation with a Memory* [1]. It documented how individual actions and systemic failures could lead to lapses in safety and, in many cases, to patient harm. Of its 92 pages, only two were devoted to the impact of adverse health care events on the patients involved. Nowhere in the main body of the report, or in its list of recommendations, was any mention made of how patients (and their families) might usefully participate in safety improvement.

In this respect *An Organisation with a Memory* is typical of the patient safety movement, which has historically neither widely recognised nor understood the patients' role in patient safety. While debate has shifted towards more complex and nuanced accounts of medical error, it still generally falls short of acknowledging that patients themselves are an integral part of the safety team. This neglect may partly arise as a consequence of a medical paternalism that views patients as passive recipients of care, treatment and services. Certainly, patients are typically portrayed as the victims of medical errors and safety failures [2]. If technical expertise and skills are seen as prerequisites for informed participation in safety improvement efforts, then patients can easily be overlooked. Practical considerations might also have a bearing, including concerns that actively involving patients in patient safety could increase the likelihood of complaints or litigation, or place undue additional burdens on health workers or resources. Whatever the explanation – and it is likely to be combination of all these factors – there are many ways in which patients can make a positive contribution to the safe delivery of their care, which we outline in detail below.

Why is patient involvement important?

Increasing patient and public involvement is a major element of health policy and is central to the goal of achieving 'patient-centred' health care. Many patients want to be active participants in their health care: they want to share

Health Care Errors and Patient Safety. Edited by Brian Hurwitz and Aziz Sheikh.
© 2009 Blackwell Publishing, ISBN: 978-1-4051-4643-2.

decisions about their care and treatment, use a service that is responsive to their needs and wishes [3], and avoid making errors themselves (see Chapter 4). However, the drive towards greater patient involvement is not only about responding to public demand. There is a significant and growing body of evidence demonstrating that patient involvement can improve the appropriateness and outcomes of care [4]. Not surprisingly, then, it has also been found to increase patient satisfaction. Additionally, the 2002 Wanless report on the future of the National Health Service (NHS) suggested that the population's 'full engagement' in health improvement was crucial to achieving long-term financial sustainability of the health service [5].

There are good reasons to expect that patient involvement may also lead to improved outcomes in the area of patient safety. Above all, patients have a strong interest in the safe delivery of their care, given that they will be directly affected by the consequences of any medical errors made. This is not to say that patients always act in the interests of safety, and may themselves contribute to adverse health care events [6]. None the less, if appropriately informed and supported, it is probable that many – if not most – patients would choose to engage in practices that promoted safety and minimised the potential for error. Additionally, patients have an important and unique perspective on safety events; as Koutantji and colleagues [2] note:

the patient is the privileged witness of events – both in the sense that they are at the centre of the treatment process and also that, unlike clinical staff who come and go, they observe almost the whole process of care.

It may sometimes, therefore, be apparent only to the patient when their symptoms have changed or deteriorated, where medications or procedures are overdue, or where there are inconsistencies in practices. Following from this, patients need to feel able to raise their concerns about possible safety issues and be reassured that their care will not be negatively affected if they do so.

With the shift towards greater community and home-based care, patients are assuming increasing responsibility for their health and health care. Self-care is especially important for the estimated 17 million people who have a chronic medical condition, and is being widely promoted in the NHS through initiatives such as the Expert Patients Programme [7]. As active participants in their own care, patients necessarily have a role to play in the quality and safety of that care. Indeed, many of the tasks that patients perform to manage their health – such as administering medicines or using medical equipment – have safety implications, particularly if not done so correctly. Patients need timely and appropriate information, education and support to ensure that they can look after their health effectively, including guidance on how to identify and respond to early warning signs. Although confidence to make autonomous decisions in situations of uncertainty may be critical, patients should also know that they can readily access professional help and advice whenever it is needed.

Recent initiatives

A number of initiatives have been launched in recent years to promote patient involvement in patient safety. The 'Patients for Patient Safety' programme is one of six action areas that comprise the World Alliance for Patient Safety, a global initiative launched by the World Health Organization in 2004 [8]. The programme aims to collate and build on work that is already underway in this area, led by organisations such as Consumers Advancing Patient Safety in the USA and Action Against Medical Accidents in the UK. 'Involving and communicating with patients and the public' is one of the National Patient Safety Agency's (NPSA) seven steps to safer health care [9]. To this end, the NPSA has produced a range of consumer fact sheets and a toolkit for health care staff to help them communicate openly and honestly with patients when errors have occurred.

Patient-focused safety campaigns tend to combine two key elements: informing and advising patients about safety-related issues, and encouraging them to voice concerns or ask for clarification when they are concerned about the delivery of their care. In the USA, there are several high profile campaigns of this kind, including the 'Speak Up' programme run by the Joint Commission on the Accreditation of Healthcare Organizations (JCAHO). This includes general guidance on how patients can contribute to their safety (Box 12.1), as well as information on specific risks associated with wrong-site surgery, organ donation, infection control and medication

---

Box 12.1: Speak Up – help prevent errors in your care (from Joint Commission on Accreditation on Healthcare Organizations)

• Speak up if you have questions or concerns, and if you don't understand, ask again. It's your body and you have a right to know
• Pay attention to the care you are receiving. Make sure you're getting the right treatment and medications by the right health care professionals. Don't assume anything
• Educate yourself about your diagnosis, the medical tests you are undergoing and your treatment plan
• Ask a trusted family member or friend to act as your advocate
• Know what medications you take and why you take them. Medication errors are the most common health mistakes
• Use a hospital, clinic, surgery centre or other type of health care organisation that has undergone a rigorous on-site evaluation against established, state-of-the-art quality and safety standards, such as that provided by the Joint Commission
• Participate in all decisions about your treatment. You are the centre of the health care team

mistakes [10]. Similar initiatives have been developed by the US Department for Health and Human Services, the National Patient Safety Foundation and the Agency for Healthcare Research and Quality (AHRQ) (see Box 1.5, p. 14). In the UK, a series of information and advice sheets for patients, parents and relatives have been produced by the NPSA as part of their 'Please Ask' campaign [11]. This follows on from the NPSA's 'Clean your hands' initiative, which encouraged patients to ask health workers whether they had washed their hands if they thought that hygiene standards were not being maintained.

A review of five leading US-based patient-focused campaigns, including the JCAHO's 'Speak Up' campaign, questioned the merits of this approach and suggested that the advice given could do more harm than good [12]. Specifically, it found significant gaps in the content of the patient information materials; that patients were given little practical advice to carry out the recommended actions; and that in some cases there appeared to be an inappropriate shifting of responsibility for safety onto patients. One explanation offered for this was the general lack of patient involvement in developing or evaluating campaign materials, which resulted in them having a strongly provider-oriented perspective. The campaigns were felt to have a restrictive focus on changing the attitudes and behaviours of patients, while neglecting possible barriers to patient participation embedded in the prevailing organisational or professional culture.

As the researchers on the study also noted, patients may feel uncomfortable directly challenging staff over what may be sensitive safety issues. This is borne out by the findings of a survey of patients who were treated in hospitals that were serving as pilot sites for the NPSA's 'Clean your hands' campaign. While 71% of respondents felt that they could help staff to comply with hand hygiene, only 26% were prepared to raise concerns about hand washing in practice [13]. Patients' willingness to act can be influenced by the perceived status or approachability of the individual concerned. To illustrate, patients participating in a hand hygiene initiative in a hospital in Oxford, UK, raised the issue of hand washing with every nurse they were seen by, but with only one-third of doctors [14].

The drive for greater patient involvement must work alongside and complement, rather than act as a substitute for, efforts focused on influencing professional attitudes and behaviours or implementing systems change. Patients can be encouraged to raise concerns about safety or ask questions about their care, but meaningful involvement can only be achieved within a culture that appreciates the value of patient contributions, and is supportive of these. A culture of this kind will be developed by promoting the principles of openness and honesty, and by building trust and communication between clinicians and patients. Just as patients will need high-quality information and the opportunity to develop new competencies, so health professionals may benefit from preparation and training to support patients and work with them towards the goal of safer health care.

Opportunities for patient involvement in patient safety

In the above section, we described two ways in which patients are already being encouraged to take a more active role in ensuring their safety: observing and checking care processes, and participation in hand hygiene initiatives. Throughout the patient's health care journey, there are many more potential opportunities for them to contribute to safety and reduce the likelihood of error, to which we now turn.

Making informed choices about health care providers

During many recent high-profile medical scandals – including that involving cardiac surgery on babies at the Bristol Royal Infirmary – it has emerged that colleagues had been aware of lapses in patient safety long before official action was taken. This information was also known to professional bodies, but was not publicly disclosed. Had the parents concerned been aware of the potential risk to their child's safety, they could have chosen to go to a different provider. Patients can make safer choices when comparative information on the quality and safety of care is produced for their use. Such information has been publicly available for some time in the USA, where organisations like The Leapfrog Group gather and report performance data to help patients make informed decisions about where to receive their care [15]. Based on evidence linking the number of procedures conducted and the quality of outcomes, the AHRQ advises patients to choose hospitals and doctors that are high-volume providers [16]. Similar moves to make performance information available to the UK public are underway, including the launch in April 2006 of a website with information on the outcomes of adult cardiac surgery.

Helping to reach an accurate diagnosis

The information that patients can provide to clinicians – about the onset and duration of symptoms, and their medical and treatment history – is important in establishing early and accurate diagnosis. As with all types of medical error, poor communication and the misunderstandings that can arise from this are a major cause of error in diagnosis (see Chapter 9). Not listening to what a patient has to say about their health problems, or dismissing their concerns too hastily, can lead to misdiagnosis, which in turn can cause delayed or incorrect treatment. A patient-centred consulting style increases the likelihood that important information will be shared. For most patients this means a sympathetic clinician, who listens and encourages them to discuss their problems [17]. However, research has shown that consultations are not always consistent with patients' preferences. Respondents to the NHS patient surveys in England have reported problems in this regard: in 2004, 26% of emergency patients said staff did not always listen carefully to what they were saying; 32% of outpatients said they had not received a clear explanation of treatment risks; and 32% of inpatients and 47% of primary care patients said they would have liked more involvement in decisions about their care [18].

Barriers to effective communication relate not only to clinicians' and patients' communication styles, interpersonal skills and attitudes towards sharing information with each other. Organisational constraints, in particular the restricted time available for consultations, also hamper the full and open exchange of information between clinicians and patients. There is evidence to support a number of strategies designed to facilitate patient participation in consultations, including coaching in how to raise issues and prompt sheets to guide patients in asking important questions [19]. What is needed now is a concerted effort to implement these strategies, supported by specific training for health workers at all levels on patient communication skills.

Sharing decisions about treatments and procedures

When deciding on the best way to treat or manage a condition, the aim is to maximise the likelihood of desired health outcomes and minimise the chance of undesired consequences. Where there is more than one possible course of action, it is important that the patient is informed about the potential benefits and harms of each option, and that their values and preferences guide the decision. This shared decision-making approach improves patient adherence to treatment, leading to better health outcomes [20]. Decision aids have been developed to provide patients with information about their options – including benefits and harms – and guide them through the decision-making process. Patients using decision aids have more realistic expectations about their care, tend to opt for less invasive and risky procedures, and are more likely to receive medical screening and other preventive treatment [21]. Conversely, failure to involve patients in this way can lead to unrealistic demands, over-treatment (with consequent increased risks) and ultimately to disillusion. If patients are encouraged to believe there is an effective pill for every ill, or that surgery is risk free, it is no wonder that they sometimes find the reality disappointing.

Contributing to safe medication use

Medication errors are a leading cause of adverse health care events. Between July 2005 and July 2006, more than 40 000 medication errors were recorded by the 173 NHS trusts in England, with 2000 cases of moderate to severe harm to patients and 36 deaths [22]. It is for this reason that strategies to reduce medication errors form a major part of most patient safety initiatives (see Chapter 11). In hospital settings, patients can contribute to such strategies if they are kept informed about medication management, and are encouraged to tell a member of staff if they notice changes in the way they are given or respond to their medicines [2] (see Chapter 10). The patient's role is particularly important at home, when they may be responsible for the self-administration of prescription medicines or self-treating with over-the-counter remedies. While patients need accessible and reliable information to use their medicines safely, the current quality of patient literature in this area is variable and often poor. A review of the mandatory patient leaflets accompanying prescription medicines found that they made excessive use of technical and medical jargon, were poorly written and designed, and contained too much – and sometimes conflicting – information [23]. A key step in overcoming these problems is to involve a range of patients in the development and review of medicines information that is produced for their use.

Checking the accuracy of medical records

Until recently, medical records were seen as the property of the clinician, rather than the patient. Few patients saw their notes and those that asked to do so were often actively discouraged or reprimanded. Attitudes are slowly changing, but patient-held records are still a rarity. Studies examining the effects of giving patients access to their records have generally produced positive results [24,25]. Holding their records and reading them can increase patients' knowledge of their health and their sense of shared responsibility for their own health care. It can also help to increase the accuracy of the records. One British general practice discovered errors in more than 30% of medical records when patients were encouraged to review their notes [26]. Accurate records are a prerequisite for safe care.

Direct reporting of adverse health care events

One of the key principles of patient safety is that, while it is not always possible to prevent adverse health care events, much can be learned from reporting and analysing their occurrence. An understanding of the incidence, nature and causes of medical errors leading to adverse events is essential to their prevention [1] (see Chapters 15 and 16). A number of systems for reporting adverse drug reactions have been established, including the UK Medicines and Healthcare products Regulatory Agency's (MHRA) Yellow Card Scheme. However, the usefulness of such systems is weakened by the generally low levels of reporting to them. This problem will hopefully improve now that patients themselves are able to submit reports directly. There is evidence that patients report suspected adverse events far earlier than health professionals, which suggests that patient involvement may reduce the time taken to identify and respond to drug safety problems [27]. Patients are also more likely to report potentially embarrassing or distressing side effects to an anonymous scheme than directly to a health professional, which may also improve detection rates [28]. Longstanding schemes for patient reporting of suspected adverse drug reactions operate in Sweden, the USA and Denmark, while the Yellow Card Scheme was extended to patients and the public in the UK in January 2005.

Practising effective self-management

For people living with chronic health problems, they themselves are generally the person responsible for the day-to-day management of their care. Self-management incorporates a variety of health maintenance and monitoring activities, for which assistance, education and/or skills development may be essential. If patients are appropriately supported, then self-management can lead to better health and improved safety. For example, patient self-monitoring has been shown to improve the quality of oral anticoagulation treatment and is associated with fewer bleeding and thromboembolic events [29,30]. This finding is particularly significant given that an estimated half a million people in the UK are prescribed oral anticoagulation therapy each year. Complications after discharge from hospital can be minimised if time is taken to explain to patients how they can monitor their progress and response to treatments, and when they can resume their normal activities. Discharge planning should begin at the earliest possible opportunity and be based on the individual's specific needs and circumstances. Health care providers need to anticipate any problems that might occur following discharge and educate patients about appropriate courses of action. Safe discharge can also be encouraged by supervising patients in self-administration of medicines or the use of medical devices during their hospital stay.

Shaping the design and improvement of services

A 2003 report by the UK's Department of Health and Design Council considered the significance of service design to improving patient safety [31]. If potential sources of error are not anticipated and addressed when services are being planned, as has often been the case, then patient safety problems are effectively 'designed into' the system. Placing safety considerations at the centre of service design may not always prevent errors, but it can help to make errors visible when they do occur, or mitigate their effects when they are not identified and intercepted. Such an approach, as the Department of Health/Design Council report highlighted, must be informed by a thorough understanding of the views and experiences of all those who interact with and use health care facilities. This can help to achieve a better understanding of the complex environments in which care is delivered and errors occur, as well as ensure that solutions are guided by and responsive to the needs of the different groups involved.

Conclusion

Patients have an important role play in ensuring the safety of their care, with opportunities for patient involvement in safety improvement across the health care continuum. There will be challenges for both patients and health workers in working towards a partnership approach, not least in building open and effective communication around sensitive safety issues. Patients may not always want or feel able to play a more active part, and some situations – such as critical and intensive care – are less suitable for patient involvement than others. The patient's preferences should be respected and individuals should be encouraged to participate in safety initiatives, but not required to do so. However, it is also important to recognise that during routine situations, patients frequently act in ways that can enhance or detract from the safety of their care. It is not a case of whether patients contribute to patient safety, but

how and to what effect. Given this, a joined-up approach to patient involvement should focus on equipping patients with the knowledge and skills to
promote their safety wherever possible and appropriate.

References

1 Department of Health. *An Organisation with a Memory: Report of an Expert Group on Learning from Adverse Events in the NHS.* Stationery Office, London, 2000.
2 Koutantji M, Davis R, Vincent C, Coulter A. The patient's role in patient safety: engaging patients, their representatives, and health professionals? *Clinical Risk* 2005; **11** (3): 99–104.
3 Coulter A. *The Autonomous Patient.* Nuffield Trust, London, 2002.
4 Coulter A, Ellins J. *The Quality Enhancing Interventions Project: Patient-focused Interventions.* The Health Foundation, London, 2006.
5 Wanless D. *Securing Our Future Health: Taking a Long-term View.* HMSO, London, 2002.
6 Vincent C, Taylor-Adams S, Stanhope N. Framework for analysing risk and safety in clinical medicine. *British Medical Journal* 1998; **316** (7138): 1154–7.
7 Department of Health. *Supporting People with Long Term Conditions. An NHS and Social Care Model to Support Local Innovation and Integration.* Department of Health, London, 2005.
8 World Health Organisation. *Patients for Patient Safety* (online). WHO, Geneva, c. 2006. Available at http://www.who.int/patientsafety/patients_for_patient/en.
9 National Patient Safety Agency. *Seven Steps to Patient Safety: a Guide for NHS Staff.* National Patient Safety Agency, London, 2003.
10 Joint Commission on the Accreditation of Healthcare Organizations (JCAHO). *Speak Up Initiatives* (online). JCAHO, c. 2006. Available at http://www.jointcommission. org/PatientSafety/SpeakUp.
11 National Patient Safety Agency, Please Ask website: http://www.npsa.nhs.uk/pleaseask.
12 Entwistle V, Mello M, Brennan TA. Advising patients about patient safety: current initiatives risk shifting responsibility. *Joint Commission Journal on Quality and Patient Safety* 2005; **31** (9): 483–94.
13 National Patient Safety Agency. *Achieving our Aims: Evaluating the Results of the Pilot CleanyourHands Campaign.* National Patient Safety Agency, London, 2004.
14 McGuckin M, Waterman R, Storr IJ et al. Evaluation of a patient-empowering hand hygiene programme in the UK. Journal of Hospital Infection 2001; **48** (3): 222–7.
15 The Leapfrog Group website: http://www.leapfroggroup.org.
16 Vincent C, Coulter A. Patient safety: what about the patient? *Quality and Safety in Health Care* 2002; **11**: 76–80.
17 Britten N, Stevenson FA, Barry CA, Barber N, Bradley CP. Misunderstandings in prescribing decisions in general practice: qualitative study. *British Medical Journal* 2000; **320**: 484–8.
18 Picker Institute Europe. *Is the NHS getting Better or Worse? An In-depth Look at the Views of Nearly One Million Patients between 1998 and 2004.* Picker Institute Europe, Oxford, 2005.
19 Griffin SJ, Kinmonth AL, Veltman MW, Gillard S, Grant J, Stewart M. Effect on health-related outcomes of interventions to alter the interaction between patients and practitioners: a systematic review of trials. *Annals of Family Medicine* 2004; **2** (6): 595–608.
20 Mullen PD. Compliance becomes concordance. *British Medical Journal* 1997; **314**: 691.

21 O'Connor AM, Stacey D, Entwistle V et al. Decision aids for people facing health treatment or screening decisions. *Cochrane Database of Systematic Reviews* 2003; **2**: CD001431.

22 Boseley S. 40 000 drug errors logged in a year. *Guardian* 11 Aug. 2006.

23 Consumers Association. *Patient Information Leaflets: Sick Notes?* Consumers Association, London, 2000.

24 Drury M, Yudkin P, Harcourt J et al. Patients with cancer holding their own records: a randomised controlled trial. *British Journal of General Practice* 2000; **50** (451): 105–10.

25 Elbourne D, Richardson M, Chalmers I, Waterhouse I, Holt E. The Newbury Maternity Care Study: a randomized controlled trial to assess a policy of women holding their own obstetric records. *British Journal of Obstetrics and Gynaecology* 1987; **94** (7): 612–19.

26 Pyper C, Amery J, Watson M, Thomas B, Crook C. *ERDIP Online Patient Access Project.* Bury Knowle Health Centre, Oxford, 2001.

27 Egberts TC, Smulders M, de Koning FH, Meyboom RH, Leufkens HG. Can adverse drug reactions be detected earlier? A comparison of reports by patients and professionals. *British Medical Journal* 1996; **313** (7056): 530–1.

28 van Grootheest K, de Graaf L, de Jong-van den Berg LT. Consumer adverse drug reaction reporting: a new step in pharmacovigilance? *Drug Safety* 2003; **26** (4): 211–17.

29 Douketis JD. Patient self-monitoring of oral anticoagulant therapy: potential benefits and implications for clinical practice. *American Journal of Cardiovascular Drugs* 2001; **1** (4): 245–51.

30 Heneghan C, Alonso-Coello P, Garcia-Alamino JM, Perera R, Meats E, Glasziou P. Self-monitoring of oral anticoagulation: a systematic review and meta-analysis. *Lancet* 2006; **367** (9508): 404–11.

31 Department of Health, Design Council. *Design for Patient Safety.* Department of Health, London, 2003.

PART 3

Responses to health care errors and violations

CHAPTER 13

Aftermath of error for patients and health care staff

Charles Vincent, Lesley Page

Human beings frequently make errors and misjudgments in every sphere of activity, but some environments are less forgiving of error than others. Errors in academia, law or architecture, for instance, can mostly be remedied with an apology or a cheque. Those in medicine and health care, in the air or on an oil rig may have severe or even catastrophic consequences. This is not to say that the errors of doctors, nurses, midwives or pilots are more reprehensible, only that they bear a greater burden because their errors can have greater consequences [1]. Making an error, particularly if a patient is harmed because of it, may therefore not only have profound consequences for the patient and their family, as they may have to contend with both physical and psychological trauma, but also for the staff involved, particularly if they are seen, rightly or wrongly, as primarily responsible for the outcome.

In this chapter we discuss a neglected topic in risk management and patient safety, the aftermath of errors and harm. Research is scant in this area, both in respect of patients and staff, but we provide a brief overview of some of the studies supplemented by examples from our own experiences and conversations with those affected by health care errors. Finally, we provide some suggestions as to how these events might be approached with the aim of mitigating the trauma for all concerned.

Psychological responses to medical injury

Patients are often in a vulnerable psychological state, even when diagnosis is clear and treatment goes according to plan. Even routine procedures and normal childbirth may produce post-traumatic symptoms [2,3]. When patients experience harm or misadventure therefore, their reaction is likely to be particularly severe.

Traumatic and life-threatening events produce a variety of symptoms, over and above any physical injury. Sudden, intense, dangerous or uncontrollable events are particularly likely to lead to psychological problems [4]. Awareness under anaesthesia is an example of such an event. When people

Health Care Errors and Patient Safety. Edited by Brian Hurwitz and Aziz Sheikh.
© 2009 Blackwell Publishing, ISBN: 978-1-4051-4643-2.

experience such a terrifying, if short lived, event they often later suffer from anxiety, intrusive and disturbing memories, emotional numbing and flashbacks. Almost everyone experiences such memories after stressful events, such as a divorce or bereavement and, while unpleasant, they gradually die down. However, they can be intense, prolonged and cause considerable suffering.

The full impact of some incidents only becomes apparent in the longer term. A perforated bowel, for example, may require a series of further operations and time in hospital. The long-term consequences may include chronic pain, disability and depression, with a deleterious effect on family relationships and ability to work [5]. Depression appears to be a more common long-term response to medical injury than post-traumatic stress disorder [6], although there is little research in this area. Whether people actually become depressed and to what degree will depend on the severity of their injury, the support they have from family, friends and health professionals and a variety of other factors. When a patient dies the trauma for those left behind and for staff involved is obviously more severe still, and may be particularly severe after a potentially avoidable death [7]. For instance, many people who have lost a spouse or child in a road accident continue to ruminate about the accident and what could have been done to prevent it for years afterwards. They are often unable to accept, resolve or find any meaning in the loss [8].

Death in childbirth may be particularly hard to bear. Childbirth is usually a time of new life starting and is anticipated with joy. When the baby dies in pregnancy or labour and birth or the early weeks of life, the loss is not only of the baby but also of this promise of a new life and family. The death of a mother in childbirth leaves the baby as an orphan with the attendant practical problems of raising the child for the partner and family left behind. If both mother and baby die, grief may be unendurable [9]. Nowadays in industrialised countries the risk of death of the baby or the mother is very low. However, when death does occur the prior expectation of a healthy outcome may make the aftermath for both family and staff very difficult. Often it may be genuinely difficult to know whether or not death or disability could have been avoided; this seems to be particularly hard for all to bear. A continued search for a cause or for somebody to blame may interfere with the ability to mourn and to find healing and resolution. Morbidity following childbirth, including cerebral palsy arising from asphyxia occurring in labour and birth, may be accompanied by legal action as the family use litigation as a way of finding financial support for their disabled child. Legal processes that usually take years to complete will prolong grief and guilt for the family and staff involved.

Experiences of injured patients and their relatives

The impact of a medical injury differs from most other accidents in some important respects. First, patients have generally been harmed, unintentionally, by people in whom they placed considerable trust, and so their reaction may be especially powerful and hard to cope with. Second, they are often cared for by the same professions, and perhaps the same people, as those involved in the original injury. As they may have been very frightened by what has happened to them, and have a range of conflicting feelings about those involved, this too can be very difficult, even when staff are sympathetic and supportive [1].

Patients and relatives may also suffer from the injury in two distinct ways. First from the injury itself and second from the way the incident is handled afterwards. Many people harmed by their treatment suffer further trauma through the incident being insensitively and inadequately handled. Conversely, when staff come forward, acknowledge the damage and take the necessary action, the support offered can ameliorate the impact both in the short and longer term. Injured patients need an explanation, an apology, to know that changes have been made to prevent future incidents, and often also practical and financial help [10]. When we think about the trauma of medical injury therefore we have to consider not only the original incident, but the way in which it was handled afterwards.

Reports of studies have helped us understand the main effects of injury to patients, but it is still difficult to grasp the full extent of the trauma that people sometimes face. Appreciating and understanding their experiences is essential if one is going to provide individually appropriate and practical help. This means that one must endeavour to see the story from the perspective of the patient and family rather than from the perhaps more familiar clinical perspective. From the clinical side, the patient's view may seem incomplete and insufficiently appreciative of the limits of medicine and the ordinary human frailty of practitioners. From the converse perspective, clinicians have to try to understand the total incomprehension of the patient and family that people who were trying to help have in the end caused great additional suffering.

Two true stories retold here (Boxes 13.1 and 13.2) illustrate some of the themes of the chapter, illustrating both physical and psychological trauma, which encompass the impact of the initial event and the 'second trauma' that may result from poor handling by the organisation concerned. The first example comes from a series of interviews with patients whose care had been seriously deficient and, while it may seem extreme to some, it is actually chosen as a fairly typical account of serious surgical complications as experienced by the patient. In the second example, a personal communication to one of the authors, the deaths may well not have been avoidable but, in spite of the efforts of the clinicians, the delayed, defensive and thoughtless response of the wider organisation caused much additional suffering and triggered legal action which could certainly have been avoided.

Trauma may disable a person and their family in a number of different ways. A combination of grief and disabilities may affect the person involved

Box 13.1: Perforation of the colon leading to chronic pain and depression (adapted from Vincent & Coulter [6])

A woman underwent a ventrosuspension – the fixation of a displaced uterus to the abdominal wall. After the operation she awoke with a terrible pain in her lower abdomen which became steadily worse over the next 4 days. She was very frightened and repeatedly told both doctors and nurses about it, but they dismissed it as 'wind'. On the fifth day the pain reached a crescendo and she felt a 'ripping sensation' inside her abdomen. That evening the wound opened and the contents of her bowel began to seep through the dressings. Even then, no one seemed concerned. Finally, the surgeon realised that the bowel had been perforated and a temporary colostomy was carried out.

The next operation, to reverse the colostomy, was 'another fiasco'. After a few days there was a discharge of faecal matter from the scar, the wound became infected and the pain was excruciating, especially after eating. She persistently asked if she could be fed with a drip but the nursing staff insisted she should keep eating. For 2 weeks she was 'crying with the pain, really panicking – I just couldn't take it any more'. She was finally transferred to another hospital where she was immediately put on a liquid diet.

A final operation to repair the bowel was successful but left her exhausted and depressed. She only began to recover her strength after a year of convalescence. Three years later she was still constantly tired, irritable, low in spirits and reported that 'I don't enjoy anything any more'. She did not welcome affection or comfort and felt that she was going downhill, becoming more gloomy and preoccupied.

Her scars remain uncomfortable and painful at the time of her periods. Her stomach is 'deformed' and she feels much less confident and attractive as a result. As her depression has deepened, she has become less interested in sex and more self-conscious about the scar. Three years later, the trauma of her time in hospital is very much alive. She still has nightmares and is unable to talk about it without breaking into tears. She feels very angry and bitter that no one has ever apologised to her or admitted that a mistake was made.

very directly but may also have an effect on the relationships within the family, and marital break up is common as the result of looking after a disabled child or as the result of a change in bodily functions or illness (Box 13.1). These difficulties may be compounded by a conflict with organisations that do not respond to error appropriately. For example, a healthy woman who can no longer control her bladder or bowel following childbirth will find

---

Box 13.2: The unexpected death of a mother and her baby

A pregnant woman was admitted to hospital in labour. She and her unborn baby appeared to be healthy and no problems were anticipated. Within a few hours her unborn baby died; she then became very unwell and died soon after despite emergency treatment. The mother had suffered from a very rare condition that affected both her and her baby. The risk of mortality from the condition was high, although there was a slight chance that early detection may have saved the baby.

First responses to the deaths were timely and appropriate. The widower and father of the baby was seen by senior clinicians who gave an honest account of what had happened. They expressed their sorrow and their commitment to a thorough investigation with a promise of honest feedback. This seemed to help the father who was given the name of two senior members of staff to contact should he feel the need at any time. Enquiries were started immediately by the managers and risk manager and staff were supported.

This was, quite naturally, seen as a very serious outcome with serious potential consequences for the hospital, including the possibility of litigation. While the investigation that was undertaken by clinicians in the service happened in a timely manner there were considerable delays in the process of approval at a higher organisational level. There was also anxiety about sharing the report with the widower that led to severe delay. It was clear from direct contact with him that this delay was adding to his grief and he was becoming extremely angry.

Eventually the detailed report was provided. By then, however, relationships with the father were strained and trust had been eroded. Soon after this he started legal proceedings. It was clear that, however difficult it may have been to know that his wife and baby may have been saved, receiving a full report would have helped him. The father's grief was intensified and rather than being supported by the organisation he found himself in conflict with it. In fact, care of his wife and baby had been good on the whole, but the failure to be honest and open in a timely way coloured his view of the care.

---

difficulty in everyday activities as well as in her sexual relationship. She will find mothering far more difficult. If these problems are accompanied by the failure of the health care organisation to make an apology or to hold a good and transparent enquiry or to admit error, the struggle to achieve justice may add to all the other difficulties. There may be feelings of grief for the lost healthy self, mixed with extreme anger. It may also be difficult to talk about these personal problems with family and friends. If there is a protracted battle with the health service or through the courts, potential support from within and outside of the family may eventually fade away. As time moves on there is a lack of resolution of either the complaint or of psychological issues. Life may become a continued fight to gain an apology.

Principles for helping patients and their families

Every injured patient has their own particular problems and needs. Some will require a great deal of professional help, while others will prefer to rely on their family and friends. Some will primarily require remedial medical treatment, while in others the psychological effects will be to the fore. The trauma for patients harmed by treatment can be greatly reduced if certain basic principles are borne in mind. Some of the most common recommendations, discussed in detail elsewhere [1], are as follows:

• Believe people who say their treatment has harmed them, at least in the first instance. The patient may have information the care giver lacks. If fears are groundless a complete and sympathetic explanation is essential therapy. Being ignored is frightening for the patient and may delay remedial treatment.

• Be honest and open about what has occurred, and what is being done to prevent recurrence. The lack of an explanation, and apology if appropriate, can be experienced as extremely punitive and distressing and can be a powerful stimulus to complaint or litigation.

• Ensure continuity of care and maintain the therapeutic relationship. After an injury, patients and families need more support not less, though both patient and clinician may feel a natural wish to distance themselves from what has happened.

• Ask specific questions about emotional trauma, especially about the patient's anxieties about future treatment. Psychological treatment may be needed when reactions are severe.

• Provide practical and financial help quickly. Relatively small sums of money can make a major difference to the impact of an injury when spent wisely on childcare, disability aids or to alleviate temporary financial hardship.

• Sometimes a very simple action will help, for example going through the medical records so the patient can structure the order and timing of events that may have become jumbled and confused in their memory.

A patient harmed by treatment poses acute and painful dilemmas for the staff involved. It is natural to avoid that pain by avoiding the patient, yet the staff's response is crucial to the patient's recovery. When patients think that information is being concealed from them, or that they are being dismissed as trouble makers, it is much more difficult for them to cope with the injury. A poor explanation fuels their anger, may affect the course of their recovery and may lead patients to distrust the staff caring for them. They may then avoid having further treatment – which in most cases they very much need. In contrast, an honest explanation and a promise to continue treatment may enhance the patient's trust and strengthen the relationship.

Patients, whether or not they have suffered an adverse event, would generally like to be fully informed about any significant error. Both qualitative and quantitative studies have found that doctors generally underestimate the information that patients would like about errors and adverse outcomes [11] (see Chapter 12). Being defensive and failing to explain after adverse outcomes is a major cause of litigation and a source of bitterness and anger from patients. Conversely, being open with patients can dramatically alter their reaction and promote a climate of trust. When there has been a significant error or a bad outcome doctors should take the initiative to seek out the patient and/or family and discuss the situation openly and honestly. James Pichert and Gerald Hickson [12] have provided a thoughtful but practical discussion of communication after adverse events (Box 13.3).

Very often staff and managers are frightened to apologise to patients if there is a risk of litigation in case this is seen as an admission of guilt. However, a genuine expression of sympathy and saying sorry for what has happened is possible without admitting possible negligence or incompetence. Role modelling by senior clinicians and training in this area will help staff support patients and their relatives without being encumbered with fear of admitting culpability. It may be particularly difficult for clinicians who have made a serious error to inform and support the patient or family afterwards. However, if there is a good working professional relationship this communication may be very important to both parties; sharing the

---

Box 13.3: Communication after an error or adverse outcome
(adapted from Pichert & Hickson [12])

- Give bad news in a private place where the patient and/or family may react and you can respond appropriately.
- Clearly deliver the message. The adverse outcome must be understood: 'I'm sad to report that the procedure resulted in x and, as you may recall, that means y'.
- Wait silently for a reaction. Give the patient/family time to consider what has happened and formulate their questions.
- Deal with the reaction(s). The usual reaction to bad news is a mixture of denial, anger, resignation, shock, etc. Listen. Acknowledge feelings.
- Resist the urge to blame or appear to blame other health professionals for the outcome.
- Discuss transition support. Tell the patient/family what steps might come next to provide medical, social or other forms of support.
- Finish by reassuring them about your continued willingness to answer any questions they might have. Discuss the next step. Afterwards, document a summary of the discussion.
- Consider scheduling a follow-up meeting. Some patients will want to talk only after the crisis has subsided.

results of a subsequent investigation may be a particularly important point of resolution. Sometimes, however, the patient or their family does not want to see the people who may have been responsible for errors and this wish should be respected. Ensuring that the patient and family have another person in the organisation with whom they are officially linked is crucial here.

The initiatives of individual clinicians and risk managers must be strongly supported by board-level policy and directives. It is quite unreasonable to expect any clinician to be honest and open about problems that have occurred if they will later face sanctions from senior management. All health care organisations need a strong proactive policy of active intervention and monitoring of those patients whose treatment has caused harm. Clearly there is an ethical imperative to inform patients of adverse outcomes, but the fear of legal action and media attention can act as a major disincentive. Nevertheless, those organisations that have followed the path of open disclosure have not been overwhelmed by lawsuits and have argued strongly for others to follow [13,14]. Open disclosure is now a recommended practice by organisations such as England's National Patient Safety Agency and the Australian Safety and Quality Council [15] (Box 13.4).

Box 13.4: Patient information sheet on open disclosure (adapted from Australian Safety and Quality Council [15])

When we need to visit a health care professional we can expect to receive the safest health care available. But sometimes things may not work out as expected. For example, a patient may be given the wrong dose of medicine. Or there may be complications after surgery that mean the result is not as good as expected. Most adverse events are minor and do not result in harm. When a patient is harmed they have a right to know what has happened and why.

If an adverse event occurs the hospital needs to follow a process of open disclosure. This means that the patients and their family or carers are told, as soon as possible after the event, what has happened and what will be done about it. An important part of the process is finding out exactly what went wrong, why it went wrong and actively looking for ways to stop it happening again.

What can I expect if something goes wrong?
If something goes wrong during your hospital visit, a member of the hospital staff will talk to you and your family and carers about what happened. You can also discuss any changes to your ongoing care plan because of the adverse event.

In this situation you have the right:
• To have a support person of your choice present at the discussion.
• To ask for a second opinion from another health care professional.
• To pursue a complaints process.

(Continued p. 187)

Box 13.4: (Continued)

• To nominate specific people (family or carers) who you would like to be involved.

• To make the process easier we will ask you to nominate someone (a member of your family, close friend or hospital patient advocate) to support you during your stay in hospital.

Who at the hospital will speak to me?

The person who talks to you about what happened is likely to be one of the health care team that is looking after you. However, if you have difficulty talking to this person you can nominate someone else. Ideally this will be someone who:

• You are comfortable with and can talk to easily.

• Has been involved in your care and knows the facts.

• Has enough authority to begin action to stop the problem happening again.

Who else will be present?

The person who will be discussing what happened is also able to have someone there to assist and support them. When something goes wrong it is distressing for the patient and their carers, but is also traumatic for the health care team involved. Sometimes discussion after the event can become quite emotional or heated. Having someone there who is not as closely involved can help you to make the discussion more constructive. This is likely to assist you as well as the health team member.

What will happen afterwards?

As part of the open disclosure process, if something does go wrong, steps are taken to prevent it from happening again. The hospital will investigate what went wrong. You will be informed of the results and the changes that will be made to prevent the same thing from happening to someone else. If the investigation takes a long time, you will be kept up to date with its progress. If you wish, a meeting will be arranged for you to discuss the results of the investigation when it is finished.

Impact on staff

Reactions to error and adverse outcomes in medicine are greatly magnified because so much can be at stake. Few other professions face the possibility of causing the death of another person with such regularity, although the likelihood of this varies hugely in different areas of health care. The typical reaction has been well expressed by Albert Wu in his aptly titled paper 'Medical error: the second victim' [16]:

Virtually every clinician knows the sickening feeling of making a bad mistake. You feel singled out and exposed – seized by the instinct to see if anyone has noticed. You agonize about what to do, whether to tell anyone, what to say. Later, the event replays itself in your mind. You question your competence but fear being discovered. You know you should confess, but dread the prospect of potential punishment and of the patient's anger.

When a patient is harmed those involved are more likely to blame themselves than if an error occurred and no harm resulted. However, the causes of adverse events are complex. Many could not have been prevented: some are the result of genuine uncertainty in diagnosis and decision making. Even where errors have occurred, they are often only part of a chain of events inseparable from a web of organisational background causes. Seldom, after close analysis, is it possible to lay the blame for an adverse outcome solely at the door of one individual, however tempting this may be. Junior doctors, for instance, may find themselves forced to deal with events that are well beyond their competence. Even senior clinicians will be more likely to make errors of judgment and wrong diagnoses where resources are inadequate and systems are ineffective. Where many decisions need to be made at once, for example in intensive care or emergency departments or labour wards, the wrong decision is more likely. Moreover, people are particularly vulnerable to error at times of stress. It is difficult for the clinician not to feel guilty and responsible for the error despite extenuating circumstances. For those staff in the front line who may be the inheritors of problems elsewhere in the organisation, to then take responsibility and shoulder all the blame may be unwarranted and personally damaging.

There is very little research in this area and the extent and nature of reactions to error among doctors, midwives, nurses and others is not well understood. However, it is clear that reactions can be profound. In a series of 11 in-depth interviews, Christensen and colleagues [17] discussed a variety of serious mistakes, including four deaths. All the doctors were affected to some degree, but four clinicians described intense agony or anguish as the reality of the mistake had sunk in. The interviews also identified a number of general themes: the ubiquity of mistakes in clinical practice; the infrequency of self-disclosure about mistakes to colleagues, friends and family; the emotional impact on the physician, such that some mistakes were remembered in great detail even after several years; and the influence of beliefs about personal responsibility and medical practice. After the initial shock the clinicians had a variety of reactions that had lasted from several days to several months. Some of the feelings of fear, guilt, anger, embarrassment and humiliation were unresolved at the time of the interview, even a year after the mistake.

Sometimes it may be difficult to know exactly why somebody has died or suffered injury. In this situation the clinician may go over the incident doubting judgments made and decisions taken. Guilt is a part of grief and just as the family may feel guilty about the death or illness or injury of their loved ones, professionals may suffer a grief reaction that involves feelings of guilt that may not be justified. The knowledge that you may have caused the death or disability of another is very hard to bear. It should be recognised also that when there has been a poor outcome, whether or not an error has been made, that the staff involved may not be able to work effectively. For instance, in a recent example, a midwife was very shaken after caring for a baby who was born unexpectedly in very poor condition with the distinct possibility of long-term sequelae. Rather than being given a chance to recover she was sent immediately to look after another woman in labour who needed highly complex care, thereby also increasing the risk to the second woman.

The reaction of the patient and their family may be especially hard to bear, particularly when the outcome is severe and if there has been a close involvement over a long period of time. The reaction of colleagues, whether supportive or defensive and critical, may be equally powerful. Finally, clinicians, like everyone else, vary in temperament, resilience and attitude to their own errors. For a highly self-critical person, errors and mistakes will be particularly disturbing [18]. The high personal standards of excellent clinicians may in fact make them particularly vulnerable to the impact of mistakes. This tendency may be reinforced during medical training, in that the culture of medical schools and residencies imply that mistakes are unacceptable and, when serious, indicate a failure of effort or character [19].

Feelings of guilt and recrimination in the professional involved in a medical error may be difficult for others – both family friends and colleagues – to understand. In the worst circumstances the professional feeling guilt and suffering depression may be cut off from potential support, and these reactions may affect the family of the professional, even if they are not clear what the problem is. It is invaluable to have a trusted and experienced colleague go through the case helping to view the situation in a balanced way. Expert professional counselling is crucial, and it may be helpful to extend this to the family of the professional too.

The impact of errors and mistakes is compounded and deepened when followed by a complaint or litigation, the incidence of which have become increasingly common in the last 20 years. Patients now demand much more of the doctor or other health professionals, and may be less forgiving when their own expectations of outcome are not fulfilled, though are rightly angry when no apology or explanation is given. Litigation can clearly be very unpleasant, and occasionally traumatic [20,21], but the impact of litigation should not be overstated. Often, when the case is clear-cut and the harm not severe, or at least not permanent, it may be little more than tedious. In the UK at least, very few cases ever reach trial, almost all being settled by lawyers and risk managers, sometimes with little involvement of the clinical staff (which is sometimes welcome and sometimes not).

Staff who have been involved in a medical accident or poor outcome will be helped by knowing that the organisation is able to conduct the enquiry from a basis of natural justice. The result of an internal enquiry may indeed be a life sentence if the reputation, confidence and competence of the professional is at stake. Professionals should have the right to similar standards of investigation that apply in the legal system. This involves avoiding prejudice and using balanced arguments and consideration of the evidence, in the same way that is expected in a court of law. It should be recognised that there is an inherent conflict in both supporting staff and investigating potential errors or professional negligence or incompetence. Providing experienced counselling from outside the department or the organisation for staff who are the subject of an internal investigation is particularly important.

Finally, we should just step back for a moment and reflect, from the perspective of both clinician and patient, on why litigation has to happen at all. Although some people will always complain, and a few unpleasant or deluded characters delight in litigation, in fact very few patients sue. This is partly because, whatever the rights and wrongs of the case, it is a deeply wearing experience in which they constantly have to recall experiences they would much prefer to forget. When they do sue it is for explanations, apologies, to bring about change in the system and, to a widely varying extent, for money [10]. As was said earlier, for most of the deserving cases all of these things could be provided by proactive health care organisations without litigation, and in fact without the need for legislation on no-fault compensation. This in turn would make life a great deal easier for the staff involved – when care had been substandard, they would know the patient and family were being supported. When care had been satisfactory, and a case had to be defended, they would have the organisation firmly on their side.

Supporting staff

Understanding that mistakes will always occur, and that reacting to them is ordinary and in fact necessary for learning, is a first step. Being understanding of others when they are in that unenviable position is a vital step towards a more open, indeed a safer, culture. Individual clinicians can do a great deal here, whatever their profession or seniority, to promote a more constructive and supportive approach to errors. However, there is no doubt that the wider organisation and context play a large part in the way a health care professional will react to an error or harm to a patient. Just as systems thinking is needed to understand how harm comes about, it is also needed to appreciate how things unfold afterwards. Many initiatives that are aimed to help patients, such as a policy of open disclosure, can also be a considerable help to staff. Supporting patients and supporting staff are not separate activities, but inextricably intertwined.

The culture of medicine does not make it easy for either doctors or nurses to ask for or receive the support they need after a major incident [22]. In one of the few studies of the aftermath of serious incidents, Newman found that doctors recognise the likely effects on their colleagues but, for various reasons, found it difficult to offer support [23]. News of a major incident spreads rapidly. Those directly involved, in addition to feeling anxious and

ashamed, may also feel isolated. However, a number of things can be done to limit the damage and support those involved:
• Be open about errors and their frequency. Senior staff talking openly about past mistakes and problems is particularly effective.
• Accept that a need for support is not a sign of weakness. Clinicians are resilient people but almost all are grateful for the support of colleagues when disaster strikes.
• Provide clear guidelines for the discussion of error with patients backed up by board-level policy on open disclosure.
• Offer training in the difficult task of communicating with patient and families in the aftermath of an adverse event.
• Provide basic education in the law and the legal process, which should reduce some of the anxiety about legal action.
• Offer support to staff after major incidents. This may simply be informal support from a colleague. For a particularly profound reaction, perhaps to the death of a child, formal psychological intervention may be valuable.

Conclusion

We suggested at the beginning of this chapter that the aftermath of error and harm has been much neglected in risk management and patient safety. There is little research on the aftermath of error, and you will seldom hear it discussed at conferences, except in the context of avoiding litigation. There are certainly many people, patients, nurses, doctors, lawyers and others, working for a more humane approach to the people affected by errors and harm, but it is still very much an uphill battle. We suggest, however, that given the avowed aim of patient safety to reduce the harm caused by health care, that the aftermath is one of the most important and potentially most fruitful areas for both research and action.

References

1 Vincent C. *Patient Safety*. Elsevier Churchill Livingstone, Edinburgh, 2006.
2 Clarke DM, Russell PA, Polglase AL, McKenzie DP. Psychiatric disturbance and acute stress response in surgical patients. *Australia and New Zealand Journal of Surgery* 1997; **67** (2/3): 115–18.
3 Czarnocka J, Slade P. Prevalence and predictors of post-traumatic stress symptoms following childbirth. *British Journal of Clinical Psychology* 2000; **39** (1): 35–51.
4 Brewin CR, Dalgleish T, Joseph S. A dual representation theory of post-traumatic stress disorder. *Psychological Review* 1996; **103** (4): 670–86.
5 Vincent CA, Pincus T, Scurr JH. Patients' experience of surgical accidents. *Quality in Health Care* 1993; **2** (2): 77–82.
6 Vincent CA, Coulter A. Patient safety: what about the patient? *Quality and Safety in Health Care* 2002; **11** (1): 76–80.
7 Lundin T. Morbidity following sudden and unexpected bereavement. *British Journal of Psychiatry* 1984; **144**: 84–8.

8 Lehman DR, Wortman CB, Williams AF. Long-term effects of losing a spouse or child in a motor vehicle crash. *Journal of Personality and Social Psychology* 1987; **52** (1): 218–31.

9 Parkes CM. *Bereavement: Studies of Grief in Adult Life*. Penguin, London, 1988.

10 Vincent C, Young M, Phillips A. Why do people sue doctors? A study of patients and relatives taking legal action. *Lancet* 1994; **343** (8913): 1609–13.

11 Gallagher TH, Waterman AD, Ebers AG, Fraser VJ, Levinson W. Patients' and physicians' attitudes regarding the disclosure of medical errors. *Journal of the American Medical Association* 2003; **289** (8): 1001–7.

12 Pichert J, Hickson G. Communicating risk to patients and families. *In*: Vincent CA, ed. *Clinical Risk Management: Enhancing Patient Safety*. BMJ Books, London, 2001: 263–82.

13 Kraman SS, Hamm G. Risk management: extreme honesty may be the best policy. *Annals of Internal Medicine* 1999; **131** (12): 963–7.

14 Lamb RM, Studdert DM, Bohmer RM, Berwick DM, Brennan TA. Hospital disclosure practices: results of a national survey. *Health Affairs* 2003; **22** (2): 73–83.

15 Australian Safety and Quality Council. *What is Open Disclosure?* Australian Safety and Quality Council. Sydney, Australia, 2004. Available at http://www.safetyandquality.org.

16 Wu A. Medical error: the second victim. *British Medical Journal* 2000; **320** (7237): 726–7.

17 Christensen JF, Levinson W, Dunn PM. The heart of darkness: the impact of perceived mistakes on physicians. *Journal of General Internal Medicine* 1992; **7** (4): 424–31.

18 Firth-Cozens J. Stress, psychological problems and clinical performance. *In*: Vincent CA, Ennis M, Audley RJ, eds. *Medical Accidents*. Oxford University Press, Oxford, 1993: 131–49.

19 Leape LL. Error in medicine. *Journal of the American Medical Association* 1994; **272** (23): 1851–7.

20 Charles SC. The doctor–patient relationship and medical malpractice litigation. *Bulletin of the Menninger Clinic* 1993; **57** (2): 195–207.

21 Bark P, Vincent C, Olivieri L, Jones A. Impact of litigation on senior clinicians: implications for risk management. *Quality in Health Care* 1997; **6** (1): 7–13.

22 Ely JW. Physicians' mistakes. Will your colleagues offer support? *Archives of Family Medicine* 1996; **5** (2): 76–7.

23 Newman MC. The emotional impact of mistakes on family physicians. *Archives of Family Medicine* 1996; **5** (2): 71–5.

CHAPTER 14

Significant event auditing and root cause analysis

Mike Pringle

Until the middle of the 19th century, delineation of individual cases and series of cases constituted a great deal of the medical evidence base. Descriptions were founded on careful history taking, observation, clinical examination, case discussion on ward rounds and the findings of postmortem examination.

While this system was not perfect, relying as it did on the perceptions and clinical distinctions of individual doctors concerning particular cases it successfully created the greater part of the classification of diseases still in use today. A similar paradigm now operates for significant event auditing and root cause analysis. Rigorous reflection on individual patients or small groups of patients can increase understanding of patient experience, quality of care, origins of harm and the ways of providing better, safer health care.

Over the past 150 years a different but complementary approach to quality assurance also developed. Although the use of statistics to report on causes of death was commonplace many years before, it was the audits conducted by Florence Nightingale in the Crimea [1] that started the modern interest in quantitative surveys. As we shall see, general practice in the UK, as elsewhere, largely developed its quality assurance methods in the cohort audit mould using statistics based on substantial populations.

Much of the recent interest in case-based auditing originated from analyses of adverse events, often in hospitals in the USA [2]. This re-emergence of case-based auditing has rebalanced the portfolio of quality of care studies. Neither cohort nor case-based audits is intrinsically superior to the other and both have drawbacks. But when used together they can be complementary, in developing a culture in which opportunities for quality of care are maximised.

This chapter looks at case-based auditing, its background, its uses and its effects. In primary care, case-based auditing is often referred to as significant event auditing, and one of the techniques within it is the rigorous analysis of causes of error and harm, called root cause analysis.

Health Care Errors and Patient Safety. Edited by Brian Hurwitz and Aziz Sheikh.
© 2009 Blackwell Publishing, ISBN: 978-1-4051-4643-2.

Background

In 1901 a massive inscribed stone was found in the hills of Iran bearing the Code of Hammurabi (king of Babylon between 1795 and 1750 BC) [3]. Among other laws, this code stipulated the loss of a surgeon's hand that caused the loss of life or limb in a patient. While draconian, this must have focused the physicians' minds on individual cases rather than key performance indicators.

Seminal descriptions of diseases, perhaps most eloquently by Osler [4] in the late 1800s, were based on single cases or small series. Freud built his general observations on singular cases, illustrating perhaps both the power of case studies and the risk of their mis- or overinterpretation.

While the clinical tradition in British hospitals, despite the work of Nightingale, developed around the clinical presentation of individual patients, a crisis in New York's hospitals demonstrated the value of auditing cohorts of patients, as in Codman's pioneering work [5]. Codman's heir was Avadis Donabedian, who coined the triad for cohort auditing – structure, process and outcome [6]. From the early part of the 20th century case-based observation was retained as a foundation of teaching and clinical decision making, but evidence and quality assurance was increasingly undertaken through the analysis of cohorts of patients.

As general practice developed in Britain, especially as it was re-energised by the 1965 GP Charter [7], it naturally looked to quantitative audit methodologies. This has persisted through to the Quality and Outcomes Framework of the 2004 General Medical Services Contract, which financially rewards general practitioners according to the results of detailed computerised surveys of their care – the audit cycle is completed with the re-surveying annually with financial incentives for improved performance.

It was not, of course, that clear-cut. Balint groups were using individual patients' stories to create generalisable verities [8]. Random case analysis was used extensively in monitoring the care of young doctors' vocational training for general practice from the late 1960s onwards [9]. Confidential enquiries, such as the first ones into maternal deaths [10,11] and anaesthetic deaths [12], created a system around case-based auditing, combining it with some of the merits of cohort auditing.

Inception of significant event auditing to the present day

Significant event auditing did not arise in a vacuum. The value of reflecting on individual cases was being discussed [13–17] and reservations identified [18]. The first description of significant event auditing – the systematic use of single cases for quality assurance – was in 1994 by Pringle and Bradley [19]. They went on to undertake and report a randomised controlled trial of significant event auditing in 20 British general practices, demonstrating its feasibility and effectiveness as part of a portfolio of auditing methodologies [20].

It has become clear that case-based auditing has a strong link to behavioural change. It has been shown that people change their behaviour after one big message or three medium-sized ones [21]. While conventional evidence sources, such as articles in the literature or reports from conventional audits, by and large operate at a cerebral level, significant event auditing operates at both a cerebral and emotional level. Since change is both an intellectual and an emotive event, it is not surprising that case-based auditing achieves change.

Many teams value the discussions involved during the course of significant event auditing which help members to understand each other's values and behaviours. Peer assessment, accreditation, contracts and regulation are additional motives for taking part in significant event auditing [22].

At first the extent of support from the National Health Service (NHS) was the creation of Medical Audit Advisory Groups (and their successor organisations) in every Family Health Services Authority area [23]. In time the Department of Health began, largely through the leadership of the Chief Medical Officer, Sir Liam Donaldson, to develop policies and systems to support quality enhancement. These have included clinical governance [24], the recognition of patient safety through *An Organisation with a Memory* [25] and the formation of the National Patient Safety Agency [26]. The secure place of significant event auditing in UK general practice is illustrated by its inclusion as a quality marker in Fellowship by Assessment of the Royal College of General Practitioners and in its inclusion within the terms of the 2004 General Medical Services Contract.

What is significant event auditing?

Significant event auditing is a process applied in general practice and community care [27] comprising systematic examination and reflection on individual cases. It is not referred to in the same way in other settings, except the related context of prison care [28], and there is no reported use of the methodology in hospital care – although case conferences and confidential enquiries fulfil a similar role. It appears to be a predominantly UK concept, although there are some reports of its use from Australia [29,30].

The purpose of significant event auditing is to learn lessons and improve patient safety through the regular and methodical assessment of the care experienced by individuals [31,32]. Box 14.1 examines the nomenclature in this area, placing significant event auditing in context.

Significant event auditing can be used for any event that occurs in health care. The event might be clinical, such a new diagnosis of breast cancer, or administrative, such as a referral not being made. It can be noted by any member of the practice team or be prompted by a patient through a comment or complaint. The essence is that at least one member of the team thinks that the event might offer worthwhile insights. Before describing types of significant event auditing, there are generic ground rules that apply to all types that need to be understood and followed (Box 14.2).

Box 14.1: The definition of some terms used in case-based auditing focusing on patient safety

• A *patient safety incident* is any unintended or unexpected incident that could or did lead to harm for one or more patients receiving health care [33]. It includes adverse health care events and near-misses.
• An *adverse health care event* is an event or omission arising during clinical care and causing physical or psychological injury to the patient [25]. One of these is also referred to as a *critical incident*.
• A *health care near-miss* is a situation in which an event or omission, or a sequence of events or omissions, arising during clinical care fails to develop further, whether or not as a result of compensating action, thus preventing injury to a patient [25].
• A *significant event* is a patient safety incident (including therefore adverse health care events and near-misses), an expected adverse outcome, a patient-defined outcome (such as a complaint) or a circumstance that can be used to reflect on the quality of care.
• In *significant event auditing* individual cases in which there has been a significant occurrence (not necessarily involving an undesirable outcome for the patient) are analysed in a systematic and detailed way to ascertain what can be learnt about the overall quality of care and to indicate changes that might lead to future improvements [20].
• *Root cause analysis* is a process for investigating and categorising the underlying causes of adverse health care events [34] – finding and dealing with the real cause of the problem rather than simply continuing to deal with the symptoms. It can be part of a significant event audit that throws up a complex problem.
• *Risk management* is the process of ensuring that the learning from case-based auditing is embedded into systems and practice to reduce the chance of future harm [35].
• *Clinical governance* is the process for ensuring that all elements – auditing, root cause analysis and risk management – are occurring effectively.

Models of significant event auditing

There are several models of significant event auditing described in the literature, clustered around the following themes:
• Mortality.
• Patient safety incidents, including critical incidents, adverse health care events and near-misses.
• Random case analysis.
• Marker conditions.
• Mixed methods.
Mortality is a particular example of a marker, but with a sufficient tradition to be considered separately. Growing out of postmortems, perinatal mortality

---

Box 14.2: The ground rules for significant event auditing

Although these rules are not mandatory, following them should increase the probability of a successful outcome. If they are impractical – for example, where there is no trust between team members – significant event auditing may not be possible or desirable.

1 There needs to be protected quality time put aside.

2 It should be conducted in an atmosphere of honesty, openness and trust, without blame allocation. This is not a method for identifying culprits or dealing with poor performance.

3 Although a team member or several team members may have made an error or delivered suboptimal care, any member of the team might equally have done so. There needs to be a culture of learning from the experience of others and changing systems to prevent recurrence – a culture that benefits all the team members.

4 The team members most involved in an event should be asked to present it and reflect on it, recognising shortfalls in care, before others contribute.

5 Other team members should ask questions to clarify the information, delving deeper if necessary, but to do so positively, offering constructive suggestions that they themselves might act on.

6 A period of information gathering and analysis before decision making is often valuable. An event may be discussed at several meetings before resolution.

7 Decisions on root causes and on actions to take should be based on available evidence and best practice.

8 Agreed actions should be proportionate to the risk and the severity of effect of recurrence.

---

meetings and confidential enquiries, teams have looked at terminal care [36], asthma deaths [37], suicides [38] and deaths following accidents [39]. It was natural that early applications of significant event auditing in primary care should look at an outcome that was well defined, easily identified and dramatic in its implications. Case-based discussions concerning deaths were among the early publications [40–43] and they continue to be used, often as a starting point.

Some teams have chosen to look at events that may indicate that harm has occurred, or might have occurred. The implication is that some harm is avoidable, and there are lessons from these that need to be learnt, but some harm is inevitable. We accept that even under the most ideal circumstances some patients will experience side effects of their medication, or develop a deep vein thrombosis after surgery. The art is to identify those events in which there was an avoidable element and to decide on a proportionate response.

A team can either wait until a team member has identified such an event and convene a discussion, or can identify circumstances in which adverse health care events are most likely to be found. Some have focused on patient complaints [46] and litigation [47], waiting times after referrals for potential cancer [48], difficult prescribing decisions [49] or the use of investigations [50].

Random case analysis is used educationally and in the assessment of clinicians – for example for Membership by Assessment of Performance and Fellowship by Assessment of the Royal College of General Practitioners, or in the General Medical Council's performance procedures – but is not described as an effective auditing tool in the literature. Despite that, there are practices that have used random case analysis as an entrée into significant event auditing, as a way to develop mutual trust and confidence.

Significant event analysis should use all these techniques, but with an emphasis on two sources of cases. The first is those events or circumstances where a team member thinks that an adverse health care event has happened. The second is the routine listing of a number of marker conditions. This is a mixed approach that maximises the chances of a systematic problem being revealed. In the first category a general practice team might wish to identify for potential discussion anything that occurs that raises questions of patient safety: from a serious prescribing error through to a problem with the rota that led to understaffing on a particular day. However, these cases are supplemented by lists of all cases with a number of marker conditions (usually generated through computer searches) such as in Table 14.1.

Process of significant event auditing

There are many ways to conduct significant event auditing, and every team will evolve its own methods [51]. However, here I will describe one approach that can be adapted to individual circumstances.

One of the recurrent objections to taking part in significant event auditing is the lack of time. There are a number of arguments against this – we should never be too busy to care about improving quality, but the most powerful is two-fold. First it takes far less time to do significant event auditing with a far greater yield than the time and effort put into conventional auditing. The second argument is that significant event auditing is genuinely enjoyable. It may seem daunting to discuss a case where you failed to respond to an abnormal pathology result when it first crossed your desk, but the mutual support and exploration of how it can be prevented from happening again should be genuinely energising.

Most practices put aside 1 hour every month either at lunchtime or at the end of the day. Practices report anecdotally that these are the meetings with the best attendance and the most buzz. It is ideal if the patient's electronic health record can be projected or displayed on a big screen so everybody can follow case presentations. It is for each practice to decide who is invited. Many would automatically include the doctors, nurses (practice and

Table 14.1 Events in the life of a general practice team that might be routinely listed for potential discussion in a significant event audit meeting.

Marker events	Reason for listing
All new diagnoses of cancer (except basal cell carcinoma)	To audit opportunities for prevention and early detection, the process of care (waiting times, interventions, etc.) and psychological and social support
All new diagnoses of ischaemic heart disease and stroke	To audit opportunities for prevention (smoking, blood pressure, weight, cholesterol), the process of care (acute or emergency care) and continuing care (including nursing)
All episodes of meningitis, measles, mumps, rubella, whooping cough and bacterial gastroenteritis in children	To audit immunisation and the advice offered, the process of care (acute or emergency care, public health interventions) and psychological and social support
All positive cervical smears or mammography results	To audit opportunities for prevention (including previous tests and advice given), the process of care (waiting times, interventions, etc.) and psychological and social support
All unexpected deaths (i.e. those discussed with the coroner's office)	To audit opportunities for prevention and intervention, and psychological and social support
All palliative or terminal care cases	To audit the process of care and psychological and social support
All unplanned pregnancies	To audit contraceptive care offered and delivered
All emergency visits or admissions for acute asthma, epileptic fit or parasuicide	To audit prevention and emergency care
All prescribing or dispensing errors or administrative errors (home visit not done, breach of confidentiality, etc.)	To audit the process of care and management of the risk
All informal or formal complaints or suggestions from patients	To audit the sources of complaint or comments

community) and senior managers and receptionists. Some practices are more inclusive, but there has to be a balance between all those who can contribute to an honest discussion and creating such a large group that discussion of sensitive issues, such as errors, is inhibited. One practice has been reported to have included a patient representative at meetings to discuss significant events: this might be more common than I think.

Since each meeting is minuted, a significant event audit meeting should start with looking at agreed actions from the last or previous meetings. Minutes do not have to be exhaustive but if a significant event yields an important discussion, the key elements of that discussion need to be captured. Agreed actions with the people to take them forward and a timescale should be meticulously recorded. Patients should only be identified by practice or NHS number in the minutes.

Cases potentially identified for discussion should be identified by initials and number, and be allocated to a key team member to lead on in the description of what happened. Each person present can then be asked to choose one case, rotating around the room until everybody has had a chance to present a case. If there is time, a second trip around the room can occur. Each person can choose a case allocated to them or to someone else if they were involved. The person should choose an event that they think offers the best chance of a useful discussion. If there is no obvious case, then a random one from the list is chosen. For each case, the person (or persons) most involved in the event gives the story aided by the medical records or other material. They are given a chance to reflect on the event, drawing out issues for discussion. Then the event is open for group discussion. After sufficient time to explore the event, the action points, if any, are agreed.

The outcome (or outcomes) of a significant event discussion come within these categories:

1 *Congratulations and recognition of good care.* This is a real strength of significant event auditing. Although errors and adverse events are discussed, many events discussed reveal good care that was previously unrecognised. It may be an astute or early diagnosis, prompt and effective care in a crisis or a particularly caring approach to a patient or their family. Recognising and acknowledging excellence may be rare but can be a major outcome of this process.

2 *There are no lessons to be learnt.* Often case discussions reveal a perfectly normal process of care with no special issues to be picked out. These discussions are usually very short – maybe a minute or so – and the baton moves on to another person and another event.

3 *Immediate action must be taken.* This should be an outcome that is used with caution, but it is often appropriate. For example, if a doctor reports that she discovered that an injectable drug was out of date, then a system for regularly checking doctors' bags should be agreed.

4 *A learning need must be met.* An event may reveal a learning need for the team member most involved, but the learning need may be shared.

A patient's sudden collapse on the surgery premises might reveal that the nurse and doctor involved need retraining in cardiopulmonary resuscitation. Other team members might agree they need it too.

5 *A learning point is agreed.* Often everybody knows what they should do and how a system should work, but they just did not do it or they did not apply the system correctly on that occasion. Sometimes the lesson learnt is just to be alert to the risk and to be aware of the need to avoid it.

6 *Information and evidence is needed.* Often there will be issues of fact ('What time was the ambulance called?') or of evidence ('What dose should have been given?'). A team member will be asked to report back to the next meeting. Often the evidence is a conventional audit. If an event shows that a patient had failed to attend for review of their warfarin, a cohort audit is needed to find out if this is an isolated occurrence or is common.

7 *A fuller investigation is required.* This is termed a root cause analysis (see below) and a team member might wish to consult people outside the practice team to help achieve an understanding of exactly what is the underlying problem and what solutions may be required.

8 *A new policy, protocol or guideline.* The end result of a significant event, or more usually a number of events, is a new policy which contains statements within it that are auditable either through cohort audit or through significant event discussions.

The last two elements in the significant event process are monitoring and reporting. Where a change or action is agreed, it must be followed through. If a nurse identifies a learning need, there must be a tracking tool to ensure it is met, such as a spreadsheet that records dates, the need is identified, how it can be met and when it has been met.

Every year the team should ask for a report on the previous year's significant event auditing. This is a chance to reflect on the range of issues identified and to highlight those actions which have not been carried though. Sometimes this is because, on reflection or in the light of further evidence, the action was subsequently agreed to be inappropriate. Some actions take time to be completed. Most teams find such a review reinforces their confidence in significant event auditing, builds their culture of quality improvement and, by inclusion in their practice report, shows patients and others that the practice team is striving for excellence.

Root cause analysis

A root cause analysis is one possible important outcome from a significant event discussion. It is an attempt to get beyond a superficial action designed solely to prevent an event recurring towards an understanding of the causal problems and the actions needed for resolution. It may require one team member to do some sleuthing, or it may involve a team being convened with meetings and reports. Sometimes it involves bringing in outside 'experts'.

Three case studies illustrate root cause analysis (Box 14.3). In each of these cases a superficial approach, addressing the presenting problem, might have been considered sufficient. However, sometimes the real problem is much more deep seated and can only be established through systematic investigation. Where such an enquiry is thought to be useful, a clear mandate needs to be given. But despite that, root cause analysis can provoke strong emotions and these need to be handled sensitively. Often these analyses reveal long-standing organisational issues, personal foibles or behaviour which some team members will resist changing.

Box 14.3: Examples of root cause analyses

Example 1

The practice manager presented an informal patient complaint – a remark made to a member of the patient participation group which was passed on – to the significant event audit meeting. The 'complainant' had tried to make an appointment for her elderly mother one Tuesday afternoon. She said she had specifically mentioned chest pain but had been offered an appointment for the next morning. During the evening her mother had deteriorated and had been admitted to hospital. While a heart attack had been excluded and the problem was found to be a chest infection, the daughter felt that her mother should have been seen on the afternoon that she phoned.

The practice team might have decided that the manager should check receptionist understanding of the reception triage protocol that instructs them to alert the doctor on call if someone requests an urgent appointment complaining of certain symptoms including chest pain. But when she spoke to the receptionists on duty that afternoon a pattern became apparent. There had been another similar event several months before. Tuesday and Thursday afternoons are 'clinic afternoons' when the diabetes clinic, asthma clinic, family planning and cytology clinic, and the well person clinics run. A nurse and the practice manager were asked to look into the problem.

When they reported back a month later they had found that a problem with these clinic afternoons was well known to the reception staff. They are scheduled at a popular time for elderly patients and the consultations are often booked up several days ahead. At this time few routine consultations are available because doctors and nurses are involved in clinics. On that particular Tuesday the receptionists had been reluctant to increase the surgery sessions to accommodate urgent cases because they knew that the two doctors consulting were the trainer and the registrar and they had a regular teaching session at 4:00 pm after surgery. If surgery time ate into teaching time the trainer would be very 'grumpy'. The team agreed with the practice manager's recommendation that the nurse practitioner should see urgent cases starting mid-afternoon on Tuesdays and Thursdays.

(Continued)

Box 14.3: (Continued)

Example 2

A practice found that its relationship with the local primary care trust (PCT) was proving difficult. Community nursing rotas were changed without consultation; upgrades to the computer were difficult to get agreed and were slow to be implemented; and recently their prescribing had been criticised by the PCT – they felt unfairly. The practice partners discussed these events and each time had written to the PCT; in consequence, they felt they were being deemed to be a 'problem practice'.

When a PCT-appointed team undertook a routine visit to the practice, the partners seized the chance to talk to the leader of the visiting team, a local general practitioner (GP), who offered to mediate. In discussions with both sides it emerged that the practice manager considered himself considerably more skilled and qualified than the managers in the PCT, whom he treated condescendingly and aggressively. Through sensitive discussion the practice manager acknowledged the problem and relations improved. However it was not until the practice manger moved to another post a year or so later that the relationships between practice and PCT fully healed.

Example 3

At a significant event audit meeting, the case of a man recently diagnosed with malignant melanoma was presented. While the clinical care had been unremarkable, an issue with the referral process was reported by the practice manager. The patient had been referred routinely when clearly a cancer had been suspected and the fast-track procedure should have been used. In fact, the practice secretary had noticed it and raised it with the GP and the patient had been fast tracked and therefore no time had been lost. The meeting commended the secretary for her alertness and all clinicians agreed to be careful to use the right referral channel in future.

One of the GPs and a practice nurse, however, were still concerned about the matter. The doctor making the referral had been a retired partner whom the practice employed from time to time as a locum. They felt that nobody had wanted to discuss this in the meeting because the practice was grateful for her availability.

The GP and the practice nurse made some enquiries and presented their concerns at the next significant event audit meeting. Several other instances of potentially worrying problems with the locum's work had emerged; it was felt that she was not keeping up-to-date and was doing too little clinical work. It was decided not to use this doctor as a locum in future.

Almost all the use of locums was on a Wednesday due to one partner's role in a research project at the local university. The practice manager was asked to review the GP and nurse rotas as a result of which she was able to change the Wednesday cover to ensure that locums would no longer be required.

Conclusion

Significant event auditing is one element, and only one element, of a learning organisation. It is not an end in itself and if it were the only quality enhancement strategy adopted by a team it would be relatively ineffective. However, it can be an essential driver in a number of related activities and systems, both internal and external to the practice. Internally, the links to conventional cohort auditing and routine data collection for monitoring quality must be clear. The educational agenda for individual team members, groups and for the whole practice should be fed by significant event discussions, and education should inform the discussions within the significant event meetings [52,53].

The current contractual incentives for both the demonstration of care to cohorts and the undertaking of significant event auditing bring financial and quality drivers together. Significant event auditing can, of course, throw light on why some targets are not being met.

Annual appraisals have been introduced for all NHS doctors, and other health professionals will, in time, find that regular appraisal changes from being a voluntary, professional activity to being mandated. A formative appraisal looks at professional values, importantly at reflection, personal growth and education. Taking part in significant event auditing provides a great deal of the evidence required to fuel the appraisal discussions.

Soon doctors will experience periodic revalidation to demonstrate that they are up to date and fit to practise. A key element in being up to date is likely to be the demonstration of clinical audits, and one methodology for that will be significant event auditing.

Local clinical governance processes are the NHS mechanism for assuring the quality of patient care and patient safety. If clinical governance is to be effective, it must examine risk management and an important aspect of that is significant event auditing [54].

References

1 Baly M. *Florence Nightingale and the Nursing Legacy*. Croom Helm, London, 1986.
2 Brennan C, Leape L, Laird N. Incidence of adverse events and negligence in hospitalised patients. *New England Journal of Medicine* 1991; **324**: 370–4
3 http://englishatheist.org/hamcode.shtml.
4 Hinohara S, Niki H. *Osler's 'A Way of Life' and Other Addresses*. Duke University Press, Durham, NC, 2001.
5 Codman E. *A Study in Hospital Efficiency*. Thomas Todd, Boston, 1916.
6 Donabedian A. *Explorations in Quality Assessment and Monitoring. Vol. 2: The Criteria and Standards of Quality*. Health Administration Press, Ann Arbor, 1982.
7 British Medical Association. A new contract for general practitioners; a charter for the family doctor service. *British Medical Journal* 1965; **3138**: 89–91.
8 Balint M. *The Doctor, his Patient and the Illness*. Pitman Press, Tunbridge Wells, 1964.
9 Buckley G. Clinically significant events. *In*: Marinker M, ed. *Medical Audit in General Practice*. MSD Foundation, London, 1990, pp. 1–14.

10 Department of Health and Social Security. *Report on Confidential Enquiries into Maternal Deaths in England and Wales 1979–1980*. HMSO, London, 1986.
11 Hibbard B, Milner D. Reports on confidential enquiries into maternal deaths: an audit of previous recommendations. *Health Trends* 1994; **26**: 26–8.
12 Lunn J, Musher W. *Mortality Associated with Anaesthesia*. Nuffield Provincial Hospitals Trust, London, 1982.
13 Bailey T. The critical incident technique in identifying behavioural criteria of professional nursing effectiveness. *Nursing Research* 1956; **3**: 52–64.
14 Hughes J, Humphreys C. *Medical Audit in General Practice: A Practical Guide to the Literature*. King Edward's Hospital Fund for London, London, 1990.
15 Irvine D. Standards in general practice: the quality initiative revisited. *British Journal of General Practice* 1990; **40**: 75–7.
16 Marinker M. Principles. *In*: Marinker M, ed. *Medical Audit in General Practice*. MSD Foundation, London, 1990, pp. 120–43.
17 Lyons C, Gumpert R. Medical audit data: counting is not enough. *British Medical Journal* 1990; **300**: 1563–6.
18 Bradley C. Turning anecdotes into data – the critical incident technique. *Family Practice* 1992; **9**: 98–103.
19 Pringle M, Bradley C. Significant event auditing: a user's guide. *Audit Trends* 1994; **2**: 20–4.
20 Pringle M, Bradley C, Carmichael C, Wallis, H, Moore A. *Significant Event Auditing. A Study of the Feasibility and Potential of Case-based Auditing in Primary Medical Care*. Occasional Paper No. 70. Royal College of General Practitioners, London, 1995.
21 Allery L, Owen P, Robling M. Why general practitioners and consultants change their clinical practice: a critical incident study. *British Medical Journal* 1997; **314**: 870–4.
22 Bowie P, McKay J, Dalgetty E, Lough M. A qualitative study of why general practitioners may participate in significant event analysis and educational peer assessment. *Quality and Safety in Health Care* 2005; **14**: 185–9.
23 Department of Health. *Medical Audit in the Family Practitioner Services*. Health Circular No. (90)8. HMSO, London, 1990.
24 Scally G, Donaldson L. Clinical governance and the drive for quality improvement in the new NHS in England. *British Medical Journal* 1998; **317**: 61–5.
25 Department of Health. *An Organisation with a Memory*. HMSO, London, 2000.
26 National Patient Safety Agency: http://www.npsa.nhs.uk/.
27 Robinson L, Drinkwater C. A significant care audit of a community-based elderly resource team – an opportunity for multidisciplinary teams to introduce clinical governance? *Journal of Clinical Governance* 2000; **8**: 89–96.
28 Fox M, Sweeney G, Howells C, Stead J. Significant event audit in prison healthcare: changing a culture for clinical governance – a qualitative study. *Journal of Clinical Governance* 2001; **9**: 123–8.
29 Bhasdale A, Miller G, Reid S, Britt H. Analysing potential harm in Australian general practice: an incident monitoring study. *Medical Journal of Australia* 1998; **169**: 73–6.
30 Diamond M. A critical incident study of general practice trainees in their basic general practice term. *Medical Journal of Australia* 1995; **162**: 321–4.
31 Pringle M. Preventing ischaemic heart disease in one general practice: from one patient through clinical audit, needs assessment and commissioning into quality improvement. *British Medical Journal* 1998; **317**: 1120–3.
32 Westcott R, Sweeney G, Stead J. Significant event audit in general practice: a preliminary study. *Family Practice* 2000; **17**: 173–9.

33 National Patient Safety Agency. *Seven Steps to Patient Safety: A Guide for NHS Staff.* National Patient Safety Agency, London, 2003.

34 Rooney J, Vanden Heuvel L. Root cause analysis for beginners. *Quality Progress* 2004; **37** (7): 45–53.

35 Vincent C. Risk, safety, and the dark side of quality. *British Medical Journal* 1997; **314**: 1775–6.

36 Bennett I, Danczak A. Terminal care: improving teamwork in primary care using significant event analysis. *European Journal of Cancer Care* 1994; **3**: 54–7.

37 Mohan G, Harrison B, Badminton R, Mildenhall S, Wareham N. A confidential enquiry into deaths caused by asthma in an English health region: implications for general practice. *British Journal of General Practice* 1996; **46**: 529–32.

38 Matthews K, Milne S, Ashcroft G. Role of doctors in the prevention of suicide: the final consultation. *British Journal of General Practice* 1994; **44**: 345–8.

39 Hussain L, Redmond A. Are pre-hospital deaths from accidental injury preventable? *British Medical Journal* 1994; **308**: 1077–80.

40 Robinson L, Stacy R, Spencer J, Bhopal R. Use of facilitated case discussions for significant event auditing. *British Medical Journal* 1995; **311**: 315–18.

41 Khunti K. A method of creating a death register for general practice. *British Medical Journal* 1996; **312**: 952.

42 Holden J, O'Donnell S, Brindley J, Miles L. Analysis of 1263 deaths in four general practices. *British Journal of General Practice* 1998; **48**: 1409–12.

43 Berlin A, Spencer J, Bhopal R, van Zwanenberg T. Audits of deaths in general practice: pilot study of the critical incident technique. *Quality in Health Care* 1992; **1**: 231–5.

44 Britt H, Miller G, Steven I et al. Collecting data on potentially harmful events: a method for monitoring incidents in general practice. *Family Practice* 1997; **14**: 101–6.

45 Bhasale A. The wrong diagnosis: identifying causes of potentially adverse events in general practice using incident monitoring. *Family Practice* 1998; **15**: 308–18.

46 Pietroni R, de Uray-Ura S. Informal complaints procedure in general practice: first year's experience. *British Medical Journal* 1994; **308**: 1546–8.

47 Ritchie J, Davies S. Professional negligence: a duty of candid disclosure? *British Medical Journal* 1995; **310**: 888–9.

48 Holden J, Pringle M. Delay pattern analysis of 446 patients in nine practices. *Audit Trends* 1995; **3**: 96–8.

49 Bradley C, Riaz A. Barriers to effective asthma care in inner city general practice. *European Journal of General Practice* 1998; **4**: 65–8.

50 Robling M, Kinnersley P, Houston H, Hourihan M, Cohen D, Hale J. An exploration of GP's use of MRI: a critical incident study. *Family Practice* 1998; **15**: 236–43.

51 Harrison P, Joesbury H, Martin D, Wilson R, Fewtrell C. *Significant Event Audit and Reporting in General Practice.* School of Health and Related Research (SCHARR), Sheffield: 2002.

52 Care W. Identifying the learning needs of nurse managers: application of the critical incident technique. *Journal of Nursing Staff Development* 1996; **12**: 27–30.

53 Holmwood C. How do general practice registrars learn from their clinical experience? *Australian Family Physician* 1996; **26**: 36–40.

54 Stead J, Sweeney G, Westcott R. Significant event audit – a key tool for clinical governance. *Clinical Governance Bulletin* 2000; **1**: 13–14.

CHAPTER 15

Patient safety — epidemiological considerations

Richard Thomson, Alison Pryce

Despite growing interest in the safety of patients, there is still widespread lack of awareness of the problem of adverse events.... Understanding and knowledge of the epidemiology of adverse events – frequency, causes, determinants and impact on patient outcomes, and of effective methods for preventing them – are still limited.

Sir Liam Donaldson, Chief Medical Officer, England [1]

How safe is health care? Whilst safety has been a driving force for many years in other complex industries, such as aviation, nuclear fuel and rail transport, health services have arrived late at the conference. However, there has been a considerable increase in interest in patient safety, driven to an extent by major national reports including the Institute of Medicine's report, *To Err is Human* [2], and the UK Chief Medical Officer's report, *An Organisation with a Memory* [3]. These influential reports drew upon earlier published studies, particularly the Harvard Medical Practice Studies [4–6], which at the time of their publication had had relatively limited impact, but which have since become classic papers. Extrapolating from the Harvard data, the Institute of Medicine's report [2] suggested that there were 44 000 to 98 000 deaths each year in the USA as a result of safety incidents. Subsequently, similar studies from around the world have shown how common such phenomena are in all developed health care systems. However, despite the passage of 15 years since the Harvard studies were published [4–6], a recent report criticised the UK National Health Service (NHS) for 'the lack of accurate information on serious incidents and deaths' [7].

Yet, in order to monitor and reduce the impact of adverse effects in health care, there is clearly a need to be able to quantify and characterise the size of the problem, and to understand the causal factors and hence identify means of preventing avoidable harm. This is the core role of epidemiological study, whether it is in its classic form in investigating the distribution and causes of disease, or in describing the size and preventability of iatrogenic problems.

Health Care Errors and Patient Safety. Edited by Brian Hurwitz and Aziz Sheikh.
© 2009 Blackwell Publishing, ISBN: 978-1-4051-4643-2.

Epidemiological study requires established and robust definitions and the application of high-quality observational methods. The epidemiology of safety is a newly developing field of enquiry requiring a flexible and innovative use of a range of study methods.

Definitions

Whilst many studies have taken place worldwide in an attempt to identify, quantify, understand and learn from health care errors and adverse events, this field of research has, to an extent, been hampered by a confusing range of definitions and a lack of standardised terminology. There is ongoing debate about the concepts and terms used in patient safety, with varying levels of agreement on definitions. The recognition of this problem has recently led the World Health Organization's World Health Alliance for Patient Safety to support a project to develop an international patient safety event classification [8].

A number of terms have been used (often interchangeably) in the epidemiology of patient safety, the most common being (health care) error, adverse event, critical incident and patient safety incident.

The most widely quoted studies (the Harvard Medical Practice Studies [4–6]) sought to establish the number of adverse events, and then analysed these data further in order to establish what proportion of them occurred as a result of negligent or substandard care. An *adverse event* was defined as 'an injury that was caused by medical management (rather than the underlying disease) and that prolonged the hospitalization, produced a disability at the time of discharge, or both' [4] and negligence was defined as 'care that fell below the standard expected of physicians in their community' [4].

The National Patient Safety Agency (NPSA) has defined a *patient safety incident* as 'any unintended or unexpected incident which could have or did lead to harm for one or more patients' [9]. This definition incorporates the concept of a *near-miss* – 'any incident that had the potential to cause harm but was prevented, resulting in no harm' [9], although this is a term of variable definition. Other definitions of near-miss include 'a situation in which an event or omission, or a sequence of events or omissions, arising during clinical care fails to develop further, whether or not as a result of compensating action, thus preventing injury to a patient' [3] (see Chapter 1 and Appendix 1.1, pp. 17–18 for further discussion and definition of key patient safety terms).

Recent case note review studies have retained the concept of an adverse event as incorporating harm, whilst including the concept of a *clinical incident*, where an error occurred but no harm ensued [10].

Terminology is further complicated by the concept of *error*. Error has been defined as an occasion when 'a planned sequence of … activities fails to achieve its intended outcome', and identified as being of two broad types: unintentional and intentional [11]. Unintentional error includes slips and lapses, where the problem lies in the incomplete or erroneous pursuit of a correct plan, and mistakes, where the problem lies in the selection of an inappropriate or incorrect plan. Intentional errors, also called violations, are deviations from formal or informal rules and may be routine (as in cutting corners), necessary/situational (the only way to get the job done) or optimising (for personal gain).

Clearly there is considerable overlap between different terms. Some adverse events and patient safety incidents are the unavoidable consequences of health care. Adverse events can occur in the absence of error, for example in the case of an unpredictable drug reaction, whilst error can (and often does) occur in the absence of harm. Patient safety incidents may be preventable but not strictly related to human error, for example, patient falls are common and may occur as a result of remediable design problems in hospital layout, not as a result of a human error in care. These differences led to the distinction between latent errors or conditions and active failures [12]. Active failures are the unsafe acts that occur in health care at the sharp end of care, whilst latent errors may precipitate or encourage active failures. For example, staff shortages (latent) may mean that a ward nurse distributes patient medication alone rather than with a colleague, thus violating policy, and as a result gives Mrs Smith's tablets to Mrs Jones (active failure).

How big are these problems and how preventable are they?

There is a wide range of methods for identifying and reviewing adverse events and patient safety incidents, each with its own strengths and weaknesses. Furthermore, the great majority of studies have been undertaken in acute general hospitals, with very few done in other settings such as mental health and primary care. Some methods are better at estimating the size of the problem, others are more useful for helping to understand why things happen and what might be done to prevent incidents. The different methods have been reviewed and grouped into broad categories [13] and some are discussed below; Table 15.1 is an adaptation of these categories.

Case note reviews

The studies most widely referred to as identifying the incidence of error in health care are case note review studies. The most frequently cited of these is the Harvard Medical Practice Study [4,14]. This was the first major study to show that health care may cause significant harm to patients, much of which is potentially preventable. Case note review studies vary in their methods and definitions but the great majority use a two-stage process of screening records for possible events (usually done by nursing staff) and then reviewing screen-positive notes in more detail (usually done by medical staff).

The Harvard Medical Practice Studies involved clinical staff in the review of 30 121 randomly selected case notes from 51 acute care (non-psychiatric)

Table 15.1 Advantages and disadvantages of methods used to measure errors and adverse events in health care (adapted from Thomas & Petersen [13]).

Error measurement method	Advantages	Disadvantages
Morbidity and mortality conferences and autopsy	Can suggest latent errors Familiar to health care providers	Hindsight bias Reporting bias Focused on diagnostic errors Infrequently and non-randomly used
Case analysis/root cause analysis	Can suggest latent errors Structured systems approach Can include recent data from interviews	Hindsight bias Tend to focus on severe events
Malpractice claims analysis	Provides multiple perspectives (patients, providers, lawyers) Can detect latent errors	Hindsight bias Reporting bias Non-standardised source of data
Staff interviews and questionnaires	Can explore latent errors	Hindsight and recall bias Reporting bias
Incident reporting systems	Can suggest latent errors Provide multiple perspectives over time Can be a part of routine operations	Reporting bias Hindsight bias
Administrative data analysis	Uses readily available data Inexpensive	May rely upon incomplete and inaccurate data Data are divorced from clinical context
Case note review	Uses readily available data Commonly used	Judgments about adverse events are not reliable Expensive Medical records are incomplete Hindsight bias
Electronic medical record	Inexpensive after initial investment Monitors in real time Integrates multiple data sources	Susceptible to programming and/or data entry errors Expensive to implement Not good for detecting latent errors
Observation of patient care	Potentially accurate and precise Provides data otherwise unavailable Detects more active errors than other methods	Time consuming and expensive Difficult to train reliable observers Potential Hawthorne effect Potential concerns about confidentiality Possible to be overwhelmed with information Potential hindsight bias Not good for detecting latent errors
Active clinical surveillance	Potentially accurate and precise for adverse events	Time consuming and expensive Not good for detecting latent errors

hospitals in New York State. This found an adverse event rate of 3.7% of all hospitalizations [4]. It also identified that a substantial proportion of these adverse events were due to negligence (27.6%), and that a significant proportion (13.6%) resulted in death [4].

Further adverse event studies have since been undertaken, notably in Australia [15], Colorado and Utah in the USA [16,17], the UK [10], Denmark [18], New Zealand [19], Canada [20], France [21] and Spain [22]. They provide estimates of adverse events in hospital care, ranging from 3.7% to 16.6% of hospital admissions, and suggest that between 27.6% and 56.0% are preventable. A comparison of the key findings of these studies is given in Table 15.2.

Whilst the figures vary from study to study (and this variation is undoubtedly in part due to the use of differing methods and definitions), they all describe significant levels of error and harm associated with health care and they all imply that there is much that can be done to make health care safer and to protect patients from the adverse effects of care. They have been highly influential in creating the impetus for national programmes of patient safety. These studies are dependent upon the sensitivity and specificity of the screening and in-depth review methods, and the reliability of judgments on causation and preventability. These are themselves dependent upon the skills of the reviewers (training is essential) and the quality and completeness of the medical records.

Reporting systems

More recently much emphasis has been given to incident reporting systems [24,25]. Incident reporting systems clearly rely on individuals' willingness and confidence to report an incident. Indeed a recent report [7] suggested that on average an estimated 22% of incidents and 39% of near-misses are not reported (these figures are derived from perceptions – it is not easy to know what is not reported). It was felt that medication errors and incidents which subsequently result in serious harm were the least likely to be reported [7].

Reporting of patient safety incidents not only varies by type of incident, but also between types of staff. There is evidence to suggest that nurses are more likely to report than other staff groups [26]. However, it has also been suggested that there is a perception amongst non-medical staff that they risk suspicion if they report a serious incident [7] (see Chapter 7). None the less, incident reporting systems are less costly than case note reviews [27], and at a local level the majority of NHS organisations rely on incident reporting within their own local risk management systems as the main source of information on patient safety issues.

In addition to reporting incidents at a local organisational level, there may be a requirement for specific types of incidents to be reported at a regional level or higher. For example, strategic health authorities in England are required by the Department of Health to report information on serious untoward incidents from all NHS trusts within their respective boundaries. Such incidents extend beyond patient safety and there are difficulties in agreeing and applying a common definition of a serious untoward incident.

Table 15.2 Key findings from international adverse event studies.

City/country	Study design	Frequency	Preventability	Patient outcomes	Characteristics
New York State, USA: The Harvard Medical Practice Study [4]	1984 data Retrospective case note review n = 30 121 51 acute care (non-psychiatric) hospitals	Adverse events = 3.7% of hospitalizations (95% CI = 3.2% to 4.2%)	Proportion of adverse events due to negligence = 27.6% (95% CI = 22.5% to 32.6%)	Deaths = 13.6% Permanent disability = 2.6%	Associated with: • older patients (≥ 65 years) • vascular surgery (16.1%); thoracic and cardiac surgery (10.8%); neurosurgery (9.9%); general surgery (7.0%)
Australia: Quality in Australian Health Care Study [15]	1992 data Retrospective case note review n = 14 179 28 hospitals	Adverse events = 16.6% (10.6%*)	Proportion of adverse events with a high degree of preventability = 51.2%	Deaths = 4.9% Permanent disability = 13.7%	–
Utah and Colorado, USA [16]	1992 data n = 15 000 (non-psychiatric) hospitals	Surgical adverse events = 3.0% (95% CI = 2.7% to 3.4%)	Surgical adverse events = 54.0% (95% CI = 48.9% to 58.9%)	Surgical adverse events = 5.6% (95% CI = 3.7% to 8.3%)	Significantly elevated surgical adverse event rate. Abdominal aortic aneurysm repair 18.9% (95% CI 8.3% to 37.5%)
Utah and Colorado, USA [17]	1992 data n =14 565 (non-psychiatric) hospitals	2.9% (3.2*%)	Utah: • preventable: 54.0% • attributable to negligence: 32.6% Colorado: • preventable: 56.0% attributable to negligence: 27.4%	Deaths = 6.6% (6.9% of preventable adverse events; 8.8% of negligent adverse events)	Associated with operative procedures (45%)

		Adverse events	Proportion preventable	Outcomes	Associations
London, UK [10]	1999–2000 data Retrospective case note review n = 1014 Two acute hospitals	Adverse events = 10.8% (11.7% when multiple adverse events were included)	Proportion of adverse events that were preventable = 47.3%	Deaths = 8.2% Permanent impairment = 6.4%	Associated with older patients
Denmark: The Danish Averse Event Study [18]	1998 data Retrospective case note review n = 1097 17 acute hospitals	Adverse events = 9.0%	Proportion of adverse events that were preventable = 40.4%	Resulting in permanent disability or death = 26.3%	–
New Zealand [19]	1998 data Retrospective case note review n = 6579 13 hospitals	Adverse events = 12.9% of hospital admissions	Proportion of adverse events that had high preventability = 37.1%	Deaths = 4.5%	Associated with: • older patients (>65 years) • occurrence prior to admission (51.4%)
Canada: The Canadian Adverse Events Study [20]	2000 data Retrospective case note review n = 3745 20 teaching and community hospitals (excluding obstetric and psychiatric admissions)	Adverse events = 7.5% of hospital admissions (95% CI = 5.7% to 9.3%)	Proportion of 'highly preventable' adverse events = 36.9% (95% CI = 32.0% to 41.8%)	Deaths = 20.8% (95% CI = 7.8% to 33.8%); 9.0% of which were judged to be 'highly preventable'	Associated with: • older patients • surgical procedures (34.2%) • drug- or fluid-related events (23.6%)

(Continued p. 214)

Table 15.2 (Continued)

City/country	Study design	Frequency	Preventability	Patient outcomes	Characteristics
France [21]	2002 data Retrospective, prospective and cross-sectional case note review n = 778 Seven hospitals	Adverse event rates: • for retrospective method = 14.5% (95% CI = 10.4% to 18.7%) • for prospective method = 15.4% (95% CI = 12.2% to 18.7%) • for cross-sectional method = 9.8% (95% CI = 6.8% to 12.8%)	Preventable adverse event rates: • for retrospective method = 27.7% (95% CI = 20.2% to 36.6%) • for prospective method = 41.7% (95% CI = 33.2% to 50.6%) • for cross-sectional method = 35.5% (95% CI = 25.7% to 46.7%)	–	–
Spain: ENEAS [22]	2005 data Retrospective case note review n = 5624 24 hospitals	Adverse event rate = 9.3% (95% CI = 8.6% to 10.1%)	Considered preventable adverse event rate = 42.8%	Deaths = 4.4%	Associated with older patients (>65 years) Common causes: • medication-related (37.4%) • nosocomial infection-related (25.3%) • procedure-related (25.0%)

CI, confidence interval.
*A subsequent study involved American and Australian investigators harmonising the inclusion criteria and definitions and re-analysing the data [23].

Enhancing patient safety and reducing errors are also key priorities at a national level, for example in the UK NHS, particularly since the publication of *An Organisation with a Memory* [3]. *Building a Safer NHS for Patients* [28] recommended the establishment of a national reporting system to record, analyse and learn from incidents. The NPSA was subsequently established in July 2001. It has implemented the National Reporting and Learning System (NRLS): an electronic incident reporting system designed to collect and collate patient safety incident reports from all NHS organisations in England and Wales.

At the end of June 2006, the NRLS was receiving 50 000 to 60 000 reports of incidents per month from all care settings [29]. In terms of the degree of harm reported, approximately 0.4% of incidents were associated with death, 0.9% with severe harm, 5.4% with moderate harm, 24.9% with minor harm and 68.3% with no harm (Chapter 16 discusses methodological challenges posed by analysis of the highly diverse and complex data which incident reporting systems generate). The majority of patient safety incidents continue to be reported from acute trusts [29]. The first report from the NRLS [30] estimated that there would be 572 000 reported patient safety incidents from acute hospitals per year. The average reported incident rate for acute trusts regularly submitting data to the NRLS was 4.9% of admissions (range just under 2% to over 12%). This figure is lower than the estimates from case note review studies. The explanations for this are likely to be due largely to two factors. First, there is under-reporting of incidents. Second, incidents identified in adverse event studies using case note review and those identified from reporting systems differ. Adverse events and patient safety incidents are best thought of as being overlapping rather than directly comparable events (see later).

A survey by the National Audit Office [31] of acute, ambulance and mental health trusts in England in 2004/5 found that there were 974 000 reported incidents and near-misses over the year reported to local risk management systems.

Building a Safer NHS for Patients [28] also envisaged the NPSA developing an understanding of a range of data sources to develop a comprehensive picture of patient safety. The approach taken by the NPSA has been to establish the Patient Safety Observatory [30], which draws upon a wide range of data and intelligence (Figure 15.1).

To this picture of UK reporting should be added the need to inform other agencies in accordance with the appropriate national guidance: for example, notification to the Medicines and Healthcare products Regulatory Agency (MHRA) in the case of equipment failure and the Health Protection Agency (HPA) in cases involving healthcare associated infections.

Observation of clinical practice

Direct observation of practice has been used to attempt to quantify the frequency of adverse events, usually in selected patient groups or clinical settings. One study used direct observation of clinical practice by trained

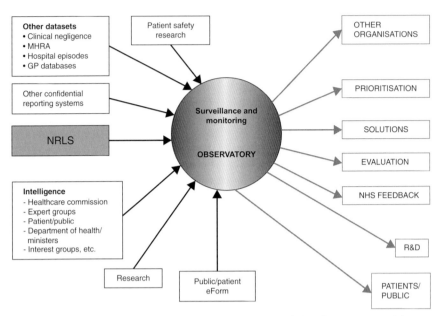

Figure 15.1 The National Patient Safety Agency (NPSA) Patient Safety Observatory model. MHRA, Medicines and Healthcare products Regulatory Agency; NRLS, National Reporting and Learning System.

ethnographers, whose observations were undertaken on two intensive care units and one surgical care unit [32]. The study reported that 17.7% of patients experienced at least one serious adverse event although the definition of a serious event is unclear and ranged from temporary physical disability to death [32]. A further prospective observational study of general surgery patients found a similar proportion of patients suffered complications deemed potentially attributable to error (18.1%), but these included low harm events [33].

Observational studies have also proven valuable in quantifying medication error. For example, a study where a trained and experienced pharmacist observed nurses during intravenous drug rounds in selected hospital wards identified one or more errors in 49% of 430 observed doses; these were potentially severe only in three doses (1%) and potentially moderate in 126 (29%) [34]. Such methods are now being applied in other settings, such as medication use in nursing and residential homes [35].

A recent observational study of paediatric cardiac surgery identified 366 minor failures and seven major failures in 24 paediatric cardiac operations [36]. The minor failures were of 29 different types, with the most frequent being failures of communication and coordination, absences from theatre and equipment problems. Conditions or situations that threatened specific tasks were the most prominent source of failures. As part of the same study, in 20 orthopaedic cases, a total of 421 minor failures and one major failure were observed [36]. The most frequent types of minor failure included distractions, equipment management failures, safety consciousness failures and coordination and communication failures. Cultural and organisational problems were the most frequently observed threats and non-technical errors were more frequent than technical errors. In both parts of the study, all but one major failure was associated with an accumulation of minor failures in higher risk operations. The authors concluded that adverse events in surgery were likely to be associated with a coincidental accumulation of a number of minor recurring failures.

Whilst direct observation has strengths there are also weaknesses, not least the cost of observational study, as well as the need for trained observers and the potential impact of observation on behaviour. Whilst valuable, such studies are likely to have a limited role in determining the overall incidence of events.

Interviews and questionnaires

Some studies have used staff interviews and/or questionnaires in order to gain a greater understanding of health care errors. These tend to have been in individual specialties or specific areas such as medication error and have some value in understanding types of events and their potential causes and prevention [37–42]. However, they have limited value in addressing the frequency of events since they suffer from bias of recall and subjectivity. Thus this approach is not ideal for quantifying incidents, but may be useful for identifying probable underlying causes. Professional views on key safety issues within individual specialities may also be helpful when set alongside other sources of data. It seems likely that clinical experts with frontline experience may well be very aware of key issues, some of which may not be readily apparent through reporting for example.

Case studies

Case studies of various types, including morbidity and mortality meetings, significant event audits and root cause analysis have much to offer in understanding the underlying causes of incidents, but less in quantifying incidence. These are discussed in Chapter 14.

Patient safety indicators

Another approach to shining a light on the potential size of the problem of health care safety lies in the use of routine datasets to derive patient safety indicators. Both the US Agency for Healthcare Research and Quality (AHRQ) and the Organisation for Economic Co-operation and Development (OECD) have programmes of work related to indicator development and use [43–46]. This approach seeks to develop measures of safety using diagnostic, health care utilisation and demographic data from (predominantly) acute hospital data systems. Only some are direct measures of safety; rather they act as indicators to raise questions and support local investigation. Such indicators include, for example, postoperative hip fracture, death in low-mortality diagnostic-related groups, foreign body left during procedure, decubitus ulcer, postoperative sepsis, and obstetric trauma with third-degree lacerations.

None the less, despite appropriate caveats – the most important of which are likely to relate to data completeness and the potential perverse impact of using such measures to assess and compare performance – such data may be of value in epidemiological studies of the incidence and consequences of incidents. For example, analysis in the USA has looked at the event rate per 1000 discharges at risk and has found obstetric trauma in around 300 in every 1000 discharges, whilst a foreign body left inside a patient during a procedure is recorded in only 0.09 in every 1000 at-risk patients [43]. This work has also demonstrated that patients displaying certain indicators have increased length of stay and mortality rates compared with those not experiencing such events [43]. However, it is early days in the using and understanding of such measures and they should be approached with caution.

Other data sources: examples
Litigation data
It has been suggested that analysis of claims made against health care organisations can contribute to our understanding of the distribution and causes of incidents. There have been several key studies of closed claims data. For example, the closed claims project of the American Society of Anesthesiologists extracts data from claims and enters them into a specially designed database [47]; it has proven an important source of information on rare events (such as the risk of sudden cardiac arrest during spinal anaesthesia) [48]. However, it is clear that claims represent a highly selected subset of incidents and as such can not provide representative epidemiological data. A recent study of claims in the UK in four specialities concluded that analysis does shed some light on patterns of litigation and the specific characteristics of cases that come to litigation, and may draw attention to important clinical issues. However, such an approach is unlikely to be the method of choice for assessing the incidence of patient harm from safety events.

Other reporting systems
Even where there are established patient safety incident reporting systems, there are commonly other reporting systems that sit alongside them which may collect a different profile of incidents. For example, in the UK, data are reported on healthcare associated infections to the HPA [49]; adverse drug reactions and problems with medical devices are reported to the MHRA [50]; deaths and severe injury to patients should be reported to the Health and Safety Executive [51]; and the Department of Health has a separate system for reporting serious untoward incidents, not all of which are patient safety incidents.

Developing an overarching surveillance and monitoring system: the Patient Safety Observatory model

It is clear that no one source of data and no single method of data collection provide a clear analysis of the frequency and causation of patient safety incidents. Whilst case note review studies come closest to a means of determining frequency of incidents, they are limited by what is available within the patient records. In particular, they are likely to miss no-harm events, which are rarely included in the medical notes, and they are limited in their capacity to understand and extract underlying causes. They are expensive and time consuming and their breadth also may limit their value. For example, we are still unclear about the actual epidemiology of deaths from incidents since these form a small proportion of incidents picked up by random case note review and hence any extrapolations are likely to be unreliable. For a good discussion of the issues see Hayward and Hofer [52].

Furthermore, an increasing number of studies demonstrate that, at different levels in the health care system, different data sources reveal different profiles of incidents, with variable degrees of overlap. Several studies have shown that serious incidents are not always picked up by local risk management systems and that the overlap between case note review and incident reporting may be limited, with each picking up a different profile of incidents [27,53–56]. A recent study undertaken on behalf of the NPSA also confirms these suspicions and suggests that local hospitals should employ a range of data sources to provide them with information to improve safety [57]. Seven key data sources (clinical incident database, health and safety incident database, complaints database, claims database, inquest database, the patient administration system and case notes) were assessed. The study found that case notes have the potential to identify the largest number of incidents and provide the richest source of information on such incidents. However, the seven data sources identified different types of incidents with differing levels of patient harm and there was little overlap between incidents identified by different sources. Thus, triangulating information from more than one source can identify a broader range of incidents and provide additional information related to the professional groups involved, the types of patients affected and important contributory factors.

Thus it is clear that we need a wider system of data collection at all levels, such as that used for the surveillance of communicable diseases. In order to address this at a national level, the NPSA in the UK has set up a Patient Safety Observatory in collaboration with a number of partners from both the NHS and elsewhere [30]. These partners include key national organisations, for example the Healthcare Commission (the independent regulator of health services in England), the Office for National Statistics, the MHRA (which regulates medicines and medical devices in the UK), patient organisations such as Action against Medical Accidents, the NHS Litigation Authority and medical defence organisations.

The primary function of the Patient Safety Observatory is to quantify, characterise and prioritise patient safety issues in order to support the NHS in making health care safer. The Observatory supports access to a wide range of data and intelligence as a basis for identifying and monitoring patient safety incident trends, highlighting areas for action and setting priorities. Figure 15.1 outlines the inputs and outputs of the Patient Safety Observatory with examples of the possible sources of information that feed in to it. This allows the findings from incident reporting to be considered alongside a range of data and intelligence, including the published literature, clinical experts, medical record reviews, hospital episode statistics, death certification data, complaints, prospective risk assessments, patient safety indicator studies, observational research, confidential enquiries, and audits and reviews of health care organisations. Triangulating information from different data sources should enable a fuller picture of the nature and severity of patient safety incidents to be obtained.

Conclusion

Most of the current data on incidents are based on studies undertaken in hospitals. However, adverse events also occur in other settings: primary care, community pharmacies, residential/nursing care and patients' own homes, but few studies have been undertaken on the frequency and nature of errors in these settings. A recent review identified 12 relevant studies in primary care, with just four reporting an error/adverse event rate [58]. One study found 3.7 adverse events per 1 000 000 primary care clinic visits, and the remaining three studies reviewed prescription error rates (which ranged between 0.8% and 4.3%). Given the increasing trend in moving care out of hospitals and closer to the patient, primary care is likely to become an increasingly important area for epidemiological study.

There is a considerable variety of sources of information on patient safety within health care at all levels of the health care system and there is no perfect method for identifying and quantifying adverse events [59]. Different methods of identifying incidents/errors in patient safety support differing perspectives on the problem and any individual method is likely to underestimate its true size [60]. None the less, patient safety is a global problem and one common to all health care systems. It is increasingly clear that a proper picture of the scale and preventability of the problem requires the use of a range of data sources within a coordinated surveillance and monitoring model at whatever level in the health care system we are interested.

References

1 Donaldson L. Patient safety: a global perspective. In: *International Hospital Federation Reference Book 2005/2006*. Ferney Voltaire, International Hospital Federation, 2006. Available at http://www.ihfpublications.org/pdfs/World%20alliance%20for.pdf.
2 Kohn LT, Corrigan JM, Donaldson MS, eds. *To Err is Human: Building a Safer Health System*. National Academics Press, Washington, 2000.
3 Department of Health. *An Organisation with a Memory: Report of an Expert Group on Learning from Adverse Events in the NHS*. HMSO, London, 2000.
4 Brennan TA, Leape LL, Laird NM et al. Incidence of adverse events and negligence in hospitalized patients: results of the Harvard Medical Practice Study I. *New England Journal of Medicine* 1991; **324**: 370–6.

5 Leape LL, Brennan TA, Laird NM et al. The nature of adverse events in hospitalized patients: results of the Harvard Medical Practice Study II. *New England Journal of Medicine* 1991; **324** (6): 377–84.

6 Localio AR, Lawthers AG, Brennan TA et al. Relation between malpractice claims and adverse events dues to negligence: results of the Harvard Medical Practice Study III. *New England Journal of Medicine* 1991; **325** (4); 245–51.

7 House of Commons Committee of Public Accounts. *A Safer Place for Patients: Learning to Improve Patient Safety (Fifty-first Report of Session 2005–06)*. HMSO, London, 2006.

8 World Health Organisation. *World Alliance for Patient Safety: Project to Develop an International Patient Safety Event Classification – the Conceptual Framework of an International Patient Safety Event Classification (Executive Summary)*. WHO Document Publication Services, Geneva, 2006. Available at http://www.who-ipsec.org/.

9 National Patient Safety Agency. *Seven Steps to Patient Safety*. National Patient Safety Agency, London, 2003.

10 Vincent C, Neale G, Woloshynowych M. Adverse events in British hospitals: preliminary retrospective record review. *British Medical Journal* 2001; **322**: 517–19.

11 Reason J. *Human Error*. Cambridge University Press, Cambridge, 1990.

12 Reason J. Human error: models and management. *British Medical Journal* 2000; **320**: 768–70.

13 Thomas EJ, Petersen LA. Measuring errors and adverse events in health care. *Journal of General Internal Medicine* 2003; **18**: 61–7.

14 Lilford R, Stirling S, Maillard N. Citation classics in patient safety research: an invitation to contribute to an online bibliography. *Quality and Safety in Health Care* 2006; **15**: 311–13.

15 Wilson RM, Runciman WB, Gibberd RW et al. The Quality in Australian Health Care Study. *Medical Journal of Australia* 1995; **163**: 458–71.

16 Gawande AA, Thomas EJ, Zinner MJ et al. The incidence and nature of surgical adverse events in Colorado and Utah in 1992. *Surgery* 1999; **126**: 66–75.

17 Thomas EJ, Studdert DM, Burstin HR et al. Incidence and types of adverse events and negligent care in Utah and Colorado. *Medical Care* 2000; **38** (3): 261–71.

18 Schioler T, Lipczak H, Pedersen BL et al. Incidence of adverse events in hospitals. A retrospective study of medical records. Ugeskrift for Laeger 2001; **163**: 5370–8.

19 Davis P, Lay-Yee R, Briant R et al. *Adverse Events in New Zealand Public Hospitals: Principal Findings from a National Survey*. Occasional Paper No. 3. Ministry of Health, Wellington, 2001. Available at http://www.moh.govt.nz/publications/adverseevents.

20 Baker GR, Norton PG, Flintoft V et al. The Canadian Adverse Events Study: the incidence of adverse events among hospital patients in Canada. *Canadian Medical Association Journal* 2004; **170**: 1678–86.

21 Michel P, Quenon Jl, de Sarasqueta AM et al. Comparison of three methods for estimating rates of adverse events and rates of preventable adverse events in acute care hospitals. *British Medical Journal* 2004; **328**: 199.

22 Aranaz JM, Aibar C, Vitaller J et al. *National Study on Hospitalisation-related Adverse Events (ENEAS 2005)*. Ministry of Health and Consumer Affairs, Madrid, 2006.

23 Thomas EJ, Studdert DM, Runciman WB et al. A comparison of iatrogenic injury studies in Australia and the USA. I: Context, methods, casemix, population, patient and hospital characteristics. *International Journal for Quality in Health Care* 2000; **12** (5): 371–8.

24 World Health Organisation. *World Alliance for Patient Safety: WHO Draft Guidelines for Adverse Event Reporting and Learning Systems: from Information to Action*. WHO Document Publication Services, Geneva, 2005.

25 Giles S, Fletcher M, Baker M et al. Incident reporting and analysis. *In*: Walshe K, Boaden R, eds. *Patient Safety: Research into Practice*. Open University Press, Maidenhead, 2005.

26 Lawton R, Parker D. Barriers to incident reporting in a health care system. *Quality and Safety in Health Care* 2002; **11**: 15–18.
27 O'Neil AC, Petersen LA, Cook EF et al. Physician reporting compared with medical-record review to identify adverse medical events. *Annals of Internal Medicine* 1993; **119**: 370–6.
28 Department of Health. *Building a Safer NHS for Patients – Implementing an Organisation with a Memory.* HMSO, London, 2001.
29 National Patient Safety Agency. *Quarterly National Reporting and Learning System Data Aummary (Autumn 2006).* National Patient Safety Agency, London, 2006. Available at http://www.npsa.nhs.uk.
30 National Patient Safety Agency. *Building a Memory: Preventing Harm, Reducing Risks and Improving Patient Safety. The First Report of the National Reporting and Learning System and the Patient Safety Observatory.* National Patient Safety Agency, London, 2005.
31 National Audit Office. *A Safer Place for Patients: Learning to Improve Patient Safety.* Report by the Controller and Auditor General. HMSO, London, 2005.
32 Andrews L, Stocking C, Krizek T et al. An alternative strategy for studying adverse events in medical care. *Lancet* 1997; **349**: 309–13.
33 Wanzel KR, Jamieson CG, Bohnen JM. Complications on a general surgery service: incidence and reporting. *Canadian Journal of Surgery* 2000; **43** (2): 113–17.
34 Taxis K, Barber N. Causes of intravenous medication errors: an ethnographic study. *Quality and Safety in Health Care* 2003; **12**: 343–8.
35 Barber N. *Medication Errors in Nursing Homes – the CHUMS Study – Care Homes Use of Medicines Study.* Patient Safety Research Portfolio, Department of Public Health and Epidemiology, University of Birmingham, in progress. Available at http://www.pcpoh.bham.ac.uk/publichealth/psrp/Publication_PS025.htm.
36 Catchpole KR, Godden PJ, Giddings AEB et al. *Identifying and Reducing Errors in the Operating Theatre.* HMSO, London, 2005. Available at http://pcpoh.bham.ac.uk/publichealth/psrp/Pdf/PS012_DeLeval_%20Final_Report.pdf
37 Cooper JB, Newbower RS, Kitz RJ. An analysis of major errors and equipment failures in anesthesia management: considerations for prevention and detection. *Anesthesiology* 1984; **60** (1): 34–42.
38 Wu AW, Folkman S, McPhee SJ et al. Do house officers learn from their mistakes? *Journal of the American Medical Association* 1991; **265** (16): 2089–94.
39 Davis J, Hoyt D, McArdle M et al. An analysis of errors causing morbidity and mortality in a trauma system: a guide for quality improvement. *Journal of Trauma Injury Infection and Critical Care* 1992; **32** (5): 660–6.
40 Cohen MR, Proulx SM, Crawford SY. Survey of hospital systems and common serious medication errors. *Journal of Healthcare Risk Management* 1998; **18** (1): 16–27.
41 Cohen H, Love E, Todd A et al. Adverse incidents in blood transfusion: serious hazards of transfusion (SHOT). *Clinical Risk* 2002; **8** (4): 155–8.
42 Gawande AA, Zinner MJ, Studdert DM et al. Analysis of errors reported by surgeons at three teaching hospitals. *Surgery* 2003; **133** (6): 614–21.
43 Zhan C, Miller MR. Administrative data based patient safety research: a critical review. *Quality and Safety in Health Care* 2003; **12** (Suppl 2:ii): 58–6.
44 Elixhauser A, Pancholi M, Clancy CM. Using the AHRQ quality indicators to improve health care quality. *Joint Commission Journal on Quality and Patient Safety* 2005; **31** (9): 533–8.
45 Agency for Healthcare Research and Quality. *AHRQ Quality Indicators: Guide to Patient Safety Indicators.* Department of Health and Human Services, AHRQ, Rockville, MD, 2006. Available at http://www.qualityindicators.ahrq.gov/psi_download.htm.

46 Millar J, Mattke S, Members of the OECD Patient Safety Panel. *Selecting Indicators for Patient Safety at the Health Systems Level in OECD Countries.* OECD Health Technical Papers No. 18. Organisation for Economic Co-operation and Development, 2004. Available at http://www.oecd.org/dataoecd/53/26/33878001.pdf.

47 Cheney FW. (1999) The American Society of Anesthesiologists Closed Claims Project: what have we learned, how has it affected practice, and how will it affect practice in the future? *Anesthesiology* 1999; **91** (2): 552–6.

48 Caplan RA, Ward RJ, Posner K et al. Unexpected cardiac arrest during spinal anesthesia: a closed claims analysis of predisposing factors. *Anesthesiology* 1988; **68** (1): 5–11.

49 Health Protection Agency. *Mandatory Surveillance of Healthcare Associated Infection Report.* Health Protection Agency, London, 2006. Available at http://www.hpa.org.uk/infections/topics_az/hai/MandSurvHCAI2006.pdf.

50 Medicines and Healthcare products Regulatory Agency. *Reporting Medical Device Adverse Incidents and Disseminating Medical Device Alerts.* MHRA, London, 2007. Available at http://www.mhra.gov.uk/home/idcplg?IdcService=SS_GET_PAGE&nodeId=291 (medical devices), http://www.mhra.gov.uk/home/idcplg?IdcService=SS_GET_PAGE&nodeId=286(medicines),http://www.mhra.gov.uk/home/idcplg?IdcService=SS_GET_PAGE&nodeId=295 (serious adverse blood reactions and events).

51 Health and Safety Executive. *A Guide to the Reporting of Injuries, Diseases, and Dangerous Occurrences Regulations 1995.* Health and Safety Executive Books, Sudbury, 1995. Available at http://www.riddor.gov.uk/.

52 Hayward RA, Hofer TP. Estimating hospital deaths due to medical errors: preventability is in the eye of the reviewer. *Journal of the American Medical Association* 2001; **286**: 415–20.

53 Stanhope N, Crowley-Murphy M, Vincent C et al. An evaluation of adverse incident reporting. *Journal of Evaluation in Clinical Practice* 1995; **5**: 1–12.

54 Jha A, Kuperman G, Teich JM et al. Identifying adverse drug events: the development of computer-based monitor and comparison with chart review and simultaneous voluntary report. *Journal of the American Medical Informatics Association* 1998; **5**: 305–14.

55 Sari AB-A, Sheldon TA, Cracknell A et al. Sensitivity of routine system for reporting patient safety incidents in an NHS hospital: retrospective patient case note review. *British Medical Journal* 2007; **334**: 79.

56 Olsen S, Neale G, Schwab K et al. Hospital staff should use more than one method to detect adverse events and potential adverse events. *Quality and Safety in Health Care* 2007; **16**: 40–4.

57 Hogan H, Olsen S, Scobie S et al. What can we learn about patient safety from information sources within an acute hospital – a step on the ladder of integrated risk management? *Quality and Safety in Health Care* 2008; **17**: 209–15.

58 Sandars J, Esmail A. *Threats to Patient Safety in Primary Care: a Review of the Research into the Frequency and Nature of Error in Primary Care.* University of Manchester, Manchester, 2001.

59 Vincent C. *Patient Safety.* Churchill Livingstone, Edinburgh, 2006.

60 Walshe K. *The validity and reliability of adverse-event measures of quality in healthcare.* PhD thesis, University of Birmingham, Birmingham, 1998.

CHAPTER 16

Analysis of health care error reports

Adrian Cook, Sarah Scobie

This chapter outlines approaches that can be taken to analyse reports of patient safety incidents. We draw primarily on examples from the analysis of a national repository of incident reports for England and Wales, but similar analysis could be undertaken within individual health care organisations.

Health care providers have developed incident reporting systems following the lead of other high-risk industries [1]. In England and Wales, the National Patient Safety Agency (NPSA) was set up in 2001 to make changes at a national level that will improve patient safety in the National Health Service (NHS) in England and Wales [2]. One of the NPSA's core functions is the development of a national reporting system now known as the Reporting and Learning System (RLS). The RLS collects reports of patient safety incidents as part of a broader approach to surveillance of patient safety that brings together a range of sources of information [3], to ensure the types and causes of safety problems can be identified, the most important risks are communicated to the NHS, and that practical solutions are developed to prevent harm to patients [4].

The RLS is the primary mechanism for the NPSA to collect information on patient safety incidents from across England and Wales. Its dataset is designed to collect a notification report of a single patient safety incident soon after it occurs [5] and focuses on:

- What happened?
- When did it happen?
- Where did it happen?
- What were the characteristics of the patient(s) involved such as age, sex and ethnicity?
- What was the outcome for the patient(s)?

The dataset solicits contributory factor(s) that might have prevented harm and allows free text for further information concerning what happened in varying degrees of detail. Additional information is provided in reports involving medication and medical devices.

The RLS is the first national reporting system of its kind in the world. It collects data from across all health care settings and provides a springboard

Health Care Errors and Patient Safety. Edited by Brian Hurwitz and Aziz Sheikh.
© 2009 Blackwell Publishing, ISBN: 978-1-4051-4643-2.

for addressing patient safety problems at a national level, and for identifying priorities for the NPSA and the wider health service.

In essence the RLS is a secondary repository of incident data: although staff and patients can report directly to the NPSA via electronic reporting forms, almost 99% of incidents within the RLS come from local risk management systems [6]. Incidents are collated and investigated locally and sent to the RLS via an electronic link. Prior to connection to the RLS, the dataset used within each local risk management system has been mapped to the national dataset, to enable the information from local systems to be uploaded to the RLS without duplicating data entry. The taxonomy for patient safety incidents used by the RLS was developed through a process of consultation with NHS organisations, and builds on the experiences of other reporting systems. Mapping local datasets to the RLS is facilitated by the structure of key items of data, such as incident type and location of incident, which can be recorded at different levels. For example, the incident category 'Clinical assessment' includes subcategories for incidents related to diagnostic error, tests, labelling of specimens or test results, and patient misidentification. The NPSA is contributing to work led by the WHO to develop an internationally accepted taxonomy for patient safety events, the International Patient Safety Event Classification [7].

There are a number of purposes of incident reporting systems and the analysis of data within them. Some of the analysis undertaken by the NPSA is directed at supporting local reporting, through benchmarking and feedback [8] and monitoring uptake of patient safety interventions [9]. Here we focus on the analysis of incident reports, which might be undertaken locally as well as nationally, in order to support patient safety improvements by:

• Identifying emerging issues.
• Learning about circumstances and causes of incidents to reduce future risks.
• Prioritising patient safety issues for action.

The role of analysis in learning from patient safety incidents

The overall purpose of incident reporting systems is to improve patient safety by learning lessons from previous incidents, thereby improving systems of care and reducing future risks. Analysis of incidents is only part of the reporting process and cannot improve patient safety unless learning from the analysis of reports is fed back to reporters and then informs changes in health care delivery [10]. Incident reports are only one source of information to improve patient safety: other sources of information – such as research evidence, data from other reporting systems and contextual information about health care activity – are essential. In England, these include a number of key national organisations, for example the Healthcare Commission [11] (the independent regulator of health services in England), the Office for

National Statistics [12], the Medicines and Healthcare products Regulatory Agency [13] which regulates medicines and medical devices in the UK, patient organisations such as Action against Medical Accidents [14], the NHS Litigation Authority [15] and medical defence organisations.

The Billings model and patient safety systems

A model for how analysis fits into incident reporting is provided by Billings, based on experience of analysis of aviation incidents [16]. This model identifies primary analysis as the initial classification of incidents and secondary analysis as the synthesis of findings from incident reports (Figure 16.1). A common feature of health care reporting systems compared with those in industrial settings is the high volume of reports received. For example, the RLS receives approximately 50 000 incident reports each month from acute hospital trusts in England and Wales [17], equivalent to approximately 3000 per year from each acute trust. This necessitates a change to the basic Billings model, since primary analysis by experts becomes unfeasible. Instead, the reporter is usually required to supply categorical data items such as location of incident, staff involved and degree of harm, as well as contributory factors. From these fields, it is possible to index and to enter reports directly into a database.

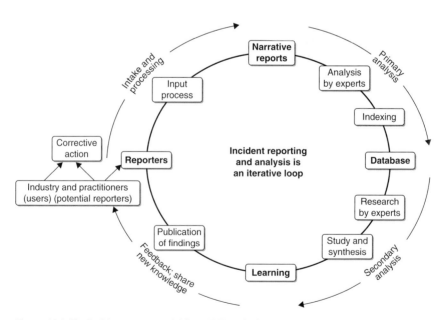

Figure 16.1 The incident report model (from Billings [16]).

Secondary analysis of all reports is similarly unfeasible, and systematic methods are required to select those reports for which secondary analysis will be undertaken. Here we will describe two methods for selecting reports: random sampling stratified by the indexed fields; and data mining using the free text incident descriptions.

Selecting reports for secondary analysis

Stratified sampling

Simple random sampling of patient safety incidents is inefficient where reporting rates vary by factors such as health care setting, type of incident or department. For example, reported incidents from acute settings are dominated by patient falls and a simple random sample may contain little else. A sampling scheme, weighted towards less common incident types, increases the likelihood of other incidents being selected for secondary analysis.

An initial breakdown of reports by incident type, care setting or other characteristics is an important starting point. Although this will identify the most common types of reported incident, it is important to remember that some types of incident are more likely to be reported than others via local incident reporting systems. For example, incidents related to infection control account for only 1% of incidents in the RLS, but we know that health care acquired infection is a factor in a substantial number of deaths each year [18], and affects a greater number of people. Incidents related to diagnostic error are also believed to be under-reported to local risk management systems, but are known to be the source of a substantial proportion of clinical negligence claims [19]. In 2005, 207 notifications of claims were made to acute trusts in England which were associated with diagnostic error and death [20]; in the same year there were 71 reports of deaths associated with diagnostic error in the RLS from acute care settings.

In order to get a better understanding of the nature of incidents reported to the RLS, the NPSA initially used a stratified sampling scheme. Thirty to 40 monthly samples of reports were selected, which were then subject to expert review. Examples of the samples of incidents that were reviewed are shown in Table 16.1. A pragmatic threshold of 150 incidents per month was selected, based on the number of incidents that can be reviewed in 1 day. Where the number of incidents is below this threshold all incidents were reviewed. Currently, all severe harm and death incidents are reviewed on a weekly basis, and monthly reviews are also undertaken of incidents with long free text descriptions, and which mention past NPSA alerts or guidance.

The NPSA also undertakes analysis in response to requests from individual clinicians and national organisations. To support scoping of patient safety issues and to inform projects to mitigate risks. During 2007, 423 responsive analyses were undertaken, of which 136 were requests from external organisations or individuals. The type and purposes of requests is summarised in Table 16.2.

Table 16.1 Examples of samples of incidents reviewed by the NPSA.

Criteria for samples of incidents	Approximate number reported/month	Sampling criteria
Severity of harm: death or severe harm	800	100%
Incident with long free text descriptions		100%
Specialty: anaesthetics	640	Random sample of 150 incidents (excluding falls)
Care setting: critical care	2600	Random sample of 150 transport incidents (excluding falls)
Topic related: correct site surgery (based on free text search, e.g. 'wrong', 'correct', 'side', 'site', 'surg*', 'op*', 'proc*', 'list', 'mark')	60	100%

Table 16.2 External requests for responsive analysis of RLS data.

	Number of requests	Examples
National organisation	48	To Support national policy or initiatives
NHS trust	47	Benchmarking local data, informing local risk management action on specific issues
Parliament, media	19	
Member of the public	18	Freedom of Information, research or study requests
Department of health	4	To inform independent enquriries

Free text data mining

Unusual incidents provide particular opportunities for learning, because they may help to identify new or emerging risks, and highlight issues that require further investigation. For example, an individual incident in which a dermatology patient died when his skin treatment of soft paraffin caught fire, has highlighted risks for patients [21]. Within the RLS, a range of automated approaches have been considered. Here we describe a method which could be tested at a local level. The method requires that the textual description of incidents be coded into a numerical dataset, from which small clusters of unusual incidents can be identified using standard statistical techniques.

To code incident descriptions, a list of key terms that may appear in the free text is needed. Such a list can be generated systematically by reading a sample of reports and reducing each to the minimum number of words that still convey its meaning (Box 16.1). In this process only word stems are

---

Box 16.1: The use of key words to code incident descriptions

Original report free text

Patient was agitated and was mobilising with her zimmer. Advice given to rest was not accepted. Patient was heard to fall and found lying on her right hand side.

Key terms

agitate mobil zimmer fall found lying.

---

retained, for example, injection, injecting and injected are all replaced by 'inject'. After doing this for 100 or so reports a key term list can be formed from the word stems that occur most frequently. The use of key terms and word stems has the added benefit of addressing a common data quality problem, since a misspelling in a report will have no effect unless it occurs in one of the stemmed words on the key term list.

In the numerical dataset the rows and columns represent incident reports and key terms, respectively. The dataset begins as a matrix of zeroes, and wherever a report contains one of the key terms the corresponding cell is changed to 1. The resulting binary matrix is thus a record of which reports contain which key terms. A segment of a matrix is shown in Table 16.3, where incident 1 is the same incident as in Box 16.1, with agitat and zimmer coded as 1 and the other terms shown coded as 0. Note the stemming of the key terms, incident 5 has 'abrasi' coded as 1 indicating that the incident report mentioned either abrasive or abrasion.

In addition to free text incident descriptions there are a number of categorical data fields such as incident type that can be used to group reports. Discriminant analysis is a technique that determines whether a set of variables can be used to distinguish, or discriminate, between groups of individuals. Therefore, with incidents grouped according to the reported incident type, discriminant analysis determines whether it is possible to distinguish between the groups using only the key term variables. For example, are medication incidents identifiable as such from their key terms alone?

The results of a discriminant analysis may be displayed in a table of reported incident type against predicted type (Table 16.4). The rows are the original incident type given by the reporter and the columns are the type predicted from the analysis. The numbers on the diagonal show how many incidents were correctly predicted, so 288 access incidents were correctly identified as such. If the key terms are chosen well then the majority of incidents should be predicted correctly. But the off-diagonal cells are perhaps more interesting, since these are likely to indicate more complex incidents that cannot be classified easily. In the data shown here there are 17 access incidents that were predicted to be disruptive behaviour incidents; these were mostly patients who were being disruptive and had access to care denied as a result.

Table 16.3 Matrix of incidents and key terms.

Incident	Key term							
	Abrasi	*Abus*	*Agitat*	*Alarm*	*Alcohol*	...	*Wrist*	*Zimmer*
1	0	0	1	0	0	.	0	1
2	0	1	0	0	0	.	0	0
3	0	1	0	0	1	.	0	0
4	0	0	1	1	0	.	0	0
5	1	1	0	0	0	.	0	0
6	0	0	1	1	0	.	0	0
etc.	.	.	.	.	.	.	.	.

Table 16.4 Discriminant analysis.

Reported type	Discriminant analysis						
	Access	*Assessment*	*Communication*	*Disruptive behaviour*	*Documentation*	...	*Medication*
Access	**288**	3	2	17	1		4
Assessment	0	**5**	0	1	0		0
Communication	1	0	**15**	3	0		0
Disruptive behaviour	19	2	5	**857**	1		5
Documentation	0	0	1	0	**9**		2
...							
Medication	2	1	0	8	1		**154**

Cluster analysis is another technique that can be used to group similar reports together, using the data in the key term matrix. It is less suited to large datasets and works best with 30–100 reports. A combination of discriminant and cluster analysis thus works well, with discriminant analysis of a large dataset identifying potentially interesting groups in the off-diagonal cells of the output matrix, and cluster analysis being used to investigate these groups in more detail.

Cluster analysis begins by calculating a measure of distance between every pair of reports. A small distance indicates similarity and if two reports contain the same key terms and no others the distance between them will be 0. Conversely, the distance between two reports with no key terms in common will be large. These distances can be displayed in the triangular grid style of road atlases, with a list of towns on the horizontal axis and the same list of towns on the vertical axis. Using the distances, the reports are then iteratively clustered. At the first iteration, a cluster is formed containing the two 'closest' reports. At the second iteration the two next closest reports are grouped together; alternatively a third report might be added to the cluster formed in the first iteration. This process continues iteratively until all reports are clustered together into one group.

The clustering process can be represented by a dendrogram, or tree diagram (Figure 16.2). Starting on the horizontal axis, each incident is shown separately by a vertical line. Moving upwards the first cluster is formed by reports 17 and 23 being joined together, so these incidents are the two most alike in respect of their key terms. The second cluster is formed from reports 21 and 27, the next most similar. At the third iteration, report 8 is joined to the cluster already containing 17 and 23. The process continues to the top of the dendrogram, at which point all the reports are contained in one cluster. From this diagram, it appears that reports 8, 17 and 23 are the most interesting, similar to one another since they are grouped at an early stage, but clearly different to the others since they remain separate until almost the last iteration. A cluster of this type can indicate an unusual incident that had occurred independently at a number of different organisations – examples being a failure to correct known bleep problems in acute settings and the abuse of fire alarms by patients absconding from secure mental health units.

Strategies for applying these techniques can be determined by the number of reports, available software and the technical expertise of analytical staff. Statistical software is required for discriminant or cluster analysis, although string searches can be used in standard database software to create the 0,1

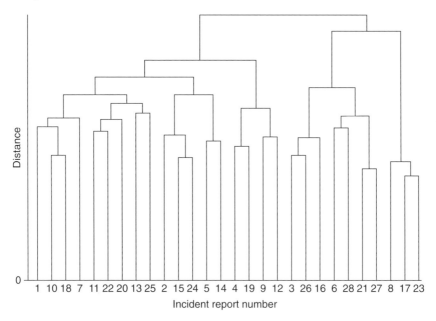

Figure 16.2 Cluster analysis dendrogram.

dataset. For small datasets cluster analysis may be used on its own, but the graphical approach described here becomes difficult with 50 or more reports. Discriminant analysis can be used to analyse several thousands of reports at one time and is thus a useful means of identifying subsets for further investigation with cluster analysis. Cluster analysis is a widely used method; discriminant analysis is not so well known but is still relatively simple and well described in introductory textbooks [22].

More sophisticated textual analysis would use context and phrases rather than short text strings, it would weight strings rather than treating all equally, and it would allow for correlation between strings rather than treating them as independent variables. However, such analysis requires much greater computing power and relies on reports that are written well. The challenge is to find methods that will cope with large databases and with data of erratic quality. The methods described here are an early attempt that can almost certainly be improved.

Secondary analysis: analysing incident descriptions

Secondary analysis should concentrate on the free text description of an incident, although reports usually contain categorical fields such as the location, specialty or degree of harm. The categorical fields in the RLS are essential for identifying subsets of incidents for more detailed analysis, but are not sufficiently detailed to support safety improvement on their own. Experience from incident reporting systems, in both health care and other sectors, shows that the description of incidents is essential to understand their causes and learn lessons from them, for example, by identifying risks or circumstances that contribute to incidents (and actions taken which reduce harm).

The analysis of incidents is complex for a number of reasons:
1 Incidents are often described using medical terminology, and may describe a series of events without stating clearly what the incident was: analysis therefore requires expert knowledge to interpret the text, and a knowledge of what best practice would be in each case, in order to identify what went wrong.
2 Descriptions rarely describe a full series of events: it may be difficult to determine what happened without requesting further information.
3 Interpretation is subjective to some extent: review of incidents by more than one reviewer is beneficial to ensure that all the salient points of an incident are identified.
4 Assessing the impact of the incident on the patient, or whether an incident was avoidable is not straightforward: for example, from case note review studies it is clear that the use of more than one reviewer does not necessarily lead to greater consistency in conclusions about which errors were avoidable or resulted in harm [23].
5 The purpose of analysis needs to be clear at the outset, and will affect analysis: for example, a review of incidents related to patient falls would have a different outcome depending on whether the review addresses environmental

or clinical factors, and on the definition of a fall used to specify criteria for which incidents were included.

A key part of the analysis of free text data is to code or categorise the text further. This makes it easier to describe the content of the free text, to identify any patterns or recurring themes in the data, and to compare incidents with different characteristics. For example, incidents were identified from the RLS by searching for incidents that used the words 'oxygen' or 'O$_2$' in the text. These were reviewed in order to get a better understanding of what types of incidents are reported to the RLS relating to oxygen therapy in acute/ general hospitals. The key themes identified related to errors in administration, equipment risks, fire hazards and other risks; sub-themes could also be identified within some of these themes (Table 16.5).

Table 16.5 Identifying risks to patients on oxygen therapy in acute hospitals: example of analysis of incidents in the RLS.

Free text	Sub-themes	Key themes
'Patient attended for chest x ray, staff member changing oxygen noted prescription for 2 litre/ min. Patient was actually on 8 litre/min'	Wrong dose administered	Administration errors
'Patient on 15 litres O$_2$ … patient desaturated. Later aqua pack found connected to air inlet and not oxygen inlet'	Wrong gas administered	
'Patient transferred from recovery to high dependency unit with insufficient O$_2$ supply (6 L via face mask). Patient blue, saturations reading 58%'	Insufficient oxygen administered	
'A patient on full ventilation was transferred from bed space one to bed space three by [staff name] assisted by [staff name 2] with no oxygen'	No oxygen administered	
'COPD patient was given 10 L to 12 L of O$_2$ when not prescribed due to breathless episode in the night'	Oxygen administered although not prescribed	
'No low oxygen flow meter available on ward'	Lack of equipment	Equipment-related errors
'… suction connected wrongly to oxygen outlet'	User error	
'Patient arrested in x ray. O$_2$ cylinder on crash trolley empty'	Cylinder not checked	
'Patient was attached to O$_2$ cylinder, which was on the bed next to him; the cylinder rolled off the bed and hit the patient leg'	Unrestrained equipment	
'Patient lit cigarette when on oxygen … burns to hand and face'	Fire risk	Fire
'In the nurse handover to the ward it was not stated that patient required oxygen'	Communication	Other

Table 16.6 Characteristics of patient falls.

Examples of information	Use of information
Buzzer/bell available within reach before fall	Highlights whether the organisation has issues in access to call bells
If a fall from bed: bed height, bedrails in use	Assess whether bed height and use of bedrails is affecting falls or injury
Floor wet/dry/talcum powder	Review cleaning regimen, need for non-slip surfaces, etc.
Footwear	Identify problems with missing or unsuitable footwear that could be addressed
Walking aid in use/not in reach	Bedside storage issues or access to walking aids for patients admitted in evenings or weekends
Mental state	Identify those patients most vulnerable to falls, through sedation, dementia, delirium, etc.
First fall this admission or repeat faller	Balance resources between preventing initial falls and secondary prevention
Culprit medication	Impact of sedative and psychotropic medication, or medication with drowsiness as a side effect may contribute to falls

Coding of incident features is important for identifying factors that contributed to the incident, in order to prioritise changes to improve patient safety. Research evidence about the causes of incidents can be used to develop initial categories to use when analysing incidents, and to provide prompts of what information to include in incident reports. The example in Table 16.6 shows factors related to patient falls that might be identified from incident reports, and for which there are evidence-based interventions which could be implemented [24].

Identifying hazards and prioritising issues for local or national action

During 2008, the NPSA has piloted and implemented an improved process to identify and prioritise risks which have resulted in serious incidents, in order to assess the risk and identify immediate actions for local organisations.

Each month, up to 1500 incidents are reviewed. These come from a range of sources, including cases of serious harm and deaths reported to the NPSA and other sources, such as Serious Untoward Incidents (SUIs) reported to Strategic Health Authorities in England[1], and coroners' reports as well as

---

[1] Equivalent Serious Patient Safety Concerns in Wales.

national and international evidence. Drawing on different data sources allows us to build as complete a picture as possible, as no single source of data will tell us everything we need to know.

Each of these serious incidents is reviewed by clinical experts. This includes detailed scrutiny of the free text within the incident report, which helps to understand the 'contributing factors' which have led to the incident (see Table 16.5). If further information about the incident is required, this is requested from the reporting organisation. At this initial stage, the focus is on identifying:

• Potential for national learning to prevent serious harm to patients.
• Issue not already covered by existing NPSA or other safety advice (such as falls prevention or anticoagulant safety).
• Potential weaknesses with the implementation of existing guidance which may require follow-up.
• There is no other agency with lead responsibility for a particular issue.

From the pool of 1500 incidents, around fifty 'trigger incidents' are taken forward each month to discuss at a weekly meeting with a range of clinical and human error experts. Decisions about priorities are made and around half of these incidents are taken forward for further scoping. This is based on the extent of harm (or potential harm) and the likely impact of national action to reduce risks to patients. At the scoping stage, evidence is sought from the wider RLS and other sources such as litigation, as well as record evidence and, importantly, views of key stakeholders on the clinical significance of the issue and what can be done. Incident reports which are not scoped further are still very valuable. These data are used to identify broad trends and patterns for feedback to local organisations and for regular review by experts in key clinical areas, such as medication safety. Further information can be found at: www.npsa.nhs.uk/nrls/alerts-and-directives/rapidrr.

Conclusion

The analysis of incident reports in health care has received relatively little attention. While hitherto health care has built on the experience of other high-risk industries, especially aviation, the volume of reports from its own sector means that there are intellectual and analytical challenges to transferring approaches to analysis of errors which have been taken elsewhere.

In this chapter, we have described the approaches taken to analysis of the RLS, and have outlined how these could be adapted to analysis at health care organisation level. These approaches have contributed to reports and alerts from the NPSA, aimed at making healthcare safer [25]. However, there is considerable scope for developing these methods, and extending their use.

Incident reporting in healthcare is a relatively new activity, and at the NPSA the approaches used to analyse and prioritise issues for action are under continuous review and development [26]. This chapter has described some approaches which have been used to analyse RLS data in the early phases of the RLS: we will be developing and refining methods in the light of experience.

Acknowledgements

The authors would like to thank colleagues at the NPSA who have contributed to the development of the methods described in this chapter, in particular Kate Beaumont, Dagmar Luettel and Frances Healey.

References

1 Barach P, Small S. Reporting and preventing medical mishaps: lessons from non-medical near miss reporting systems. *British Medical Journal* 2000; **320**: 759–63.
2 Department of Health. *Building a Safer NHS for Patients.* Department of Health, London. Available at www.dh.gov.uk/PublicationsAndStatistics/Publications/Publications PolicyAndGuidance/PublicationsPAmpGBrowsableDocument/fs/en?CONTENT_ ID=4097460&chk=gngr/O.
3 Scobie S, Thomson R. *Building a Memory: Preventing Harm, Reducing Risks and Improving Patient Safety.* National Patient Safety Agency, London, 2005. Available at http://www. npsa.nhs.uk/site/media/documents/1280_PSO_Report.pdf.
4 National Patient Safety Agency. *Seven Steps to Patient Safety.* NPSA, London. Available at www.npsa.nhs.uk/health/resources/7steps.
5 National Patient Safety Agency, National Reporting and Learning System dataset: www. npsa.nhs.uk.
6 National Patient Safety Agency. *Quarterly National Reporting and Learning System Data Summary, Winter 2006/7.* NPSA, London, 2007.
7 World Health Organisation. *International Patient Safety Event Classification.* WHO, Geneva, 2006.
8 National Patient Safety Agency. *Comparative Trust Feedback Reports.* NPSA, London, 2006.
9 National Patient Safety Agency. *Evaluation Report.* NPSA, London.
10 World Alliance for Patient Safety. *WHO Draft Guidelines for Adverse Event Reporting and Learning Systems.* World Health Organisation, Geneva, 2005.
11 Healthcare Commission: www.healthcarecommission.org.uk.
12 Office for National Statistics: www.national-statistics.gov.uk.
13 Medicines and Healthcare products Regulatory Agency: www.mhra.gov.uk.
14 Action against Medical Accidents: www.avma.org.uk.
15 NHS Litigation Authority: www.nhsla.com.
16 Billings CE. The NASA aviation safety reporting system: lessons learned from voluntary incident reporting. In: *Enhancing Patient Safety and Reducing Errors in Health Care. Proceedings of the National Patient Safety Foundation Conference.* Chicago, 1998: 97–100.
17 National Patient Safety Agency. *RLS Quarterly Data Summary, Winter 2006/7.* NPSA, London, 2007.
18 National Statistics. Deaths involving MRSA: England and Wales 2001–2005. *Health Statistics Quarterly* 2007; **33**: 76–81. Available at http://www.statistics.gov.uk/ downloads/theme_health/HSQ33.pdf.

19 Vincent C, Davy C, Esmail A et al. *Learning from Litigation: An Analysis of Claims for Clinical Negligence.* University of Manchester, Manchester, 2004. Available at http://www.mbs.ac.uk/research/groups/public-policy-management/documents/lfl-report-vol2-final-revised.pdf.

20 National Patient Safety Agency. Unpublished analysis of clinical negligence claims notified to trusts in 2005 and managed by the NHS Litigation Authority. Available at http://www.npsa.nhs.uk.

21 National Patient Safety Agency. *Skin Treatment Fire Risk.* Patient Safety Bulletin. NPSA, London, 2007. Available at http://www.npsa.nhs.uk/site/media/documents/2317_PSBulletinJan07.pdf.

22 Manly BFJ. *Multivariate Statistical Methods.* Chapman and Hall, London, 1991.

23 Hayward RA, Hofer TP. Estimating hospital deaths due to medical errors: preventability is in the eye of the reviewer. *Journal of the American Medical Association* 2001; **286**: 415–20.

24 Healey F, Scobie S. *Slips, Trips and Falls in Hospital.* National Patient Safety Agency, London, 2007.

25 National Patient Safety Agency: http://www.npsa.nhs.uk/health/alerts.

26 Carruthers I, Phillips P. *Safety First: A Report for Patients, Clinicians and Healthcare Managers.* Department of Health, London, 2006.

CHAPTER 17

Patient safety education and curriculum design

Marshall F. Gilula, Paul R. Barach

The goal of a medical education curriculum is to give physicians of the future the tools to address problems that affect the health of the public. The burgeoning complexities of health care delivery systems can amplify errors that occur. Some assume that the struggle to make patient safety a part of the medical curriculum is successful and that the battle is already won. But much evidence to the contrary suggests this is a premature conclusion. This chapter describes the challenges of assimilating patient safety curricula and identifies both positive and negative elements of safety training in medical education predominantly in the USA.

There has been much discussion in both the public and private sectors regarding ways to modify the medical education system to address the challenges raised by the 1999 Institute of Medicine (IOM) report *To Err is Human: Building a Safer Health System* [1]. The IOM's report estimated that as many as 98,000 patients die in the USA every year from preventable medical errors in hospitals, with annual costs associated with hospital-based medical errors estimated to be as high as $29 billion dollars. In the IOM's follow-up report, *Crossing the Quality Chasm: A New Health System for the 21st Century*, a strong call for change in the education and training of physicians was made in order to address the problems associated with quality, access and outcomes in the present system [2]. The Association of American Medical Colleges (AAMC) has called for a collaborative effort to ensure that the next generation of physicians is adequately prepared to recognise the sources of error in medical practice, to acknowledge their own vulnerability to error, and to engage fully in the process of continuous quality improvement (CQI). The curriculum needs therefore to contain a clear, factual and succinct statement of the ongoing safety crisis affecting patients, health care providers and teachers equally.

Although patient safety has been increasingly recognised as a key dimension of quality care, relatively little has been published in the medical education literature addressing patient safety competencies and skills that might be introduced at the undergraduate and graduate levels. Serious discussion on the design, assessment and faculty development needs of patient safety

Health Care Errors and Patient Safety. Edited by Brian Hurwitz and Aziz Sheikh.
© 2009 Blackwell Publishing, ISBN: 978-1-4051-4643-2.

education in undergraduate and graduate education has been sparse. Few schools have modified their curricula to prepare students to practise in this new environment [3].

Leape and Berwick suggested that 5 years after *To Err is Human* there was not enough substantial improvement in patient safety [4]. There have been some changes 'affecting safety at the margin, (but) their overall impact is hard to see in national statistics'. Many medical specialties can relate to the improvements that now include, for example: (i) fewer patients dying from accidental injections of concentrated potassium chloride; (ii) better management of anticoagulants in dedicated clinics; and (iii) tightened infection and glucose control procedures that have reduced serious infections. But despite continuing widespread coverage of patient safety issues in the media these changes have resulted in only minimal improvements. Although there has been improvement in knowledge and skills that are part of patient safety education, there has been very little alteration in the study and teaching of attitudes that relate to safer care. Wachter's 2001 evidence-based review [5] adopted the following definition of patient safety practice as 'a type of process or structure whose application reduces the probability of adverse events resulting from exposure to the health care system across a range of diseases and procedures'.

Our research, which predominantly pertains to the USA, and our clinical experience, points to five important challenges in making patient safety an indispensable part of the medical curriculum: (i) lack of innovation in the medical school environment; (ii) debate about course formats (as a stand-alone course or as interwoven elements within the entire curriculum?); (iii) examples of patient safety curricula in medical schools; (iv) legislative interest in best practice models of patient safety education; and (v) evidence for patient safety practices in state and national health care.

Innovation in the medical school environment

Medical education has been slow to adopt changes in curricula. Medical errors and patient safety have emerged as central public concerns in the USA and around the world. There is evidence of ongoing patient safety education in the current literature (see Chapter 12). The impact of these inroads conflicts with various 'turf wars' of established health care courses, fiscal concerns with providing clinical services, and an often prevalent attitude in health care of 'organisational silence'.

When one considers innovation of the medical school environment, it is apparent that this environment involves much more than just one institution. Challenges to both patient safety education and medical education in general include the *multidisciplinary nature* of stakeholders in today's health care. Many of the stakeholders are not only medical professionals, strictly speaking, but insurance companies, professional health care organisations and unions, pharmaceutical industries and various elements of the legal profession. Health care organisations such as hospitals, where the bulk of medical adverse errors occur, deal with a massive array of regulatory and special interest organisations in the course of their day-to-day operations. Although large organisations may prefer to pay off malpractice judgments and simply raise the costs of health care instead of identifying and ameliorating problems, this tendency can impede the teaching and implementation of patient safety principles.

A less pernicious explanation is 'organisational silence', which refers to the collective-level phenomenon of doing or saying very little in response to significant problems or issues facing an organisation or industry [6,7]. This dynamic manifests with many health care professionals who do not feel comfortable disclosing or confronting incompetence in their colleagues. One of the principles in patient safety education needs to be that of making it safer to disclose errors as well as asking for help. Many institutions perceive no political or ethical imperative for patient safety education. In fact, some educators believe that health care practitioners would resent guidelines that are 'mandated' or required. Practitioners might perceive any regulatory activity as unhelpful interference with their own professional autonomy.

Stand-alone course or interwoven curricular elements?

There is good evidence that second-year medical students at one medical school, the University of Missouri, in general benefited from a patient safety course that was integrated with an 'Introduction to patient care' course. Benefit was manifested by changes in knowledge, skills and attitude [8]. However, not all changes were sustained at the 1-year follow-up, some were not in the desired direction of reporting errors, and few of the changes were supported by self-reported behaviours. The medical students did not report errors as frequently to faculty as to residents or fellow students, and only rarely used the electronic error reporting system that had been presented during the course. Wu et al. [9] reported similar findings in which physicians in training did not feel comfortable telling their attending staff about medical errors and patient harm which ensued from their care. Vohra et al. [10] found that the exposure of physician trainees to errors and adverse events can have a negative effect on their attitudes and competencies. Exposure to adverse events and the institution's response may decrease both error reporting and willingness to adopt safety practices. But the survey and interview responses suggested that training increases perceived efficacy in dealing with adverse events.

These findings corroborate the growing support of teaching patient safety in repetitive fashion, as cardiopulmonary resuscitation (CPR) courses are taught. Should patient safety be taught as a free-standing course or as a theme that is vertically interwoven into the medical curriculum? The Barach [11] and Madigosky et al. [8] findings suggest that patient safety should be taught both ways and reinforced at regular intervals. A second-year Missouri student opined that the course needed to be taught during the first year 'before we get our God complexes'. In the turf wars involving who gives up what amount of time to patient safety, some clinicians indicate that *everything* in the medical school curriculum is about patient safety. If this were true, it would not be necessary to have a dedicated time in the curriculum for the subject. *Patient safety teaching should not be designed to supplant but to integrate with other coursework* in the health care curriculum. For example, medication events can be taught as part of the traditional pharmacology course, and patient and site identification can be taught as part of the traditional anatomy course.

Examples of patient safety courses

Literature searches in 2007 using the keywords 'patient safety course' yielded 2450 references, but only a relatively small number of actual courses that went beyond an introductory discussion of how important it is to train health care providers in patient safety competencies. A majority of the sources focus on the impact of patient safety information on health care administrative institutional policies and the policies of other educational institutions. Many of the available patient safety courses are brief introductions, half-day mini-symposia or extended update lectures on patient safety that are relevant to a particular specialty organisation meeting.

At the University of Rochester, New York, a 10-session patient safety course is offered to professionals, trainees and students at all the health care schools (medicine, dentistry, nursing, pharmacy, hospital administration, health services research). Each of the twice-monthly sessions is 90 minutes in duration. The course time includes case study discussions [12].

A six module web-based course, 'Patient safety and medical errors', was produced by the Texas Medical Association [13] in association with ten different medical institutions in Texas. Each module is designed to address 'critical issues in patient safety' and 'to provide both insight into the problem and suggest practices to reduce the incidence of errors in healthcare'.

There is a two credit hour elective patient safety course given at Creighton University, Nebraska that also provides an additional two credit hour elective student experience in focused patient safety research projects. Both the course and the textbook are interdisciplinary and interprofessional. The faculty includes professionals from the fields of business, dentistry, law, medicine, nursing, occupational therapy, bioethics, pharmacy, physical therapy and social work. The main topics of this elective course include patient–health care provider relationships, safety in health care systems, organisations and culture, safety errors and handling safety errors as they occur, along with some case-based studies [14].

Nova Southeastern University College of Osteopathic Medicine, Florida [15] has a required 20–36-hour course that is dedicated to patient safety and quality improvement and makes extensive use of health imformation technology (HIT). The course uses standardised patients (SPs), and features small group sessions with faculty members who illustrate medical fallibility by presenting and discussing their own medical errors. The students are taught to practise admitting to errors with simulated patients and are also graded by the SPs. The SPs are trained to assess how convincing the medical students are in admitting their errors and in openly disclosing resultant harm to patients.

Patient safety teaching is presented as both interwoven and stand-alone courses in the medical school curriculum. There remain inevitable worries and conflicts over which department is obliged to give up how much of their own allotted time in the curriculum so that the patient safety curricular elements can be taught. Tables 17.1–17.3 and the appendix summarise the results from our research and teaching at the University of Miami Miller School of Medicine, which are described later in the chapter.

Legislative interest in patient safety training

The Florida legislative interest in patient safety was related to better delineating the ongoing crises in medical malpractice and health care inequalities. There was bipartisan public recognition that health care was in a crisis [16]. State legislation requiring patient safety education and continuing medical education for all health care disciplines was enacted in 2004. Efforts promoting a state patient safety agency were also successful in creating the Florida Patient Safety Corporation. But these efforts have been hampered by lack of funding and leadership to help bridge the differences in legislative vision of how best to improve patient care in Florida [17].

Patient safety practices in state and national health care

Our experiences suggest that at least half of the respondents in our survey study with patient safety experts felt uncomfortable disclosing data from their own departments or institutions. One strong recommendation for reducing medical error has been the adoption of electronic medical records (EMR). The best assessment of how far health care has progressed in implementing widespread EMR was noted by one pioneer, Dr Marc Overhage: 'Don't expect too much too soon' [18]. A 7-year effort to connect hospitals and physicians' offices in the Santa Barbara, California region with interoperable e-records to share patient data across practices, with the goal of improving care and cutting costs ended recently when a $10 million grant ran out in December 2006. The health care community did not consider it worth continuing the effort to achieve interoperable e-records. The learning curve can be daunting.

Dr Marc Overhage, the director of medical informatics at Regenstrief Institute, Indiana, works with a system that has been developed over 30 years and claims a 50% reduction in adverse drug reactions. In Indiana, more than 70% of the state's hospitals and doctors use a single health data exchange created by the Regenstrief Institute, which is affiliated to the Indiana University School of Medicine [18].

Case study: the Florida experience

The Florida legislature in 2004 passed enabling legislation that created the Florida Patient Safety Corporation (a 501(c)(3) not-for-profit, state-mandated patient safety guidance organisation) [19]. The organisation was based on our previous three-part assessment of the expert and literature consensus on patient safety curricula that used a purposive sampling of patient safety experts. In January 2004, we convened a Patient Safety Curriculum Conference which brought together 80 cross-disciplinary experts to assess, collate and synthesise currently available knowledge about patient safety teaching, training and evaluation [20].

Experts from medicine, nursing, law, the pharmaceutical industry, information technology and the fields of simulation and curriculum design helped to produce a framework and recommendations for teaching patient safety in health care professional schools and continuing education courses [20]. Our study recommendations were derived from a combination of interviews, the expert conference and literature research (Table 17.1).

We found a moderate consensus on the need to create a strong state-based agency that could make and implement *recommendations* for a safety curriculum that would be integrated throughout the entire curriculum. These findings are corroborated by a recent study of 12 communities, which suggested that the Joint Commission on Accreditation of Healthcare

Table 17.1 Patient safety study recommendations.

1 Patient safety curricula should develop adaptive health care professional teams dedicated to patient safety

2 Genuine patient safety includes educating the patient and family members about their role as team members in all health care setting

3 Effective patient safety teaching uses teamwork and interdisciplinary teams that work together to create a comprehensive 'culture of safety'

4 Patient safety and improving quality should be the central features of clinical health care teaching in all disciplines

5 The knowledge, skills, attitudes and competencies that make up patient safety must be clearly defined in any curriculum

6 The core knowledge in a patient safety curriculum must be interdisciplinary and should ideally be taught in a multidisciplinary group

7 The patient safety curriculum must include an ongoing evaluation of the curriculum

8 The patient safety curriculum must include theory, practice, training and simulation in order to develop a comprehensive understanding of patient safety

9 Patient safety curricula should include learning how to manage error by means of voluntary and mandatory reporting, documenting, recovery and disclosure

10 Patient safety curricula should include learning about instruments and tools that can be utilized in causal analysis and trending of adverse events

11 Patient safety curricula should teach students how to become patient focused and help patients to be proactive about their own 'safety'

12 Patient safety curricula should teach health care students the basic knowledge required to be 'safe practitioners'

Organisations has had the most significant impact on US hospitals' efforts to improve patient safety [21]. The experts agreed that a stand-alone course was not sufficient. Components of patient safety competencies should be taught in multiple courses and reinforced daily in clinical situations. All medical professionals (i.e. nurses, pharmacists, physicians, therapists, etc.) should receive comparable integrated training. It was noted that most health care education is still conducted in a unidisciplinary manner. The experts used their own teaching and practice experience, combined with their knowledge of the relevant literature, as a basis for the following guidelines.

Challenges to implementing a patient safety curriculum are complex

There are numerous psychological, logistical and political impediments at many levels, especially at the higher administrative levels, against implementing a safety curriculum. First, physicians and educators serving as instructors, mentors and role models have limited knowledge and experience with many of the competencies required in safety education. Changing current physician behaviours related to safety and quality continues to be difficult. Most physicians believe they provide optimal patient care and that they do not make injurious mistakes. In a survey undertaken by over 1000 doctors, nurses and residents in urban teaching and non-teaching hospitals, one-third of staff members stated that they have never made an error (David Mayer, Associate Dean, University of Illinois College of Medicine, personal communication, 2006). Most denied any deleterious effects of stress on their judgment and affirmed that their decision-making skills are just as good in emergencies as in normal situations. Only one-third of the staff reported that errors are handled appropriately and over half reported that they find it difficult to discuss mistakes. Medical students and residents found it especially difficult to discuss their medical errors and subsequent patient harm [10]. Their impressions from seeing how the system addressed patient harm was that it was best for them to not talk about these outcomes. Additionally, overcoming the current medicolegal environment that favours hiding errors and near-misses instead of learning from them will continue to offer educational challenges while hindering humanistic efforts related to transparency, full disclosure and apology.

Patient safety courses should and can be taught in all health care institutions to students, practitioners and administrators alike. A longitudinal approach to safety education at the student level is needed that will be reinforced at all levels of training. The ability to reinforce and practise safety skills is a key element for curricular development. Batalden et al. defined medical education and physician development as a continuum based on the Dreyfus model that starts at the beginning of medical school and continues throughout a practitioner's professional career [22]. The Dreyfus learning model has been used by the US Air Force to describe five longitudinal stages in the development of knowledge and skills of a pilot. Similar developmental processes have been seen in chess players, adults learning a second language and adults learning to drive an automobile [23].

The model applied to health care outlines a five-stage progress from freshman medical student in the *novice stage*, junior medical student as *advanced beginner*, resident physician as *competent*, specialist physician early in practice as *proficient* and mid-career physician as *expert* [23] (Table 17.2). The first stage of the Dreyfus model (novice stage) is where basic concepts, skills and values are learned. For clinical skills, Batalden et al. notes 'this is where the beginning student starts learning how to take a medical history through memorization of the chief complaint, history of the present illness, review of systems, and family and social history' [22]. In the second stage, known as the advanced beginner stage, students begin to experiment with limited applications. It is in this second stage that 'the third year medical student begins to appreciate common situations, such as those facing hospitalized patients (admissions, rounds, discharge) that can only be learned through experience. The remaining three stages continue through residency and mid-career, where the recognition of patterns and the use of intuition are the major work drivers' [22].

A basic understanding of the concepts and values of patient safety and quality care should be introduced early in the curriculum, preferably in the first 2 years of medical education. This would be followed by the supervised experimentation and application of these skills during clinical clerkships. The competencies needed to support safe patient care – skills, knowledge and attitudes – can be learned at the novice stage but must be continuously reinforced at all stages of expertise. *Teaching of elements in the lifelong learning chart must be repeated at each stage of professional development*. Most aspects of patient safety can be taught to beginning medical students, but the training needs to be reinforced periodically (Table 17.2).

Educational strategies in patient safety curricula

Educational strategies in patient safety curricula must involve both innovative content and methods. There are a number of different strategies and educational modalities that could be utilised in addressing patient safety education at the student level. These tools include plenaries, small group learning sessions, experiential learning, simulation, standardised patient role plays, case-based learning, individual and team learning, multimedia micro-simulations and other supportive audiovisual material. Students seeking a deeper awareness of, and knowledge in, patient safety and quality care initiatives should have access to more intensive educational opportunities before graduation.

Educational content

Educational content addressed in a longitudinal patient safety curriculum for students is presented in a learning matrix of patient safety domains (see Appendix 17.1). Interprofessional (interdisciplinary) teamwork should be a mandatory cornerstone of the patient safety student curriculum. Grumback and Bodenheimer summarise research on patient care teams suggesting that cohesive teams, where physicians and other health care professionals work

Table 17.2 Patient safety and lifelong learning, with regular reinforcement of core values (adapted from Dreyfus [7]).

	Stage				
	1	2	3	4	5
I *Attitudes*					
Honesty, trust and respect; professionalism; accepting fallibility	+	+	+	+	+
Patient-centeredness; awareness of families as systems		+	+	+	+
II *Skills*					
Active communication (clarity, disclosure, transparency)	+	+	+	+	+
Multidisciplinary teamwork; learning competence and values		+	+	+	+
Analysis and managements of both errors and near-misses		+	+	+	+
III *Knowledge*					
History and driving forces of the patient safety movement	+	+	+	+	+
Types of health care errors, error theory, taxonomies of error		+	+	+	+
System, design, individual errors, adverse events, near-misses		+	+	+	+
Types of quality problems: overuse, underuse, misuse		+	+	+	+
Epidemiology of medical errors			+	+	+
Common cause/types of errors (medication, wrong site surgery)		+	+	+	+
Common locations of errors (surgery, paediatric ICU, ER)			+	+	+
Comparison to high reliability organisations	+	+	+	+	+
Ethical, legal, professional issues and 'culture of medicine'		+	+	+	+
Ethical principles: honesty, non-malfeasance, AMA ethics code	+	+	+	+	+
Legal and Malpractice issues medicolegal alternatives	+	+	+		
Culture of health care with hierarchies and power		+	+	+	+
Expectations of perfection/infallibility, intolerance of error	+	+	+	+	+
Steps in handling error; mandatory vs voluntary reporting		+	+	+	+
Root cause analysis and recovery from error		+	+	+	+
FMEA (failure mode and effects analysis)			+	+	+
Bar coding of drug packaging; automated prescription services		+	+	+	+
Handwriting; use of confusing abbreviations; dose calculations			+	+	+

AMA, American Medical Association; ER, emergency room; ICU, intensive care unit.
1, novice; 2, advanced beginner; 3, competent; 4, proficient; 5, mastery.

together, are associated with improved patient outcomes [24,25]. Improved teamwork skills and greater collaboration between professions have also been linked with safe and effective health care [26]. Students need to be made aware of the outcome improvements as well as other positive effects of teamwork. 'Interprofessional learning consists of more than sharing the same learning environment as others: it involves acquiring an understanding of the knowledge base, values and ethos of like-minded individuals and developing respect for each other's contribution to the learning process' [27].

Despite growing agreement in theory, today's health care educators are not yet putting theory into practice. *Safety science must be taught beginning at entry level for all health care trainees* (see Table 17.2). Safety science needs to be constantly re-learned on a periodic basis just in the same way that we recognise the need to do this with CPR and other protocols. One major difference, though, is that the attitudes need to be periodically reinforced. As health care training progresses, the competing attitudes that are learned from the commercial marketplace are often in direct opposition to the attitudes of mutual cooperation, fallibility and transparency which are necessary for safeguarding the health care of the patient.

There is still an ambivalent unanimity in the way educators perceive the urgency of patient safety problems. Health professional students will report errors, when it becomes safe for them to admit mistakes or errors openly and immediately without consequence. Extreme honesty at the expense of the provider can be difficult to practise [28]. While the practising provider has the threat of litigation and peer criticism, the student has an additional threat of receiving low evaluations or, in worst cases, failing a course or a rotation. Teaching and learning improvement science by studying error reduction strategies can be a partial remedy to this problem. Creating safe environments that are non-punitive to the student and the provider will go a long way to ensuring a culture of safety.

It is imperative that a critical mass of faculty becomes motivated and trained to incorporate patient safety into their teaching. A key factor for inculcating a safety culture is addressing the 'hidden curriculum' which students learn in the hallways and other informal gathering places away from the wards and laboratories [29–32]. A robust curriculum promoting altruism, patient-centredness and team values is vital for creating a safety culture in which the health care provider teaches safety culture values to patients by precept. In the public health sector, students majoring in health care systems have the option of focusing their efforts on patient safety. Additionally, health care administrative courses are beginning to integrate instruction in systems thinking and quality improvement methodology.

The metrics for assessing curricula are still unsatisfactory. Mechanisms for evaluating curricular effectiveness can be accomplished in at least two ways: (i) indirectly, by measuring the impact of teaching on the knowledge, skills and attitudes of the learner; and (ii) directly, by assessing the entire health care 'system' for fewer errors and improved safety. Skill acquisition could be assessed by using micro-simulations (as with interactive computer-based patients), clinical skills exams using SPs and by encouraging students to design research projects exploring this topic [33].

Simulation has proven effective in aviation, nuclear power and the military, to maximise training safety and minimise risk. Since health care and related professions are hazardous disciplines, the use of simulation in health care is logical. Trainees should use simulation models before taking on patient care responsibilities. Simulated standardised and atypical patients and computer-driven mannequins not only help assure optimal treatment of patients, they help students develop knowledge, skills and attitudes while protecting live patients from unnecessary risk [34].

Simulators are considered very efficient for teaching how to handle problems and prepare for examinations featuring simulation, but the absence of well-designed studies and robust data showing effective transfer of learning *from* the simulation and simulator *to* the real life situation is still concerning. Recent research on the use of virtual reality methodology strongly suggests that the fidelity and reliability of simulated carotid stent placement by trainees is equivalent to practising on patients [35–37]. The carotid stenting trial that began in 2004 trains physicians 'to an objectively established level of proficiency on a virtual reality simulator prior to performing stenting in a patient'. The stenting training was followed up in a randomised double-blind trial by Grantcharov, and demonstrated that training by virtual reality significantly reduces objectively assessed intraoperative errors in laparoscopic cholecystectomy [38]. This is one of many examples underscoring the value of simulation in reducing cost, decreasing the time required to achieve competencies and also reducing organisational hazards when compared to present modes of teaching invasive procedures.

Assessing changes in attitude is more difficult. The current educational model is driven by individual performance on examinations that predominantly reward memorisation and recall of factual knowledge versus application. Kenneth Shine, past president of the US Institute of Medicine, concluded that [39]:

In the areas of self-governance and quality, I think we have largely failed. We have failed because we equate quality with how much an individual physician knows. We do an examination and we look at the knowledge base, as opposed to looking at quality as something that has to do with how well patients are cared for.

Assessment strategies will also need to be modified to reflect the importance of patient safety education. A recent article by Kachalia et al. on the incorporation of safety knowledge and skills into board exams is encouraging [40]. Changing the culture from a physician-centred to a patient-centred culture must occur. Dr Shine also noted [39],

The 21st century paradigm is that of physicians who understand teamwork and systems of care in which they can provide leadership. Solo practice was the paradigm of the late 19th century and the first part of the 20th century, whereas in the 21st century it will be systems of care in which individual physicians or groups of physicians play key roles that will determine the outcomes of care and health. Fallibility should be replaced by an approach to multidisciplinary problem solving.

The University of Miami patient safety curriculum was designed around the patient safety competencies shown in Appendix 17.1. The material was subsequently used in three different lecture series with medical students and house staff physicians during 2004–2005. We developed 30 multiple choice questions for a knowledge assessment test that could be administered before and after patient safety courses. An attitude assessment from a previous study of medical student attitudes [10] towards sentinel events was also designed to be co-administered online with the multiple choice questions [41]. We have developed a web-based patient safety overview and a streaming video presentation of the same overview [42]. Web-based presentations and such online pre- and post-teaching surveys can estimate both knowledge and attitude change [43].

Despite a number of robust, ongoing challenges to the incorporation and integration of patient safety coursework with establish medical curricula, there have already been many inroads formulated about how to teach these elements and what these elements should be. One bottom line we have learned about in the progression of information technology and EMRs is 'Don't expect too much too soon' [18]. But other aspects of patient safety, like hand washing, may not be so difficult to see already happening.

Yet putting into practice the more difficult aspects of what has been taught and learned is also vital. Honesty and straightforwardness in disclosing to patients when something adverse has happened has already been shown to have significant benefit [44]. Recent evidence from the University of Michigan, highlighted by Senator Clinton and President-elect Obama in the *New England Journal of Medicine*, support an aggressive disclosure policy [45]. In 2002, the University of Michigan Health System launched a program with three components: (i) acknowledge cases in which a patient was hurt because of medical error and compensate these patients quickly and fairly; (ii) aggressively defend cases that the hospital considers to be without merit; and (iii) study all adverse events to determine how procedures could be improved. Before August 2001, the organisation had approximately 260 claims and lawsuits pending at any given time. As of August 2005, the number of lawsuits had dropped to 114. The average time from the filing of a claim to its resolution was reduced from approximately 21 months to less than 10 months; annual litigation costs dropped from about $3 million to $1 million.

Conclusion

Medical errors and patient safety have emerged as concerns in the provision of quality health care. If we are to change the current health care culture, many believe it is important that students begin to understand, appreciate and demonstrate appropriate skills related to medical errors and patient safety early in their professional education. Tremendous opportunity exists to influence the safety of health care delivery profoundly by changing the educational environment, teaching methods and health professional curricula. Adoption of patient safety knowledge by leading health care education groups has been slow. There are elements such as 'organisational silence' and unrecognised 'hidden curriculum' teaching that can impede effective implementation of patient safety education. Information systems and technologies are available that can improve significantly the educational process, but they have yet to be fully implemented. Simulation, successfully employed for years in the military and aviation industry, can facilitate patient safety teaching. Team-based teaching, in simulated or controlled real-time situations, emphasises cooperation and clear communication in a context of systems-based care. Fostering trust, honesty and respect between consumers and providers, patients and health care professionals, and among the health care disciplines, empowers patients and health care providers alike.

There is a critical leadership role needed for improving the knowledge, skills and attitudes of health professionals in order to provide safer health care. Specific implementation steps include conducting an in-depth assessment of existing curricula in health professional schools *as an important first step* (Table 17.3).

Table 17.3 Specific implementation steps and recommendations.

1 *In-depth assessment of existing curricula in health professional schools*

An in-depth analysis of existing curricular approaches among health-provider schools should be commissioned. This analysis would ideally include the following characteristics:
• Solicitation of curricula
• Prioritisation of medical and nursing education
• Interviews with chairs of curriculum committees and a sample of medical residency directors
• Surveys of trainees at various stages of training (e.g. first-year medical students, residents, fellows) to establish baseline
• Identification of key curricular components and proposed sample content
• Identification of barriers to development and/or implementation of curricula
• Development of strategies to address barriers (including external incentives, funding and regulatory approaches)

2 *Development of a core curriculum for all health practitioner education programmes*

Given the recent growth in available curricula on a national basis, this activity should yield results within 2 years, contingent upon sufficient funds being appropriated to sponsor this. Characteristics of this curriculum development project would include:
• Review of existing curricula identified in point 1 above, and nationally available models, to identify priority content areas for inclusion, specifying those which are shared across all disciplines and those which are discipline specific
• Review of possible implementation models and instructional design modalities to provide a range of implementation options for health professional schools
• Development of online modules as well as classroom-based courses
• Design of an evaluation/monitoring strategy to track dissemination and impact of courses
• Presentation of the results at a state-wide conference, ideally convened in partnership with the relevant professional societies (e.g. Medical Association, Nursing Association, Pharmacy Association, etc.) to present the findings and gain feedback on the proposed content and implementation strategies
• Identification of at least one school in each discipline to pilot test the curriculum in the second year
• Revisions to the curricula based on the field test experience

Appendix 17.1: Matrix of patient safety training domains for health care students

Patient safety domains	Knowledge, skills and attitudes
1 Introduction: theoretical foundations	Explores the history of patient safety and contributions of different disciplines such as cognitive psychology, human factors and ergonomics, sociology, economics and management
2 Epidemiology and information	Explores the various sources of information available and methods used to study the problem of risk and safety in health care. Examples of information and methods available include: trust information systems; use of routine data for monitoring quality and safety; structured record review for assessing clinical specialties; integrated risk management systems; and quality and safety indicators
3 Interpersonal aspects and issues	Explores the domain related to the effect of clinical incidents and adverse events on patients and staff as well as prospective and proactive methods of risk reduction. These themes explore research evidence, policy guidelines and current clinical practice on: (i) how health care professionals can effectively communicate information relating to risk to patients and their families; (ii) how adverse events and clinical incidents affect patients and their relatives; (iii) how complaints and litigation are managed; and (iv) how patients and their families can facilitate clinical safety and the role of health care professionals in supporting them
4 Human factors and ergonomics	Explores various reporting systems, both within health care and in industry, and root cause analysis and other incident analysis tools for reducing risk and improving quality and safety. Other aspects of this module include documentation, continuity of care, multidisciplinary teams and team training, ergonomics and design, and safety culture
5 Medication safety	Explores the medication administration microsystems: medication errors, health information technology tools (EMR, Computer-based Provider Order Entry (CPOE) and adverse and near-miss reporting
6 Crisis management tools	Explores the roles of communication, team training, shared decision making and situational awareness
7 Simulations and simulation science	Explores the training of micro-, macro-, debriefing, immersion levels, scripting and role playing

References

1 Kohn LT, Corrigan JM, Donaldson M, eds. *To Err Is Human: Building a Safer Health System*. Healthcare Services/National Academies Press, Washington, 1999.
2 Institute of Medicine. *Crossing the Quality Chasm: A New Health System for the 21st Century*. Healthcare Services/National Academies Press, Washington, 2001.
3 Gould BE, O'Connell MT, Russell, MT, Pipas CE, McCurdy FA. Teaching quality measurement and improvement, cost-effectiveness, and patient satisfaction in undergraduate

medical education: the UME-21 experience. *Family Medicine* 2004; **36** (Suppl): S57–S62. Available at http://www.stfm.org/fmhub/fm2004/January/BruceS57.pdf (accessed 14 Feb. 2007).

4 Leape LL, Berwick DM. Five years after to err is human. *Journal of the American Medical Association* 2005; **293** (19): 2384–90.

5 Wachter RM. *Making Health Care Safer: A Critical Analysis of Patient Safety Practices.* Evidence Report/Technology Assessment No. 43. AHRQ Publication No. 01-E058. Agency for Healthcare Research and Quality, Rockville, MD, 2001. Available at http://www.ahrq.gov/clinic/ptsafety/ (accessed 14 Feb. 2007).

6 Morrison E, Milliken F (2000) Organizational silence: a barrier to change and development in a pluralistic world. *Academy of Management Review* 25(4):706–725.

7 Henrikson K, Dayton E. Organizational silence and hidden threats to patient safety. *Health Services Research* 2006; **41** (4): 1539–54.

8 Madigosky WS, Headrick L, Nelson K et al. Changing and sustaining medical students' knowledge, skills, and attitudes about patient safety and medical fallibility. *Academic Medicine* 2006; **8** (1): 94–101.

9 Wu AW, Folkman S, McPhee SJ, et al. Do house officers learn from their mistakes? *Journal of the American Medical Association* 1991; **265**: 2089–94.

10 Vohra P, Daugherty C, Mohr J et al. Housestaff and medical student attitudes towards adverse medical events. *Joint Commission Journal on Quality and Safety* 2007, **33** (9): 493–501.

11 Barach P (2000) Patient safety curriculum. *Academic Medicine* 75:141–142.

12 University of Rochester Certificate Course in Patient Safety and Prevention of Medical Errors. Available at www.abaaurp.org/module.asp?courseID=22 (Accessed 25 Sep 2008).

13 Texas Medical Association. Patient Safety and Medical Errors. Available at www.texmed.org/Template.asp?id=5440 (accessed 25 Sep 2008).

14 Creighton University Medical Center. The Office of Interprofessional Education. Available at http://www.creighton.edu/ipe/patientsafetycourse.htm (accessed 20 May 2007).

15 Nova University S.E. College of Osteopathic Medicine. Available at http://hpd.nova.edu/catalog/forms/college of osteopathic medicine catalog.pdf (accessed 10 May 2008).

16 Barach P. Florida Patient Safety Corporation 2004 – a model for other states. *Accreditation Council on Graduate Medical Education Bulletin* 2004; **2004**; 23–7.

17 Barach P. *Does New Florida Legislation Reduce Patient Safety? Perspectives on Patient Safety.* Agency for Healthcare Research and Quality, Rockville, MD, 2005. Available at http://www.webmm.ahrq.gov/perspective.aspx?perspectiveID=14 (accessed 10 June 2007).

18 McGee MK. Urgent care: diagnosis critical. *Information Week* 2007; **1** (140); 40–50.

19 Florida Patient Safety Corporation (2004) *Promoting Excellence in Health Care.* Available at http://www.floridapatientsafetycorp.com/about_us.asp (accessed 14 Feb. 2007).

20 Miami Center for Patient Safety, Department of Anesthesiology, University of Miami School of Medicine, January 2004.

21 Devers KJ, Pham HH, Liu G. What is driving hospitals' patient-safety efforts? *Health Affairs* 2004; **23** (2): 103–15.

22 Batalden P, Leach D, Swing S, Dreyfus H, Dreyfus S. General competencies and accreditation in graduate medical education. *Health Affairs* 2002; **21** (5): 103–11.

23 Dreyfus H, Dreyfus S. *Mind over Machine.* Free Press, New York, 1986.

24 Bodenheimer T, Wagner E, Grumback K. Improving primary care for patients with chronic illness. *Journal of the American Medical Association* 2002; **288**: 1775–9.

25 Baker D, Battles J, King H et al. The role of teamwork in the professional education of physicians: current status and assessment recommendations. *Joint Commission Journal on Quality and Safety* 2005; **31** (4): 185–202.

26 Wood DF. Interprofessional education – still more questions than answers? *Medical Education* 2001; **35** (9): 816–17.

27 Glen S, Reeves S. Developing interprofessional education in the pre-registration curricula: mission impossible? *Nurse Education in Practice* 2004; **4** (1): 45–52.

28 Bolsin S, Faunce T, Oakley J. Practical virtue ethics: healthcare whistleblowing and portable digital technology. *Journal of Medical Ethics* 2005; **31** (10): 612–18.

29 Hafferty FW, Franks R. (1994) The hidden curriculum, ethics teaching, and the structure of medical education. *Academic Medicine* 1994; **69** (11): 861–71.

30 Hundert EM, Hafferty F, Christakis D. Characteristics of the informal curriculum and trainees' ethical choices: plenary session. *Academic Medicien* 1996; **71** (6): 624–33.

31 Hafferty FW. (1998) Beyond curriculum reform: confronting medicine's hidden curriculum. *Academic Medicine* 1998; **73** (4): 403–7.

32 Madigosky W, Buescher J. *The Rest of the Story: Identifying our Hidden Curriculum.* Department of Family and Community Medicine, University of Missouri-Columbia, Columbia, Missouri, 2004.

33 Christensen U, Heffernan D, Barach P. Micro-simulators in medical education: an overview. *Simulation and Gaming* 2001; **32** (2): 247–58.

34 Salas E, Baker D, King H et al. On teams, organizations and safety. *Joint Commission Journal on Quality and Safety* 2006; **32**: 109–12.

35 Gallagher AG, Cates CU. Virtual reality training for the operating room and cardiac catheterization laboratory. *Lancet* 2004; **364**: 1538–40.

36 Gallagher AG, Cates CU. Approval of virtual reality training for carotid stenting. *Journal of the American Medical Association* 2004; **292** (24): 3024–6.

37 Gallagher AG, Ritter EM, Champion H, et al. Virtual reality simulation for the operating room: proficiency-based training as a paradigm shift in surgical skills training. *Annals of Surgery* 2005; **241** (2): 364–372.

38 Grantcharov TP, Kristianson VB, Bendix J et al. Randomized clinical trial of virtual reality simulation for parascopic skills training. *British Journal of Surgery* 2004; **91**: 146–50.

39 Shine KI. Health care quality and how to achieve it. *Academic Medicine* 2002; **77**: 91–9.

40 Kachalia A, Johnson J, Miller S, Brennan T. The incorporation of patient safety into board examinations. *Academic Medicine* 2006; **81**: 317–25.

41 Gilula MF, Barach PR (2004) *Evaluation of House Staff Physician Attitudes towards Adverse Medical Events at the University of Miami.* Available at http://umdas.med.miami.edu/links/housestaffphysiciansurvey/default.asp (accessed 14 Feb. 2007).

42 Barach PR, Gilula MF. *Calling for Help: Interns' Patient Safety Workshop.* 2005. Available at http://www.mindspring.com/~mgilula/ptsafety.htm (accessed 26 Sep 2008).

43 Leeders S. Future challenges of post-graduate medical education. Keynote address to the Australasian Faculty of Rehabilitative Medicine (27 Oct. 2006). *Rhaia: The Official Newsletter of the Australasian Faculty of Rehabilitation Medicine* 2006; **14** (4): 15–21.

44 Cantor M, Barach P, Derse A et al. Disclosing adverse events to patients. *Joint Commission Journal on Quality and Safety* 2005; **31**: 5–12.

45 Clinton HR, Obama B. Making patient safety the centerpiece of medical liability reform. *New England Journal of Medicine* 2006; **354** (21): 2205–8.

CHAPTER 18

Teaching and learning about patient safety

John Sandars

Patient safety is a major priority for health care. It is therefore reasonable to suggest that all health care providers are educated about patient safety. This raises two important questions: what should be learned and how should it be taught? These questions appear at first sight to be obvious but teaching and learning about patient safety offers a challenge to all health care educators. This chapter explores these challenges. It is not my main purpose here to provide a definitive or detailed syllabus but sources and frameworks for teaching and learning about patient safety are listed in Appendices 18.1–18.5 (see also Appendix 17.1, p. 251). The main aim of this chapter is to offer helpful educational insights into the challenges that face this dimension of improving patient safety.

Everyone who has a responsibility to provide teaching about patient safety will need to make choices about their approach which will be influenced in part by the wider context, whether a specific educational setting, such as an undergraduate medical course, or a health care provider organisation, where the interest is continuing professional development. Different pressures to conform to a prescribed syllabus will operate in different settings. However, whatever the context, the educator will need to address common issues.

What should be learned?

The concept of patient safety is easy to define but it is far more difficult to clearly identify the essential components since it involves a complex mix of individual and organisational factors [1]. Most threats to patient safety are not due to one cause and there is usually an inter-relationship between causal factors [2].

The typical educational approach to deciding what should be learned about patient safety is to identify the key aspects of the chosen area of interest and then derive specific objectives from them so that 'intended learning outcomes are defined'. The decision about key aspects will be usually determined by

Health Care Errors and Patient Safety. Edited by Brian Hurwitz and Aziz Sheikh.
© 2009 Blackwell Publishing, ISBN: 978-1-4051-4643-2.

the perspective on patient safety that is taken by the organisation producing the objectives. For example, a malpractice insurer is likely to produce objectives that are different from those selected by an organisation concerned with incident reporting. This could lead to a plethora of curricular objectives. Similar differences in perspective are found if health care professionals are asked to state their personal learning objectives, doctors rank medicolegal aspects of safety more highly than nurses [3]. The main difference in the lists of potential learning objectives that can be generated in these ways is that some are more specific to patient safety, such as how to perform a root cause analysis, whilst others are more generic, such as how to become an effective member of a health care team and how to develop cultural competence.

The ultimate aim of all teaching and learning about patient safety is to reduce the threats to patient safety that health care users are exposed to. Specific knowledge and skills are called for but, most importantly, appropriate attitudes too. The first step is to develop increased awareness of the extent, frequency and nature of threats to patient safety. This is not achieved merely by providing information (knowledge) of facts and figures, but also requires the development of an attitude of recognition regarding the significance of safety problems and that something needs to be done about them.

A specific aspect of patient safety is understanding of why threats to patient safety exist or happen and how they can be reduced. Knowledge is required about contributory factors, both individual and within the organisation of health care, and how they can be overcome. There are also specific skills, such as root cause analysis or significant event analysis. Another specific area is related to the fact that health care provision is always embedded within a particular health care and regulatory system and is subject to different incentives, policies and reporting procedures.

There is a wide range of generic knowledge and skills that are essential to reduce threats to patient safety. The areas include clinical decision making, communication, team working and use of evidence-based medicine. Many of these intended learning outcomes can be regarded as basic competences for any health care professional.

How should it be taught?

The approach to teaching is determined by the choice of the most appropriate method to achieve the intended learning outcomes. Emphasis is often placed on instructional methods that deliver knowledge and develop skills. However, like most educational provision, there is often scant attention paid to the wider social aspects that influence learning, especially the development of appropriate attitudes [4].

Knowledge can be provided and skills developed by a wide variety of methods that use a range of learning resources. Increasingly, electronic resources are being developed which offer interactive learning opportunities. An example is a recently evaluated interactive DVD that includes a variety of video vignettes and post-tests [5]. The vignettes do not only include patient encounters but also interactions between health care professionals.

Simulations are particularly important since they offer ethical benefits, and training in specific skills can be targeted [6]. Established and successful simulation methods include standardised patients and role plays, and virtual patients undergoing surgical procedures who may need life support procedures.

Patients are, of course, a valuable resource since they can actively participate in discussion, problem-based learning groups and interactive seminars on topics such as risk communication and dealing with the aftermath of an adverse event (see Chapter 13).

A recent systematic review of the effectiveness of continuing medical education highlights the importance of the learner being actively involved in the learning process, especially by participating in small group workshops [7]. This approach is in contrast to much of the teaching in patient safety, which is often organised by health care providers who merely offer instructional leaflets or protocols. An essential dimension of learning is the social aspect by which experiences can be shared and personal strategies developed to allow new learning to be applied to the reality of daily professional practice. Learning has to be relevant to the needs of the learner, especially the context in which the learner has to apply the new learning. [8].

Small group work can be helpful in shaping attitudes, such as individual and collective regard for safety as a positive consideration of all health care interventions [9]. There is increasing recognition that a negative approach to patient safety, in which errors are seen as wrong and blameworthy, results in rigid adherence to checklists but does not produce increased safety. A positive approach arises from awareness that all situations are inherently risky and that when entering new situations a useful question to bear in mind is: How can I make my actions as safe as possible? The answer may reside in collective not individual factors. This has been recognised in cardiothoracic surgery, where learning in groups has enabled health care workers to recognise when the behaviours and actions of colleagues are a threat to patient safety [10]. But empowering health care workers to warn colleagues of impending threats to patient safety requires each worker to begin to accept feedback from other colleagues. This approach has been extensively used in civil aviation as part of crew resource management training.

Many of their generic learning outcomes can also be covered in the curricula of undergraduate and postgraduate health care professionals. Specific sessions on patient safety can be provided, even if they only have the intention of raising awareness of safety. Many professionals have the opportunity to choose optional courses and these can have a specific patient safety focus [11].

How should the learning be assessed?

An essential part of all teaching and learning is the assessment of whether the intended learning outcomes have been achieved. The important aspects of the assessment are the choice of outcomes to be assessed and the methods that will be used to assess them. However, no assessment occurs in isolation, its purpose has to be clearly defined. In addition, assessment usually drives the learning. This includes not only the strategic approach taken by the learner in their attempt successfully to attain the required standard but it also determines the content and method of the teaching.

Miller, in his widely quoted educational pyramid, recognises that assessment is best performed in authentic work situations [12]. It is only in such situations that there can be an assessment as to whether the learner actually uses the intended learning outcomes in professional practice. This creates a challenge for all assessments, including those of patient safety. Knowledge and skills can be assessed easily, for instance performing a random case analysis, but attitudes are more difficult to assess. An important method of identifying attitudes is feedback from colleagues and patients. This is particularly important for patient safety, and the development of effective methods is a challenge to all educators [13].

How can a strategy be developed?

An important question is whether the long lists of intended learning outcomes will be comprehensive enough to ensure that patient safety is improved. There are no simple answers. The approach to the improvement of patient safety is complex and this is mirrored by the approach required to develop effective teaching and learning about patient safety. An essential first step is to agree that patient safety is a priority in the education of all health care learners, irrespective of their position in their lifelong journey of learning. A balance has to be made between specific intended learning outcomes and more generic outcomes. Specific outcomes are essential so that patient safety is recognised as an important part of overall curriculum, especially one that is already overcrowded. This approach has been taken in the new Postgraduate Medical Curriculum for General Practice (http://gpcurriculum.co.uk/contents.htm), which contains a specific curriculum statement on patient safety.

Aron and Headrick have drawn a metaphor between the filters that operate within an organisational system to maintain patient safety and those within a medical school to produce a graduate who has the necessary competence to improve patient safety [14]. These filters are the entrance requirements, the medical school curriculum, its organisational, approaches to assessment and accreditation requirements. A medical school that wishes to respond to the challenge of developing teaching and learning about patient safety has to pay attention to all of these factors.

Each type of health care learner will need learning outcomes that are specific to their own professional area, but there is an overlap between all health care learners, irrespective of where they are on their educational journey. An example of a common approach is the National Patient Safety Education

Framework produced by the Australian Council for Safety and Quality in Health Care [15]. This is supported by a detailed bibliography.

A frequent cause of threats to patient safety is poor interprofessional working, and experience from high-risk industries, such as nuclear or civil aviation, has clearly shown that joint learning about safety improves safety. The notion of 'tribalism' between the various layers of health care professionals – whether between primary care and secondary care, junior and senior staff or between doctors and nurses – highlights the tension between the various groups [16]. It is not a deficit in communication skills that produces problems although it is related to attitudes. It is essential that the opportunities for interprofessional learning are not merely paid lip-service but recognise that appropriate opportunities, often with a trained facilitator, have to be provided to allow health care professionals to meet and learn together.

The importance of the culture of a health care organisation 'the way that things are done around here' is recognised to be important in understanding how patient safety is developed and maintained [17]. Stevens recently described significant parallels between the culture of medical education and the safety culture of an organisation [18]. The relationship between the teacher and learner is fundamental in all education but, as Stevens notes, in medicine the culture is dominated by 'blame and shame'. Learners do not disclose lack of confidence or competence when facing a situation, yet both are common causes of major threats to patient safety. A hierarchical and competitive atmosphere is often present and teaching still frequently occurs by humiliation of the learner [19, 20].

Conclusion

Teaching and learning about patient safety cannot be achieved unless all those who are responsible for the education of health care professionals recognise the importance of addressing the wide range of critical factors that determine how a health care professional develops the necessary knowledge, skills and attitudes to maintain the safety of the patients that they care for.

Appendix 18.1: Sources of educational resources

- National Patient Safety Agency: http://www.npsa.nhs.uk/.
- National Patient Safety Foundation, http://www.npsf.org/
- Agency for Healthcare Research and Quality: http://www.ahrq.gov/qual/errorsix.htm.
- VA National Center for Patient Safety: http://www.patientsafety.gov/
- MEDLINE Plus Patient Safety Resources: http://www.nlm.nih.gov/medlineplus/patientsafety.html.
- BMJ Learning: http://www.bmjlearning.com/planrecord/index.jsp.

Appendix 18.2: Examples of patient safety curricula

• Australian Council for Safety and Quality in Health Care: National Patient Safety Education Framework [15]. Available at http://www.safetyandquality.org/internet/safety/publishing.nsf/Content/60134B7E120C2213CA257483000D8460/$File/framework0705.pdf (Accessed 29 Sept 2008).
• Royal College of General Practitioners: Curriculum Statement 3.2, Patient Safety. Available at http://www.rcgp.curriculum.org.uk/extras/curriculum/statementDetails.aspx?id=4 (Accessed 29 Sept 2008).

Appendix 18.3: Critical factors for teaching and learning patient safety in medical school (after Aron & Headrick [14])

• *Entrance requirements*: Selection criteria may not identify individuals with the ability to reflect on practice, work with others and continually improve their performance.
• *Curriculum*: There is often a lack of attention to the skills needed to improve individual practice, including collaboration, interdisciplinary team-work and the ability to admit and discuss error.
• *Organisational culture*: There is often an overemphasis on physician–physician interaction, chronic fatigue and other threats to professionalism.
• *Student assessment*: There is often a lack of assessment related to improvement and patient safety.
• *Accreditation standards*: These do not address sufficiently the skills needed by physicians to improve care and safety.

Appendix 18.4: National Patient Safety Education Framework: learning areas and topics (after Lyons et al. [15])

1 **Communicating effectively:**
   1.1 Involving patients and carers as partners in health care
   1.2 Communicating risk
   1.3 Communicating honestly with patients after an adverse event (open disclosure)
   1.4 Obtaining consent
   1.5 Being culturally respectful and knowledgeable
2 **Identifying, preventing and managing adverse events and near-misses**
   2.1 Recognising, reporting and managing adverse events and near-misses
   2.2 Managing risk
   2.3 Understanding health care errors
   2.4 Managing complaints
3 **Using evidence and information**
   3.1 Employing best available evidence-based practice
   3.2 Using information technology to enhance safety

4   **Working safely**
   4.1 Being a team player and showing leadership
   4.2 Understanding human factors
   4.3 Understanding complex organisations
   4.4 Providing continuity of care
   4.5 Managing fatigue and stress
5   **Being ethical**
   5.1 Maintaining fitness to work or practice
   5.2 Ethical behaviour and practice
6   **Continuing learning**
   6.1 Being a workplace learner
   6.2 Being a workplace teacher
7   **Specific issues**
   7.1 Preventing wrong site, wrong procedure and wrong patient treatment
   7.2 Medicating safely

Appendix 18.5: Key messages of the Royal College of General Practitioners Curriculum Statement 3.2, Patient Safety

• It is likely that further training on patient safety throughout a doctor's career will be required.
• General practitioners are well placed to be active members of the health care team and positively influence the safety culture within the practice and the development of the practice as a learning organisation.
• The knowledge and application of risk assessment tools must become part of a general practitioner's skills and, whatever change occurs in their environment, they should assess the effects of change and plan accordingly.

References

1 Walshe K, Boaden R. *Patient Safety: Research into Practice*. Open University Press, Maidenhead, 2006.
2 Sandars J, Esmail A. *Threats to Patient Safety in Primary Care: A Review of the Research into the Frequency and Nature of Error in Primary Care*. Department of Health, London, 2002.
3 VanGeest JB, Cummins DS. *An Educational Needs Assessment for Improving Patient Safety: Results of a National Study of Physicians and Nurses*. White Paper Report No. 3. National Patient Safety Foundation, North Adams, MA, 2003.
4 Jarvis P. *Adult and Continuing Education*. Routledge, London, 1995.
5 Sanson T, LaSalle G, Tavernero T. Patient safety video education tool. *Academic Emergency Medicine* 2006; **13**: 209–10.
6 Ziv A, Small SD, Wolpe PR. Patient safety and simulation-based medical education. *Medical Teacher* 2000; **22**: 489–95.
7 Thomson O'Brien MA, Freemantle N, Oxman AD, Wolf F, Davis DA, Herrin J. Continuing education meetings and workshops: effects on professional practice and health care outcomes (Cochrane review). In: *The Cochrane Library*, 2, 2001. Oxford: Update Software Digital Object Identifier (DOI) 10.1002/chp.1340210310.

8   Walton MM, Elliott SL. Improving safety and quality: how can education help. *Medical Journal of Australia* 2006; **184**: S60–S63.

9   Rochlin GI. Safe operation as a social construct. *Ergonomics* 1999; **42**: 1549–60.

10 Aggarwal R, Undre S, Moorthy K, Vincent C, Darzi A. The simulated operating theatre: comprehensive training for surgical teams. *Quality and Safety in Health Care* 2004; **13**: 27–32.

11 Barach P. Patient safety curriculum. *Academic Medicine* 2000; **75**: 551–2.

12 Miller GE. The assessment of clinicalskills/competence/performance. *Academic Medicine* 1990; **65**: S63–S67.

13 Stern DT. *Measuring Medical Professionalism*. Oxford University Press, Oxford, 2006.

14 Aron DC, Headrick LA. Educating physicians prepared to improve care and safety is no accident: it requires a systematic approach. *Quality and Safety in Health Care* 2002; **11**: 168–73.

15 Lyons P, Walton M, Australian Council for Safety and Quality in Health Care. National Patient Safety Education Framework bibliography. Canberra: Commonwealth of Australia, 2005. Available at: www.safetyandquality.org/internet/safety/publishing.nsf/Content/60134B7E120C2213CA257483000D8460/$File/framework0705.pdf (Accessed 29 Sept 2008).

16 Gorman P. *Managing Multi-disciplinary Teams in the NHS*. Kogan Page, London, 1998.

17 Weick K. Organizational culture as a source of high reliability. *California Management Review* 1987; **2**: 112–17.

18 Stevens DP. Finding safety in medical education. *Quality and Safety in Health Care* 2002; **11**: 109–10.

19 Kohn LT, Corrigan JM, Donaldson M, eds. *To Err is Human: Building a Safer Health System*. Healthcare Services/National Academies Press, Washington, 1999.

20 Leape LL, Berwick DM. Five years after to err is human: what have we learned? *Journal of the American Medical Association* 2005; **293**: 2384–90.

CHAPTER 19

Health care errors, patient safety and the media

Geoff Watts

Medical errors play well in the media. The biggest can make headlines for weeks or even months. Think of the six men admitted to intensive care in 2006 in the UK following an unexpected reaction to the new anti-inflammatory drug being tested at Northwick Park Hospital. Or think of the paediatrician Sir Roy Meadow and his misleading statistics on the probability of two cot deaths in one family which helped to convict Sally Clark of unlawful killing of her children, and of the subsequent court proceedings in which his reputation was thoroughly and publicly trashed. And think of the inquiry into the death rate among children who underwent heart surgery at the Bristol Royal Infirmary during the early 1990s.

Three unrelated affairs, each differing in the nature of the tasks being undertaken and the 'mistakes' that were made. But each prompted intense media scrutiny and widespread discussion in the UK. Add to these three episodes a vastly greater number of other lesser but still reported incidents – the wrong drug, the wrong dose, the wrong organ removed – and the appeal of medical error to journalists and the pubic they serve is self-evident. While there is no reason to suppose that accountants are any less error prone than doctors, a balance sheet that does not quite add up lacks the drama of a patient undergoing surgery who has not had quite enough anaesthetic.

A few years ago I was asked to speak to a group of people who handle press relations on behalf of members of the Association of Medical Research Charities. They wanted to know what makes a good (i.e. likely to be reported) press release. I began by pointing out that what the media want are stories. By way of trying to provoke what I hoped might be some constructive reflection on the issue – and also to entertain the audience while so doing – I decided to go for caricature. My aim was to get them thinking about the media from the viewpoint of those working within it. So let me outline what I said, and why I think the moral of the tale is as relevant to understanding the reporting of error as of new research.

I began by suggesting that news about medicine – indeed all news – can be categorised as 'good' or 'bad'. There is frequently more mileage in bad news

Health Care Errors and Patient Safety. Edited by Brian Hurwitz and Aziz Sheikh.
© 2009 Blackwell Publishing, ISBN: 978-1-4051-4643-2.

unless the good news is very good indeed. Either way the stories should feature people. If there are no people involved in the story it will be harder to sell. If people are involved they should be young and beautiful – or, even better, children.

So what sort of things make good news? Cures. Cure is always better than prevention which, by comparison, is dull. Cures should be quick, dramatic, unequivocal and clever. Bits of gadgetry or high tech instruments or a miracle drug never go amiss. The disease in question should, ideally, be familiar if not common. If neither familiar nor common, then it should have clear-cut and preferably devastating symptoms, either physical or psychological but not too unmentionable or revolting. As organs go the heart, brain and lungs are all reliable. The womb is not bad, but ears are less interesting than eyes. The gut can be a problem, and the male genitalia even more so. These are not to be recommended. Patients – victims – should be able to say in their own words how awful things were before the cure, and how good they are now.

An angle involving the doctors or researchers is helpful: years of dedicated toil overcoming hurdles and setbacks; personal experience of disease among members of the research team; researchers who have bravely tested the remedy on themselves. It is useful to label the work a 'breakthrough' – though not essential because the media will do this anyway. Hints of a future Nobel Prize add glamour.

On then to the most saleable bad news stories. These include the emergence of new diseases, especially if the word 'plague' can be invoked. The disease should be serious, and preferably fatal. Infectious disease is always best because of the extra frisson it provokes, especially if the microbes responsible can be described as 'flesh-eating'. Other possibilities include the major side effects of a drug, preferably a common one; the failure of a hitherto accepted treatment; rare cancers affecting children; and virtually anything negative about pharmaceuticals or radiation.

The Association of Medical Research Charities subsequently issued a guide to communicating with the media based on this talk. I still worry that its comic intent may not have been fully appreciated. That aside, the point I was seeking to make, and which applies equally to the reporting of medical error, is that the media have an agenda that is predominantly concerned with being read, listened to and watched. In other words, for commercial and other reasons they have to give people what they expect and/or want. This shapes the questions that journalists have to ask themselves when selecting stories:

• Not 'Is this of interest to health professionals?' but 'Is this going to catch the interest of my readers and listeners?'

• Not 'Is this important to an objective sociopolitical understanding of present circumstances?' but 'Will my readers, listeners and viewers think it's important?'

• Not only 'Do I, as a specialist correspondent, think this is important?' but also 'Can I persuade my editor that it's important?'

The extent and form of the coverage will depend on the outlet concerned: electronic or print, tabloid or broadsheet. Equally important is the degree of competition in any particular branch of the industry. On this point it is worth recalling that publishing has become vastly more competitive over recent decades. More and tougher competition can drive publishers to seek more dramatic and less refined means of attracting readers and audiences. More thoughtful, more restrained reporting is one likely casualty.

In parentheses it is worth recalling that while academic publishing may not have been subject to quite the same kind of pressures as those facing the *Sun*, the *Times* or television's *News at Ten*, this part of the industry has, if anything, faced even greater turmoil as the advent of on-line dissemination begins to change its entire commercial basis. Even the most scholarly journal has to earn a living.

To return to the mainstream: some doctors, policy makers and others who work in health care continue to believe that health and medical journalism exists to fulfil an educational role of some kind. This is a huge misunderstanding; journalism is not about health or medical education any more than it is about political education or arts education or foreign affairs education. It is about stories that interest people. Nor do reporters and broadcasters owe their first loyalty to the health care community; they owe it to their readers and listeners.

Within these limitations there is, of course, room for much that is socially valuable. Not least is the space available in the media for individuals who do wish to speak for the professionals' view of what is important in medicine and health care. The point is simply that such views do not and should not hold a monopoly position. Nor do I suggest that journalism should have a licence for irresponsible reporting, or that journalists should disregard the consequences of what they say and write. Few, in practice, are indifferent – and the best among them go beyond purely professional obligations in trying to illuminate the more difficult, obscure or even murky nooks and crannies of medicine. But those doctors who believe that the media exist solely to disseminate their particular view of health care and to follow their priorities will be disappointed. They should hope for much, expect little, kick up a fuss when misrepresented, and be grateful whenever media involvement in anything proves to be a force for good.

Within these limitations – the ground rules, as it were, of journalism – what do the media have to offer that may in some way assist when health systems are faced with situations involving error? You can think of what they do in terms of a set of overlapping roles: revelatory, investigatory, remedial, persuasive and even – sometimes – educational.

First and most obviously there is the revelatory role: the simple act of laying bare for public scrutiny the details of whatever it is that has gone wrong. The likelihood of any particular incident being reported will depend not only on the objective measure of its gravity, but on the extent to which it fulfils some or all of the requirements of a news story. An open society worthy of the name has an obligation to report failure as well as success. Indeed, in most non-authoritarian societies, failure occupies as much or more space than success. Foolishly, many people find this upsetting. In truth it should be a cause for celebration, not regret. One of the principal criteria by which events are deemed to be worth reporting is the extent to which they are exceptional: the minority of aircraft that crash, not the overwhelming majority that land safely. If bad things fill the time on radio and television and the space in newspapers, it is because bad things are still the exception.

The investigatory role demands much more of the media. But from Thalidomide on, and to an admittedly varying extent, journalists and broadcasters have often been prepared to pursue the sources of error whether they stem from the policy of a government, the greed of an industry or the incompetence of an individual. In some cases it is far from clear that any other agency would have had the powers or the inclination to follow the trail.

The remedial role is driven, as often as not, by the simple facts of what has been revealed – be it staff shortage, poor training, lack of money, inadequate equipment or whatever. Revealing the nature of the failure may be tantamount to revealing what has to be done. Which is not, of course, to say that it will be done.

In their persuasive role the media may seek to act on what they or others have discovered. Most media, with the debatable exception of public service broadcasters, are explicitly in the business of forming opinion. Newspapers and magazines frequently mount campaigns in favour of this or that action or policy – sometimes because the journalists involved believe in it, sometimes because proprietors believe in it, and sometimes not because anyone believes in it but because all agree it will be good for the circulation figures or the audience ratings. Divining motives for campaigns of this kind is difficult, not least because they are usually mixed. Health care professionals who approve of this or that campaign should adopt a pragmatic attitude and just be glad that an interest is being shown.

Although most of the media for most of the time are not in the business of education, they do have an educative role. Except in a few instances this is largely incidental: a by-product of non-didactic reporting. But an explicitly educative purpose may occasionally emerge, usually in the form of special supplements or features, boxed information attached to news stores, web references, lists of organisations that can be contacted for further information, and the like. Such activities may be valuable, but are seldom at the heart of the media brief. The famous BBC triad of duties (to inform, educate and entertain) are represented in widely differing proportions even in the output of the BBC itself.

From the viewpoint of people engaged in a profession like medicine (one imbued – still – with authority and whose practitioners continue to spend much of their time offering advice to others, if not actually telling them what they could or should be doing), the media have another value: a reflective one. Doctors and nurses may know how they themselves feel about errors in medicine; but how do the public view the matter? Are they angry, or inclined to be forgiving? Will a simple apology suffice, or will compensation be required? Are people generally prepared to accept a certain level of mistakes, or is it vital to pitch for an error rate of zero? The views fed back via the media may be filtered by selection and editorial bias, subjected to amplification or muffled to a whisper, and spun to suit the editorial purposes of their publisher. But without them, how are professionals to form judgments of themselves and their colleagues that range wider than the relatively small number of patients and relatives with whom they have personal dealing? The reflection they look for will sometimes be dim and distorted; but it will often be all that is available.

Having said all this, it is as well to remember that the media are no less error prone – in fact vastly more so – than the health professions. The speed with which they are required to work, often with inadequate information and little background knowledge, is hardly calculated to make for accuracy. Alas, even with no malice intended and when operating in any or all the roles listed above, media involvement can make things worse. Although the sorry tale of the measles, mumps and rubella (MMR) immunisation in the UK is not a health care error in the usual sense of that phrase, the manner of its reporting in even the most 'responsible' media illustrates what can go wrong when journalists have no particular axe to grind, and are just trying to do their job according to the usual rules.

The alleged risk posed by MMR immunisation – that it can cause a form of autism – was one of three much debated science issues chosen by the Cardiff University School of Journalism for a study of science and the media funded by the Economic and Social Research Council and carried out in 2002 [1]. Its authors wanted to explore the relationship between media coverage of these issues and public knowledge of them. From the end of January until the middle of September 2002 the researchers monitored and analysed national press, television and, to a limited extent, radio reporting on the issues. To assess public knowledge of MMR they used two national surveys, one carried out in April of that year, the other in October. The aim was look for any changes in public knowledge and opinion that had occurred.

The biggest single problem lay with the weight of evidence about the allegedly malign effect of MMR. The weight of evidence in 2007, makes a nonsense of the autism hypothesis. But even in 2002 the balance of opposing views was hardly equal. On one side, and attempting to debunk the link, were a majority of doctors including virtually all those with a special interest in the relevant areas of medicine. Against them were the principal protagonist of the MMR damage view, Dr Andrew Wakefield, a small number of other conventionally qualified doctors and scientists, and a larger group of practitioners of non-scientific forms of health care predisposed to believe anything that challenged the wisdom and supremacy of their orthodox counterparts. The emergence of each new piece of evidence casting doubt on the alleged hazards of MMR was conscientiously reported in the media – usually, in the interest of balance and fairness, with a comment from one of the individuals or pressure groups opposed to MMR. As the organisers of the Cardiff research point out,

If some media reports did point out that the *weight* of scientific evidence suggested the safety of MMR, this was not, apparently, the *impression* created by the coverage. When asked about the scientific evidence, many people (25 per cent in April, falling to 20 per cent in October) felt that Wakefield's speculative claim was actually backed (rather than contradicted) by most research, while the most popular response was to say there was 'equal evidence on both sides'.

In short, even when reports draw attention to the disparity in the relative weight of two lots of conflicting evidence, what tends to be heard and remembered is that there is a dispute.

One course of action when isolated experts are at loggerheads with a majority of their fellow professionals would be for the media to back off and wait until further studies confirm or refute the dissident opinion. This is not a stance that has much appeal to the media themselves. Journalists lose a potentially good story and, perhaps more to the point, play into the hands of conspiracy theorists who would accuse the media of covering up an issue of public interest.

This 'damned if you do, damned if you don't' predicament is not, of course, confined to the media. Official bodies of all sorts may be tempted not to announce that errors have been made if they honestly believe that the effect of these errors is of no great consequence. If the errors subsequently come to light it will, likely as not, be assumed that the officials concerned were indeed covering something up. The way to avoid this accusation is to be open and transparent and declare everything. But the very fact of making an announcement then invites the suspicion that the errors must actually be of some significance. If they were not, goes the argument, why would anyone be announcing them? It is a predicament long familiar to all involved in nuclear power safety.

The Cardiff study also draws attention to the role of emotion in reporting matters of this kind, especially when it involves a head to head debate between doctors or public health officials and – in this case – the parents of children affected by autism. Indeed, say its authors, experts 'cannot have relished debating with people who not only commanded immediate public sympathy, but whose own children were, apparently, testimony to the risks involved with immunisation'. To put it crudely but accurately, one sick child trumps any number of highly qualified experts.

Someone who has made considerable effort to rethink the business of medical journalism is Swedish doctor and journalist Ragnar Levi. In a book published a few years ago he explores the problems and pitfalls of writing about medicine, and also what he considers to be the inadequacies of much that is currently written and broadcast [2]. Balanced reporting is one of the issues that he tackles. His views of it might be described as moderately scathing. What he calls this 'he-said-she-said' reporting offers readers little more added value than could be found in opposing press releases, and leaves them none the wiser as to whether there is solid evidence supporting any of the claims:

The increased value which skilled medical reporters can add comes from the critical scrutiny of expert judgements. Critical reporters will question to what extent expert sources can support their statements, giving the audience at least a hint of the substance behind the words.

Levi himself is an advocate of what he calls 'critical medical journalism' – which means 'finding the truth, weighing the evidence, and watching for methodological "red flags"'. Reviewing this book when it first appeared, I noted that although steeped in journalistic 'best practice' – checking the facts, checking the sources, asking the difficult questions, remaining sceptical of all with power and authority – this conventional view of the journalist's duties is, for Levi, no more than a starting point. Medical science has devised a precise methodology for trying to uncover objective truth, and journalists reporting on medicine should be doing something very similar.

In Levi's view, any medical reporter worth his salt will know his randomised controlled trial from his relative risk ratio, be able to make use of Cochrane data, understand the importance of meta-analysis, be confident in asking researchers about 'numbers needed to treat', and much else. He is, in a way, asking medical journalists to become more like the editors of peer review journals. The hurdle here – even for the willing, enthusiastic and appropriately well-informed – is time. Academic peer reviewers get weeks to satisfy themselves about such matters; journalists may get days, hours or even a few minutes. So while this 'evidence-based journalism' may be a splendid ideal, its practicability is another matter.

Bodies such as the National Patient Safety Agency (NPSA) and the National Confidential Enquiry into Perioperative Deaths (NCEPOD) refer frequently to the wisdom of abandoning a culture of looking for someone to blame when something has gone wrong, and concentrate instead on finding out what can be learned that will prevent the incident happening again. Although this is not a view that most of the media would necessarily oppose, the notion of 'getting away with it' is one calculated to ring bells – and not exclusively at the tabloid end of the press spectrum. Journalists are no less prone than anyone else to looking for someone to blame when something has gone wrong. And their professional obligation to please as well as to inform cannot be dismissed. The fact is, telling your readership that a system is ill thought-out or inadequate is not half as good a story as identifying a named individual who has fouled up. As elsewhere in journalism, self-denying ordinances intended to serve the public good can be hard to maintain in the face of competitive pressure from rivals.

Levi's book [2] makes no specific reference to reporting on medical error but, applying his preferred principles, it is not hard to imagine what kind of stories would result. The less dramatic attempt to understand the systems that had gone wrong would certainly take precedence over the search for someone to blame. Against that, the experience of the airline industry with its long-established no-blame culture for improving safety is encouraging. There is little talk in the press of pilots 'getting away with it', and the arrangement does not seem to prevent occasional reports on behaviour – drunk on duty, for example – where culpability lies squarely with the individual rather than the system.

So, in the matter of medical error, does the involvement of the media makes things better or worse? Are they a help or a hindrance? Both, of course. Once the best sleeping position for babies had been identified, habits changed and the number of sudden infant deaths began to fall. As with most other pieces of health advice, the media were the biggest single conduit by which the word got out. In the case of MMR, by contrast, media publicity was disastrous: the erroneous interpretations and advice of a handful of doctors about the immunisation was rapidly spread and amplified beyond anything that would have happened if the media had shown no interest in the story.

The most important practical lesson for anyone with responsibility of any kind for dealing with the aftermath of medical error is not to give up on the media. Just as nature abhors a vacuum, so journalism can have no truck with blank pages and silent airtime. With space to be filled, airtime to be allocated and an event to be reported, a refusal by knowledgeable commentators to contribute will simply allow those with less knowledge to have their say.

References

1 *Towards a Better Map: Science, the Public and the Media*. Economic and Social Research Council, Swindon, 2003.
2 Levi R. *Medical Journalism: Exposing Fact, Fiction, Fraud*. Studenlitteratur, Lund, 2000.

Index